T0385369

PUSSY PEDIA

PUSSY PEDIA

A COMPREHENSIVE GUIDE

WORDS BY ZOE MENDELSON
ART BY MARÍA CONEJO

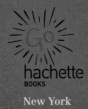

hachette
BOOKS

New York

Hachette Go, an imprint of Hachette Books
Hachette Book Group
1290 Avenue of the Americas
New York, NY 10104
HachetteGo.com
Facebook.com/HachetteGo
Instagram.com/HachetteGo

First Edition: August 2021

Hachette Books is a division of Hachette Book Group, Inc.

The Hachette Go and Hachette Books name and logos are trademarks of Hachette Book Group, Inc.

The publisher is not responsible for websites (or their content) that are not owned by the publisher.

Sister Outsider. Text © 1984, 2007 by Audre Lorde. Published in the United States by Ten Speed Press, an imprint of the Crown Publishing Group, a division of Random House, Inc., New York.

Print book interior design by Amy Quinn.

Library of Congress Cataloging-in-Publication Data has been applied for.

ISBNs: 978-0-306-92428-6 (hardcover); 978-0-306-92429-3 (ebook)

Library of Congress Control Number: 2021935099

Printed in South Korea

IM

10 9 8 7 6 5 4 3

To our grandmothers, mothers, and sisters

Table of Contents

A New Definition of Pussy

WE PROPOSE A NEW GENDER-AND-ORGAN-INCLUSIVE USE OF THE WORD THAT MEANS some combination of vagina, vulva, clitoris, uterus, urethra, bladder, rectum, anus, and—who knows—maybe some testes.

The word *vagina* comes from the Latin word for "sword holder." We are not down with the idea that vaginas exist as objects of service to penises. Also, *vagina* only refers to the canal. If we call the whole thing a *vagina*, we ignore a bunch of other important parts, including everything you see on the outside and the clitoris, which is made of the same tissues as a penis, about the same size as one, and responsible for our orgasms. (We wish we didn't have to refer back to penises to make this point about how important the clitoris is!) If we call it a *vulva*, we ignore the vagina and everything else inside. Also, there wasn't an available word that could include all of these parts plus testes, which some intersex people with pussies have! Like what if we had words for foot, shin, calf, knee, and thigh but no word for leg? We picked *pussy* because it had no prior specific definition, because you smile when you say it, it's used around the world, and because it's historically offensive, which is fun. We're taking *pussy* back cuz we like it. We hope you like it too.

A Medical Disclaimer

Foreword

I HAVE A CLEAR MEMORY OF WHAT I THINK WAS THE FIRST TIME SOMEONE TALKED plainly to me about my vulva and vagina.

My single mother often worked double shifts or night shifts. Sometimes, Ms. Smith, my sister's first-grade teacher, would spend the night with us if it was going to be an all-nighter.

One night, as we were getting into the massive nightgowns my mother liked for us (did she *want* us to get strangled in our sleep?), Ms. Smith noticed that we were leaving our underpants on. "You should really take those off when you sleep," she said. My mom grew up super Catholic—modesty was often the order of the day, so I was wary but also always interested in any potential rule-breaking.

"You've got to let it *breathe* at night," she said. "It needs to get some *air*."

Amazing.

As time went on, I learned many more things about my cunt and its cohorts from far more people and places, but what was often most impactful, what I remember the most—and I'm reaching at a point in my life where the impact of a thing is easily measured by my ability to remember it—was usually the most real. The most human and straightforward. Funny; awkward without shame. Sometimes even rude now and then, but always still smart, and never mean. Delicious, on occasion. Smelly, sometimes. Reverent, but not in a churchy way.

Like the first copy of *Our Bodies, Ourselves* on my mother's bookshelf, and then later, my own; what I'd learn from friends and from more-than-friends (what in mixed company we refer to as "field research"); the one truly excellent gynecologist I was able to encounter as a patient in public health; the street;

the feminist bookstore; smut. Also, you could honestly teach a whole—and *highly* detailed—sexual anatomy class using nothing but Irish limericks.

That's not to discount or dismiss other avenues or ways of learning about all this. I've certainly learned—and also sometimes taught—my fair share doing the kind of brainy and curious deep dives (not a euphemism) with more sciencey or clinical presentations, and fallen into the kind of research rabbit holes that led Zoe Mendelson and María Conejo to start the project that'd result in this book in the first place, and that inform so much of it so deeply and so well. I've also learned some good stuff from other, more esoteric sources.

At the end of the day, though, when the research is all done, and it's time to *just start finding out*, I feel you just can't overstate the power of plainspoken pussytalk.

Ms. Smith, bless her heart, apparently knew that and knew how to do that in 1979, and *Pussypedia* (and more to the point, its creators) is particularly great at it in 2021.

Holy areolae, the art of *Pussypedia*: you are in for a treat. María Conejo's glorious art gets at that reverence I love, and that I really want in something that's about this for-real temple (!) that is our body. But María's art isn't ever precious, nor does it feel creepily gynecological, a thing that a million clichéd pieces of truly well-meaning feminist artwork, absolutely including some of my own, easily demonstrate are very difficult balances to achieve. Delicious? Yep.

It is funny, never mean, though occasionally you might think it rude, and yes, smelly. Not literally, but—it's real in here. I think the realness manages to make it almost have an actual funk.

It is always, *always* smart. You're about to learn more than you thought you were going to when you got this book. I'm thrilled for you, to a degree that's, quite frankly, starting to get a little embarrassing for me.

The facts are here, and they are meticulously researched. *Meticulously.* Zoe and I message one another semi-regularly. Nine times out of ten that I get a message from Zoe, it opens with a research question, or, more commonly, a research frustration, usually based in the inability to find the level of support for something, or the source of a thing, she wants. Zoe is not messing around when it comes to the facts, making very sure they are the facts and then finding a whole bunch of extra facts while verifying that first bunch. I already have to fix a good ten different things in my own work this week because of things I found in this book. Thanks a lot, Zoe.

It's very, very human in this book. I think that's my favorite part.

We learn all the things that we learn about our bodies and their parts from so many different places, and one person or place would never be near enough. It's best to learn from a bunch of people, places, and situations. I think that there are some important roles filled in that. People older than you with great big boundaries who also give you good body information, like Ms. Smith up there, fill one of those roles.

Another of those important roles is a friend who knows their shit about this stuff *and* is suuuuper candid and open with you about their own personal feelings, experiences, and ideas. This friend will literally talk to you about pussy power. She will talk to you about it often.

This person is your scout, your most trusted drug (or sober) buddy, your partner on the field trip. They're your peer, but they know things you don't yet, have talked to people you haven't, or have experienced something differently from what you knew could be a thing. They're not going to talk to you like a doctor, and you'll *both* feel some vulnerability, not just you. They also are funnier and, more importantly, don't try as hard as doctors to *be* funny. (*While they have a speculum. What are they even thinking sometimes?*)

You get to know what the person giving you the facts also really thinks and feels herself. Now, you probably won't feel the same way Zoe, or everyone she interviews or quotes in this book, does. That's OK. Just witnessing someone else strongly possess and voice their own opinions, experiences, and feelings, especially about *this*, where so often the most loudly opinionated people about it don't even share this anatomy, for crying out loud, gives you so much permission to more strongly claim your *own* opinions, experiences, and feelings.

This is YOUR BODY. If there is anything for you to have strong opinions, experiences, and feelings about and to feel rightful in owning, it is this. If you want some help with that, or just some extra company in it, *Pussypedia* will make an excellent companion.

In fact, hanging out with this book and the way that it and its author engage you may put you at risk of feeling more comfortable with your body and your own thoughts and feelings about it and everything and anything related to it, and feeling in good company *with* your body. Just so you know. I think one of my favorite things about this book is also that it's pretty full spectrum as far as the life span is concerned, so if you keep this puppy in the living room, literal generations could potentially have that experience. I'm being serious with you.

We don't live in a world where we come to knowledge and comfort with our bodies—and most certainly our pussies, our cunts, our twats, our vulvas, our genitalia, whatever your favorite *nom de vajoo*—by default. So I think it's pretty fair to say that we all can often use some extra support and solidarity in being no-shame awkward, rude, smart, and real about what's real, in treating our smelly-delicious bodies with reverence, especially the parts the world treats with the least reverence, and how to just be human about . . . well, just being human.

You've got hundreds of pages of it (and so much careful, caring blood, sweat, and tears of it) in your hands right now, so who knows why you're still reading me.

¡Viva la *Pussypedia*!

Heather Corinna
February 1, 2021

A Note from María

FOR AS LONG AS I CAN REMEMBER, I'VE BEEN DRAWING MY FEELINGS. AN EMOTION, as Sara Ahmed defines it in her book *The Cultural Politics of Emotions*, "is the feeling of bodily change." It's something embodied that happens within us and doesn't exist purely in our minds but travels from our minds through our bodies. My artistic practice began with a story I developed about a female character who loses her head one day. She becomes a headless body like the iconic image of Bataille's *Acéphale*, who at first goes in search of her head but then develops a narrative of her own. She is The Body.

I believe in the power of images, of visual representation. Like with language, to depict something is to affirm its existence. The most important role that art plays in our present moment is Representation. It feels so good to see someone who looks like you somewhere besides the mirror. I have dealt with body dysmorphia my entire life and I'm still working on a more amorous and compassionate relationship with myself, and what has helped the most in recent years is art that represents the beautiful diversity of bodies that exists.

When I was five years old, I found myself one afternoon alone in my room, lit up by the last bit of golden daylight as darkness approached. I stood staring at myself in a big mirror with wonder.

I looked myself up and down, examining my head, my torso, my feet. I took in the entire shape of my body, which led me to think about the space my body took up in the room, and then about the space it took up in my house and quickly escalating to the space it took up in my country, the planet, THE

UNIVERSE! My heart quickened with anxiety. My hands began to sweat, which grounded me back in my body.

The epiphany I had in that room that afternoon has defined my whole life. It was clear to me that my body was the most important thing I owned and the only place I will inhabit my entire existence. I was never scared of it. Quite the opposite; I explored it; I liked using a mirror to look at the parts I couldn't reach with my own eyes. I wasn't afraid to stick my fingers into my pussy or wherever; I wanted to understand what it was, how it felt. It was an undiscovered land for me to explore.

My favorite things to do when I was a kid were to ride my bike as far and as fast as I could and to kick boys' asses at karate. I was the only girl in my karate class, which made me feel powerful even though most of the time I got my ass kicked too. But I really enjoyed doing those things because they allowed me to spend quality time with my body, in my body, to know its limits and its capabilities, to feel every part of it.

But my happy journey of bodily amazement didn't last forever. When I was nine, an old man harassed me on the street. It was the first time I thought of my body as something sexual. After that experience, I never wore the same clothes I was wearing that day, as if I was guilty for exhibiting my body. I remained silent. Years later, as a teenager, the nuns at my Catholic high school in Mexico would ask me to buy bigger uniforms to cover up my beautiful big butt so my classmates wouldn't get "distracted," reinforcing the message that my body was all wrong and it was drawing attention to itself in all the wrong ways. I also remained silent then.

No wonder I developed body dysmorphia in early adolescence. Those experiences, many others and also the fact I never got to speak about them with anyone, made way for all the patriarchal bullshit to take a seat at the table in my mind, letting the shame, the discomfort, the fear, and the dissatisfaction creep in. The only way I've been able to feel better has been through my work.

Drawing The Body allowed me to connect the dots between that experience I had at age five to every experience with my body since. It brought everything into full view. Seen from afar, some of those experiences looked unpleasant and unfair. I felt angry. Through The Body, I made the decision to be done with disrespect to *my* body. Enough from me, enough from everyone else. I wanted to restore my body's power, and everyone else's, too. So I made The Body the main character of all my work. I wanted it to be an invitation to others to turn their bodies into their own main characters as well. I wanted to propose that, perhaps, there is nothing wrong with having a body after all.

So I kept drawing naked bodies doing things. A lot of them. It has been challenging, to say the least, to pursue this kind of work in Mexico, a country with a deeply entrenched macho culture where internalized misogyny is rampant and 11 women get killed every day, while countless more go missing with impunity. But the response to my work has been surprisingly positive; I have been published alongside articles about feminism, gender theory, abortion, masturbation, sex, femicides in Mexico. I've made clothes, T-shirts, prints, stickers, tote bags with my drawings on them. I have aimed to spread my message however I could; forget about our preconceived notions, our bodies are the most important thing we have—let's listen to them, take care of them, enjoy them.

Now that I am 32, one of my favorite ways to spend quality time with my body is still to ride my bike as far and fast as I can. But now, instead of kicking boys' asses, I'm more interested in finding ways to have better sexual experiences with them or with other humans. And I am learning to love my body again.

So when Zoe wrote to me about doing this life-changing pussy project, it felt like a piece of the puzzle that I never knew was missing. Use my art to help spread knowledge about our bodies so people can finally enjoy their bodies, masturbate, have better sex? Fight injustice and help make this world a better, more equitable place, beginning with the Internet? And with my friend, the genius I have been wanting to collaborate with for years? Without any money at all? OBVIO! I didn't hesitate. I was sure we were going to make this a reality. And we did.

Working on *Pussypedia* has changed my life completely. I've learned a lot, not only about myself and my body but also about my community. This project has turned Zoe and me into representatives of a safe space. And that has meant that suddenly, people are very open to talking about the most personal things possible with us. I so appreciate that. This project has opened my perception to the wonderful diversity of bodies that exist in the world and to the infinite spectrum of human sexual expression. It has made me question everything I've ever been taught about my body. It has helped me understand why I was taught what I was taught. It has provided me the opportunity and the space to get to know my body for a second time. To be more compassionate with myself.

As I sat down to draw the images for this book, the most important things for me were to transmit everything I've learned and to be completely sincere. I wanted to share my wonder and amazement with you. I wanted you to understand why I believe that pleasure is the reason we all exist. I wanted to make honest, anatomically accurate images to accompany Zoe's text. I avoided using metaphors, unless necessary, because we need to see representations of our bodies and experiences exactly as they are.

I hope you enjoy this book.

I hope you enjoy your body.

María Conejo
February 1, 2021

We have been raised to fear the yes in ourselves, our deepest cravings. For the demands of our released expectations lead us inevitably into actions which will help bring our lives into accordance with our needs, our knowledge, with our desires. The fear of our deepest cravings will always . . . lead us to settle for or to accept so many facets of our oppression as women . . . For as we begin to recognize our deepest feelings, we begin to give up—of necessity—being satisfied with suffering or self abnegation or self negation and with the numbness which so often seems like their only alternative in this society, we empower ourselves to action.

—Audre Lorde, Uses of the Erotic: The Erotic as Power[1]

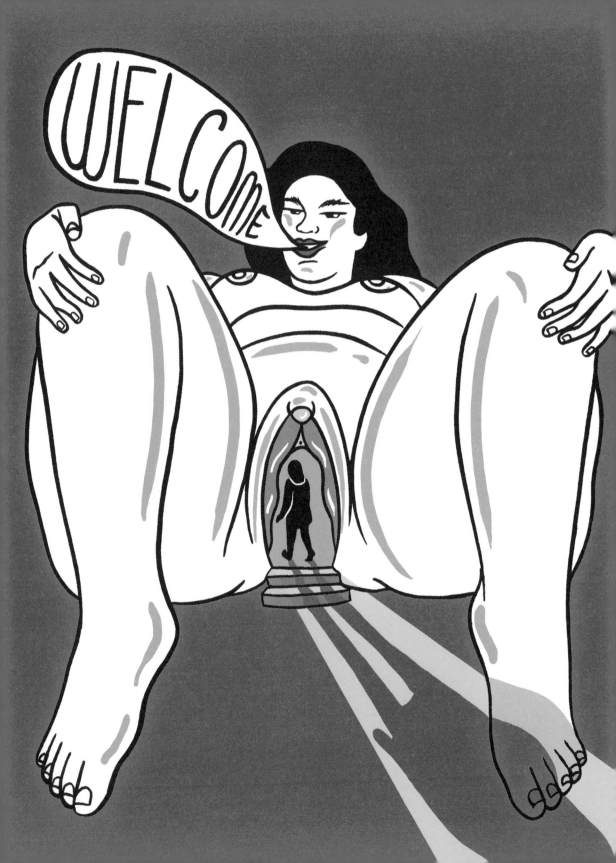

Introduction

I WAS A HORNY KID. ONCE WHEN I WAS FIVE MY MOM WAS TELLING MY LITTLE SISter not to touch her crotch in public when I interrupted, adding, "You just have to do it like *this* so nobody notices." I walked over to a doorframe, pressed my little pelvis into its corner, and started rubbing my crotch side to side.

"I do it all the time," I said.

I was the one who told all my friends how babies are made, whether they asked me or not. I asked the people sitting in the booth behind us at the diner and the guy at the photo-developing counter at Walgreens if they knew that boys had penises and girls had vaginas (fake news, turns out). In middle school, at friends' houses, I would dig around in their parents' drawers, looking for dildos, just to stare at them. I started having sex when I was 15. A lot.

Now I'm 30 and I hump doorframes way less often, but I do still talk about sex and pussies all the time—especially now that I've spent the last four and a half years creating first Pussypedia.net and then this book. This is something I never imagined for my life. I studied urban planning, made a career out of writing in emojis, and was working as a freelance journalist, researcher, and Millennial Salad internet consultant, dealing in buzzwords like *narratives!* and *content!* when one night in 2016 I googled:

"Can all women squirt?"

My search yielded what you might expect. Wildly contradictory information. Pseudoscience filled with spelling errors. Videos for men about how to make cis women squirt (*cis* means someone's gender matches the sex they were assigned at birth, i.e., they are not trans). Frustrated, I turned to medical journal articles, and *bam*. I got sucked into a vortex that I would never get out of. I could barely understand anything. I had to look up the definition of almost every word, and then look up almost every word in those definitions. But what I was finding was blowing my mind. There's only one type of orgasm?! My bladder is *where*?! I stayed up the whole night, studying diagrams and reading.

Why the hell had I lived my entire life without so much crucial information about my body? Why did I not know how exquisitely normal I was? And why was it so hard for someone without a medical background to access this information? I was furious that so many people with pussies waste precious mental space and time feeling inadequate or excessive or gross—or at least that I had.

My journey from unselfconsciously horny kindergartener to unselfconsciously horny adult was long and fucked up and honestly is still not over. I spent most of it mortified by my body. Until at least the beginning of high school, in new social situations, I would walk around with my arms crossed over my belly to hide it. Shopping for clothes almost always left me crying. I didn't wear a bikini until . . . like three years ago? I didn't participate in a single sport and often sat out PE because I was so embarrassed about the bizarre way I move my body (my best friend and my husband agree that I still walk like a drunk toddler). I was disgusted by the discharge in my panties. I was disgusted by my frequent yeast infections, which were probably caused by my habit of scrubbing between my labia with soap, trying desperately to be less disgusting (no soap in the crack, people!). I was so disgusted by my body that I didn't trust it to keep me alive, which is probably why I never learned to drive or swim. And my body would do things that would validate my distrust, like when I was 14 and one side of my labia grew into its adult form a full six months before the other. Even after they were the same size again, I felt stinging shame just for their very existence. And God, did I feel shame for being horny. So, so much.

It felt like trying really hard at a game and always losing. Finally learning about my body was like finding out that my opponent had been cheating the whole time. The Patriarchy has a lot of tricks for making people with pussies feel like shit. Suppressing information and conversation about our bodies is one of them. Knowledge *is* power, and pussy knowledge is tragically hard to come by. I say *tragically* because ignorance and ensuing shame are just phase one of The Patriarchy's evil plan to waste your MFing time! Here's how it went for me:

Shame prevented me from valuing myself and from even having any semblance of an idea what that meant. It prevented me from asking for what I wanted and needed because I didn't think my wants and needs mattered because I didn't matter because I was gross. I let yeast infections get terrible before going to a doctor because they were gross and my own fault, probably for being a "slut." I would say no to sex when I actually wanted it, to not seem like a "slut." And I would say yes to sex when I actually didn't want it, because I was so scared to disappoint people whose attention I didn't think I deserved in the first place. I let men not use condoms even though it would cause me—at best—weeks of fear and guilt and/or to have to bring myself somewhere and pay to get tested and—at worst—infections or pregnancy. Pleasure was rarely part of the equation, except the kind I often pretended to have to make sure that whoever was supplying my not-so-good time had a very good time and felt amazing about themselves.

Now, this is not to say that my roughly 15 years of biblical-and-adjacent activities have been terrible. God no. I'd say about 65% of it was bad-to-terrible, with more of the bad happening before my mid-20s, when I got a little better at saying, "NO THANKS." Even in the most casual of encounters, I felt respected enough times to learn what that felt like. I met people who made me laugh and who I could make laugh. I danced with incredible dancers. I witnessed so many different ways to think and be. There were late-night and early morning boat rides. There were blood sausages and secret concerts. There were new languages and snowmen and balconies and books and beaches. I learned what my body likes and doesn't. I learned my kinks. I made people come. They made me come, sometimes in surprising ways. I appreciated their fat rolls and freckles and innie-outies and hair textures. They appreciated mine. We helped each other feel and release and reset. I made people coffee. They made me coffee. Sometimes I saw their pain, and sometimes they saw mine. Sometimes we hurt each other but a lot of times we didn't.

At its best, sluttery can be a form of gratitude for being alive. Finding bodily pleasure through human connection, even when those connections are imperfect, is a holy act as far as I'm concerned. And in a slightly sadder but equally valid and beautiful way, sometimes it means pitching little tents together to shield ourselves, even just briefly, from the infinite solitude and terror that is life.

My best friend's partner recently joked about my lovely husband, "Wow, where did you find him?" and without skipping a beat, my best friend answered, "Well, she fucked like 1,000 assholes." I did. And I don't regret any of it, even the bad stuff.

But still, the bad stuff was really bad. I ended up googling squirting not because I was on some sex-positive fun-times learning adventure but because I was madly in love and nearly two years into a more-open-than-I-wanted-it-to-be relationship with a professor in his mid-40s who had sex with as many women in their early 20s as he possibly could because he was still hurt about and compensating for not getting laid in high school. He hated my body hair, often complained that I smelled and that I didn't dress sexy enough, threw angry tantrums whenever I didn't want to have sex, and was obsessed with making me squirt. He was sure I would squirt if I tried hard enough to RELAX. I never could. When I insisted that my body didn't do that, he argued that all women could. Cue the shame. I wanted to settle the matter so I could stop feeling inadequate or know for a fact that I was.

Thankfully, it was the former. After reading about pussies all night, shooting stars of rage were connecting dots in my brain: lack of information, shame, lack of self-worth, pleasure, health, power, why I had stayed so long in a dumpster fire of a relationship, wow, The Patriarchy.

I'm going to use the term *The Patriarchy* a nauseating number of times from here on out. The Patriarchy is the central villain of this book. So I'd like to quickly define it: The Patriarchy is just the way things are. It is a self-perpetuating system in which cis men have more power in society than everyone else. We all enact it together just by living and being in the ways we were taught to live and be.

The Patriarchy does not mean "men." When I blame The Patriarchy for Bad Things, I'm not blaming men, even if and when it is men who *do* the Bad Things. Cis men benefit from The Patriarchy, obviously, but they are also victims of it, which is a subject for a whole 'nother book, but, like, wow, I would *never* want to trade places with them. Natalie Wynn of ContraPoints could not have been more on point in her 2019 video "Men," when she said that we can't fix men or

The Patriarchy by only pointing out what's wrong with masculinity. We have to collectively imagine a healthy and positive way for men to be in the world.[2]

The Patriarchy is also white supremacist and ableist and many other -ists. For example, white cis men have more power in society than Black cis men. And here's where it gets complicated: white cis women, in most cases, do too. I'm going to demonstrate ways The (white supremacist) Patriarchy exists and works and reproduces itself throughout this book. So if you're not sure about what it is yet, that's OK. Sit tight.

Anyway, the morning after my vagina-vortex awakening, I knew exactly who I needed to talk to. I met María Conejo when I first traveled to Mexico City, where we both live, in 2014. She had briefly dated my older brother and was kind enough to let my little sister and me stay with her during our visit. She was the only person I knew when I moved here from New York City a little less than a year later. We partied together. We cried about boys and our relationships with our moms and about how terrifying it is to pursue creative careers. And we wanted to collaborate. So I texted her: "María, I've been up all night reading about vaginas. We need to do a vagina project." When I left our first brainstorming session, my body was buzzing.

Growing up, María had experiences of sexuality and shame that were not so different from mine. Except that my little hell had existed in a liberal urban bubble in Chicago (my mom's been queer since the '80s, often walked around the house naked, and always told me that magazine bodies were bullshit but still—The Patriarchy has a kind of *Final Destination*, will-find-your-ass quality), and María grew up in a small conservative town a few hours outside Mexico City, where she went to Catholic schools until college, never saw a naked "female" body, and where talking about sex was just not a Thing at all. If I had received the *YOUR BODY IS BAD* message loud and clear, María had received it through a megaphone.

Once, in high school, María was photocopying some pictures out of a magazine because she wanted to draw them. She hadn't noticed the accompanying article was about cunnilingus. When the nuns discovered her with the magazine, she was sent to the school psychologist, who promptly diagnosed her with a sexual disorder. Guess how that made her feel. Yes, you're right: horrible and ashamed.

So María did a very cool thing. She grew up and dedicated her life to making art that destigmatizes the "female" body. María's drawings and paintings are mostly bodily gestures, and with her magic powers (read: decades of hard work), she manages to convey an entire element of the human experience with each one. To me, they are the answer to art history's centuries of naked women lying seductively across rocks. They restore emotional dimension. They are the missing half's subjective.

María and I made a Kickstarter campaign for Pussypedia.net. We wanted to democratize the information I found hiding in those journal articles and academic studies. We wanted to build a free, bilingual, maximally accessible, and high-quality pussy encyclopedia. We wanted to be meticulous. We wanted to base everything on peer-reviewed, up-to-date, independently funded research. We wanted to say it all in language that would be easy to understand. And we wanted it to feel joyful to read and to look at.

We met our Kickstarter goal in three and a half days. Turns out a lot of people besides us wanted to know more about pussies. Which was awesome, except that what we had promised was, like, a comically, ginormously tall order for ourselves. It was obviously something we could not execute alone. While I felt confident in my ability to explain complex concepts with simple language (or tiny faces), I was not prepared for the complexity of medical research or the political delicacy of sex education.

Lucky for me, another one of my besties, Jackie Jahn, MPH, PhD, was at the time finishing her PhD at the Harvard T. H. Chan School of Public Health with a focus on race and gender. Dr. Jackie made a content outline for the site, which has been adapted for this book. She designed Pussypedia's research process and a very rigorous fact-checking process (available in its entirety for review in the about section of the site), and fact-checked the majority of the site herself. She wrote into our writers' guide careful instructions for responsibly paraphrasing scientific language without obscuring statistics or overstating conclusions; checking for researcher conflicts of interest and suspect funding sources; looking for the most up-to-date research; tracing each cited fact back to its original study and evaluating that study's merits, too; and a bunch more things that are tedious and super boring and hard and that I am very proud to say we actually did, both on the site and in this book. It turns out, you actually do have to read the methods sections of scientific studies. For this book, I read about 400 of them.

Most of the chapters in this book have been fact-checked by my dear friend Tarah Knaresboro, who, besides literally being a ninja (basically black belt in like every martial art ever invented [she has fact-checked this sentence as inaccurate]), studied neuroscience at Brown, has been a health-communications professional for over a decade, and is incredibly persnickety about what she lets me write based on what I read. For a few of the chapters that are more history and/or sociology than Science, I forged ahead using Dr. Jackie's fact-checking process on my own.

I was really—like, *really*—careful but, of course, there is probably at least one error in this book. The publisher of this book did not provide fact-checking. Book publishers rarely do. I can promise that we reviewed a gazillion studies and that we followed a strict verification process. And still, as a responsible reader, you should assume that all texts, including this one, have errors. Lucky for you, I've provided obsessive citations so that you can go check for yourself. Question everyone, especially anyone claiming to offer the Absolute Truth, especially if they are Some Dude on YouTube.

Another of Dr. Jackie's enormous gifts to the project was her insistence from the first discussion that gender inclusivity must be a starting point rather than an afterthought. So we hired sexuality educator and performance artist Melina Gaze, who was also my right-hand researcher and content consultant for this book, to coordinate a trans, nonbinary, intersex focus group and to create a set of inclusion guidelines for Pussypedia.net, which I have followed in this book as well. Tarah also put an enormous amount of work into keeping the language and content in this book inclusive and intelligible—especially in the dense, sciencey parts. Laura Lee Price Burks, MPP, is a grammar queen who edited the shit out of this book.

We could not be more grateful for our team of brilliant queer friends with pussies. Their skills are the result of entire lives spent working with extraordinary discipline and care. These names are here rather than in the acknowledgments because María and I are explodingly proud of the collaborative nature of this project. Between the two of us, María and I possessed about one-tenth of the skills and knowledge necessary to pull this all off. The collaboration is the point; we can take matters into our own hands and fix things (read: smash The Patriarchy) when we work together.

And speaking of working together, here it comes, the now-obligatory disclaimer: What we have created to date, in this book and on Pussypedia.net, does not (because it could not possibly) encompass the range of perspectives and experiences out there. We know that the lack of accessible information is even worse for trans, nonbinary, and intersex people and for people with disabilities. We spoke to sex experts with disabilities. We spoke to a range of trans, nonbinary, and intersex people and experts in trans, nonbinary, and intersex health. And yet, it is 100% guaranteed that our efforts will fall short. We encourage anyone to contact us at hola@pussypedia.net and let us know where, when, and how we can make our work more meaningfully helpful to more people.

Pussypedia's focus on genitalia aims to address a specific information gap, not to suggest that this part of the body defines sex or gender. Let the record show, my five-year-old self was dead wrong about "girls have vaginas and boys have penises." Many people with pussies are not women, and many women do not have pussies. That's why you won't find us using the word *women* throughout the site or this book, except when quoting statistics, another text or person, or a study that specifically looked at cis women.

I'm not sure if it's good that doing the equitable thing has acquired a social cachet. But I am sure of this: we've been chasing people with torches in the name of inclusivity when the way they've tried to do the equitable thing was unsatisfactory and doing that is at best unproductive and, at worst, absurd, morally righteous, elitist gatekeeping. Still, no matter how wrong we try to do it, inclusion is a necessary and worthwhile endeavor. Inclusive thinking has vastly improved the quality of our work on Pussypedia, not only by making it useful to more people but also by forcing us to research deeper and think harder about the nature of medical and informational injustice.

Inclusive frameworks were invented by Black people with pussies. As The Great Audre Lorde, a self-described "black, lesbian, mother, warrior, poet," put it in 1981: "I am not free while any woman is unfree, even when her shackles are very different from my own."[1] Later, the term *intersectionality* was coined by the lawyer, activist, philosopher, professor, and podcast host

Kimberlé Williams Crenshaw, JD, LLM, in 1989 when she wrote, "Because the intersectional experience is greater than the sum of racism and sexism, any analysis that does not take intersectionality into account cannot sufficiently address the particular manner in which Black women are subordinated."[3] While the word *intersectionality* may now get overused and applied in ways Crenshaw never intended, her and Lorde's insistence that analysis of and attempts to address oppression must always look at its overlapping forms were huge gifts to the world.

Making Pussypedia.net took a lot of different people caring about other people with very different shackles from their own. It would not have been at all possible without the 200+ volunteers from four continents who contributed research, writing, editing, translation, illustration, fact-checking, web development, and resource collection to the site, or without our web design and development collaborators Michael Yap and Joseph Thomas.

Pussypedia.net went live on July 1, 2019, and received over 2.3 million page views in its first year. It has since won a People's Voice Webby and a gold medal at the Mexican National Design Biennale, and reached almost every nation on earth. (One secret to our traffic success is that a lot of the visits come from people who google "pussy," probably searching for porn. The funny thing is that these visits only have a 70% bounce rate, which means 30% of horny porn-searchers stick around to read.)

The two and a half years of putting the site together with very little money was both brutally exhausting and unexpectedly healing. The outpouring of support María and I received from such a huge range of people in taking agency over our knowledge of our bodies changed us profoundly. Engaging pussy subjects with friends and strangers—not just speaking the unspeakable but picking it apart detail by detail—changed my entire relationship to them and to my body.

Also, when we went digging for information together and found exactly how little there is, when we became intimate with the scarcity and the bullshit, our shame was replaced by indignation, which fueled our work, both on the site and on loving ourselves. It becomes easier to love yourself when you are pissed about how the whole game is rigged to make that feat impossible. This truth led me to take two specific informational approaches with this book:

1. I've included a whole lot of information you never needed to know about me and my pussy. I picked up *Wow, No Thank You.* by Samantha Irby at the beginning of writing this book, and *Wow, Thank You.* Irby taught me how oversharing can be a political weapon. In her essay "Body Negativity," she lists body parts and all of The Patriarchy's absurdly high expectations for the care, treatment, and state of each and then describes how miserably she and her body seem to fail to meet those expectations. "MY BREASTS ARE SHAPED LIKE SUMMER SQUASH,"[4] she writes, caps per original. (Mine are too kinda.) And then she goes on to describe shitting on a table while getting a Brazilian. Reading Irby liberate herself by speaking her truth was liberating. I laughed so hard I cried through the whole essay while internalizing the important political message that me and my body are just fine. I felt amazing when I finished that essay. I wanted to take the book and stand on a chair and do that thing Rafiki did with baby Simba. Information is just data if it's not accessible. And information is often not accessible if an emotional state, like shame, does not allow you to process it. So I've talked about myself in detail to try to make you laugh and to try to help you receive information about things that may spark shame. And to show you that I'm at least partially fucking over it in hopes that you can be too.

2. I tried to pack in as much information *about* the information as possible, to take you with me through the research process so that you too can be healed by both facts and indignation. I hope to raise the standards for what readers consider good-quality information. I want people to expect citations. I want people to expect exploration of contradictory evidence. I want people to know that behind most facts lay long, storied debates, rich with dimension and context. I want people to know about the institutions that control knowledge, the flawed human scientists that produce it, and about the lineage of people with pussies who spent their lives digging their anatomy out of medical obscurity. I've learned a lot about the nature of information through this process, and that knowledge feels as integral to my understanding of my body and to the healing of my shame as any collection of facts.

In her TEDx Talk "A Case for Cliteracy," Sophia Wallace, artist and creator of the CLITERACY movement, pointed out that humans landed on the moon 29 years before we described with certainty the organ responsible for half the planet's orgasms.[5] The clitoris was largely missing from medical textbooks until the last few decades. Not because we didn't know it existed. We did! In 1948, the editor of *Gray's Anatomy*, which has been in print since the 1850s, took the clitoris out of the book for reasons we can only guess.[6] I'd say: it seemed profane and/or unimportant to him, and/or that he was terrified of it.

Pussy stigma and shame go at least as far back as Genesis with Adam and Eve, and they're still the reason we're not doing enough research on pussies. As recently as 2019, one study found that the research-funding applications to the National Institutes of Health (NIH) that were least likely to be granted were those characterized by the words *ovary*, *fertility*, and *reproductive*.[7] Also in 2019, eczema research received almost three times as much funding from the NIH as endometriosis research, despite the fact that most children outgrow eczema and that, among adults, up to two and a half times as many people suffer from endometriosis as from eczema.[8,9,10] Let there be light y'all, damn!

Thankfully, when God created the universe, she also created souls who would call bullshit on The Patriarchy long before my friends and I did. Sophia Wallace, whom I had the great honor of getting to know through this work, has talked to me at length about the importance of recognizing the work of people with pussies whose legacies have been systematically erased from history.

I originally learned about the true shape of the clitoris from Wallace, who is responsible for heaving, through the virality of CLITERACY, the image of the internal clitoris into the mainstream zeitgeist. Her anatomically representational work was made possible by the work of Dr. Helen O'Connell, an Australian urologist who established the internal structure of the clitoris in her famous 1998 study, "Anatomical Relationship Between Urethra and Clitoris." Dr. O'Connell's inquiry into this anatomy came about when she read *A New View of a Woman's Body* (1981) by the Federation of Feminist Women's Health Centers (FFWHC), an organization that grew out of a badass group that helped pregnant people get abortions before *Roe v. Wade*. The FFWHC's research methods involved members sitting around, spreading their legs, masturbating in front of each other, and taking notes about what they saw. And that ultimately led to the establishment of the internal clitoral anatomy!

A New View of a Woman's Body was, in turn, greatly influenced by *Our Bodies, Ourselves* (1972) by the Boston Women's Health Book Collective. One member of both projects was Rebecca Chalker, who went on to write *The Clitoral Truth* (2000), in which she explodes the possibilities and narratives around pussy pleasure and recounts how the scientific truths about pussy anatomy had to be excavated out of obscurity by non–medical professionals. She writes in the introduction, "The early editions of *Our Bodies, Ourselves* opened a tsunami of hitherto unavailable information about basic physiology and self-care, and provided sophisticated critiques of medical studies that enabled women to make truly informed choices about the diagnosis and treatment of common conditions, from yeast infections to cancer."

Both projects grew out of the consciousness-raising groups of the 1970s in which people with pussies got together simply to talk about their experiences of their bodies and social roles, which, at the time, was a super-radical act.

Another person who has worked on later editions of *Our Bodies, Ourselves* is Heather Corinna, the founder of Scarleteen, the internet's first queer, inclusive sex ed site, whom I have also had the incredible privilege of getting to know. Corinna, like Wallace, has stressed to me on many occasions the importance of ethically building one another's work, of helping to preserve one another's legacies. Scarleteen, founded in 1998, was decades ahead of its time politically and is, in my opinion, still by very far the best and most comprehensive sex ed site out there.

Corinna grew up with *Our Bodies, Ourselves*, and they explained to me that its cultural contribution goes far beyond just the information that it provides:

Before the feminist self-help health movement, nobody—I mean Western people, who I can speak for—would have privileged our own experiences in our bodies over what a doctor said was happening. Nobody would have decided they had authority on the basis of their experiences. There wasn't a tradition of believing our own or each other's experience of our bodies, of privileging that, of prioritizing that, and certainly not when the people and bodies in question were not men.

This is in no way an exhaustive account of the magnificent giants upon whose work/shoulders Pussypedia stands. It is also a terribly white list of people—not because Black people, Indigenous people, and people of color (BIPOC) have not historically contributed work to this field. As Corinna says, it's rather because "unfortunately, that's who has historically had access to publishing." This is changing.

Right now, there are a ton of BIPOC sex and pleasure educators/activists/ writers/researchers out there as well as educators/activists/writers/researchers with disabilities doing incredible work to change the way we talk about our bodies, relationships, sex, and pleasure for the better, like: adrienne maree brown; Ericka Hart, MEd, D/s; Sonya Renee Taylor, MSA; Stacey Dutton, PhD; Laura Inter; Roxane Gay, MA, PhD; Trista Marie McGovern; Alice Wong, MA; Pidgeon Pagonis, MWS; Bianca Laureano, PhD, CSES, MA;[2] and Dr. Lexx Brown-James, just to name a few. And that is an amazing and beautiful thing because sadly, access to publishing is just the tip of the systemic-racism iceberg.

As writer and medical ethicist Harriet A. Washington chronicles in her essential 2007 book, *Medical Apartheid: The Dark History of Medical Experimentation on Black Americans from Colonial Times to the Present*, the history of Medicine in the United States has involved white people preventing nonwhite people from studying medicine as well as white researchers' intellectual theft of the work of nonwhite researchers.[11] This erasure continues in the form of the (easily unnoticed) tendency not to cite BIPOC researchers' work, not to write them into history, and not to protect their legacies, as has often been the case, if to a lesser extent, for people with pussies. As late as 2015, Black researchers were still less likely to get their research proposals funded by the NIH, no matter how prestigious their institution or how long their list of academic achievements.[7]

And still, all of this is to say nothing of the centuries of horrendous abuse that went into generating so much of our medical knowledge—especially gynecological knowledge. J. Marion Sims, the "father of gynecology," did his experiments on enslaved people, which involved surgeries without consent or anesthesia. Up to 30 of those surgeries were performed on one woman, Anarcha Westcott. Sims was neither the first nor the last; Washington writes that "dangerous, involuntary, and nontherapeutic, experimentation upon African

Americans has been practiced widely and documented extensively at least since the eighteenth century."[11]

Brutal racial injustice persists. And we must always look directly at it and name it, just as we must The Patriarchy. And we must figure out what the hell to do about both because we can't take down one without taking down the other.

It has been strange, to say the least, to sit inside writing about vaginal discharge as the world at times seems to be—and at other times literally is—on fire, a revolution rages outside my window, the water runs out, democracy falls to pieces, millions of people drop dead of a plague, and the dark implications of inequality make themselves clearer than ever.

There have been moments when I have had to ask myself, *Should I really be spending this time comparing the chemical compositions of squirt juice and pee?* But then I remind myself that a lot of people have pussies and that a lot of those people live with a lot of their mental space taken up by a lot of inane patriarchal bullshit and that if we can free up even a little bit of that or restore even a little bit of pleasure or agency, then there will be more space, more joy, and more pussy power for the revolution. And the answer is always yes.

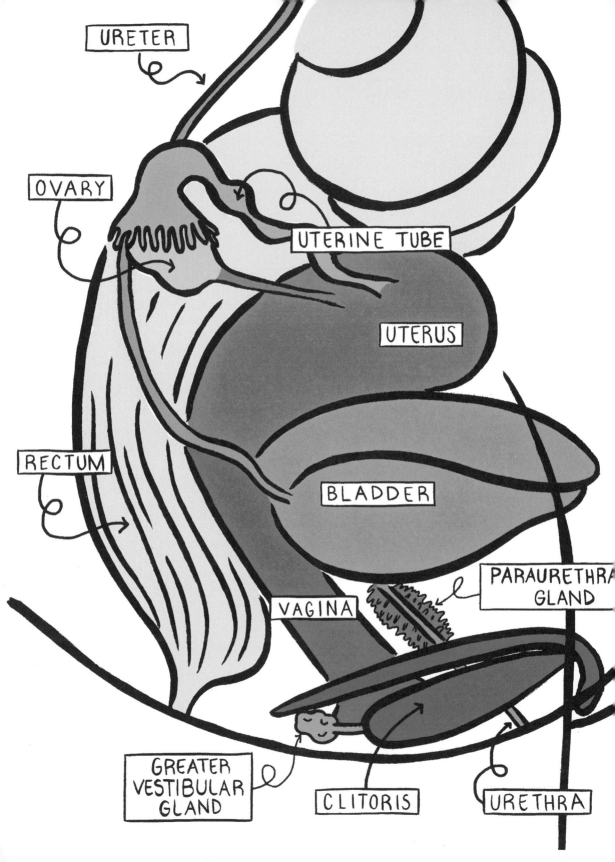

URETER

OVARY

UTERINE TUBE

UTERUS

RECTUM

BLADDER

PARAURETHRA GLAND

VAGINA

GREATER VESTIBULAR GLAND

CLITORIS

URETHRA

PUSSY PARTS

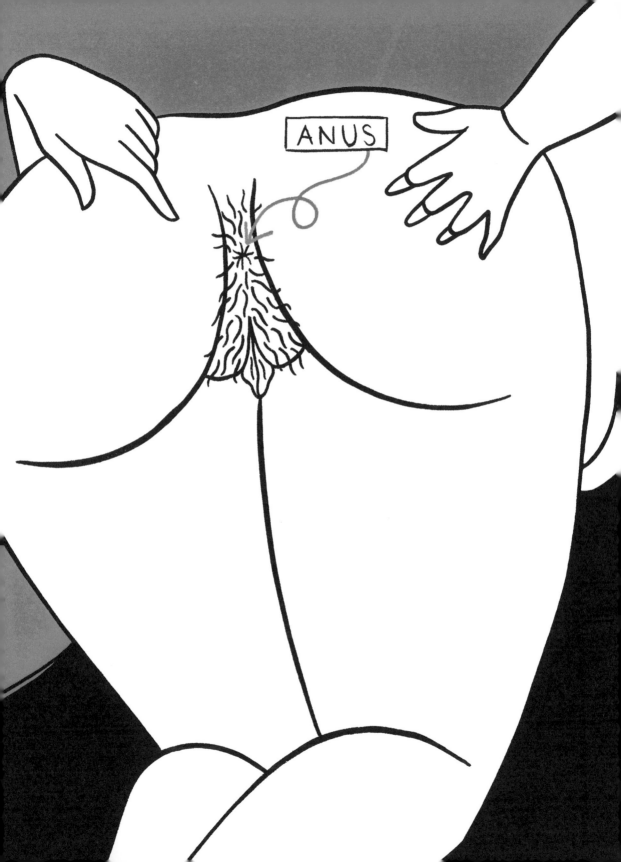

1
Anus, Ass Crack, and Rectum

I HAVE A HAIRY ASS CRACK. I MEAN, LIKE, REALLY, SUBSTANTIALLY HAIRY. YOU might have a hairy ass crack too. That's because sometimes ass cracks are hairy. Though you wouldn't know that from looking at most anatomical illustrations, which, if they show any hair at all, usually only show it going down to the bottom of the vulva. Anyway, I didn't know that it was hairier than most until I was 22 and dating an older man who told me, the first time I was in his shower, "I love your super-hairy ass crack." Shout-out to him. He meant it. He was a good one. But my super-hairy ass crack was news to me. Since then, I have 100% had sexual partners be like, "Wow, ew, I can't deal with that." And, hey, they don't have to! But neither do I.

Really, what are my options to "deal with it"? Shave it? No. Wax it? Who has time and money for that shit? Seriously. I've been stressed about money my whole life, so spending it to "fix" something that doesn't feel broken has always seemed out of the question and like a much less appealing way to spend my money than buying weed. And, even if I *were* rich, I can't imagine using my precious time on that. Here is a list of activities that seem like a better use of my free time:

- Drink beer with my friends
- Call my grandma

- Observe pigeons
- Pick up garbage around my neighborhood

Also, who would I be waxing it for? A person whose values I don't respect, like my one horrible ex who was so bothered by my ass-crack hair that he would wax it himself? No, thank you. I pretended not to mind but it hurt and felt degrading. I basically haven't thought about my ass crack hair since we broke up. My husband offered to braid it once.

Anyway, if you love waxing your ass crack, more power to ya. I just hope everyone's ass-crack-related decisions come from their own personal desires and priorities and not out of fear of being unappealing to others.

Now That We've Gotten Ass-Crack Hair Out of the Way, Here Is My Second-Favorite Anus Topic

Your rectum and anus are basically geniuses. Your rectum—the 12-centimeter tube that connects the large intestine to the anus—and your anus can feel whatever's in them and send messages to your brain about whether it's a fart or poop or diarrhea, so you won't shart.[1,2] I mean, sometimes sharts happen, but mostly not. You can thank your very smart, very sensitive anus and rectum for that.

Third-Favorite Anus Topics (A Tie)

There are two correct plural forms of *anus*: *ani* and *anuses*. That fact is tied with the fact that anuses, the very end of the human digestive tract, happen to look hilariously similar to pursed lips, which are the beginning of the digestive tract. *Lips in, lips out.* Pure poetry. (Now imagine an anus smiling.)

Fourth-Favorite Anus Topic

All people, whatever sex, whatever gender, can have prostates! The prostate is *not* part of the rectum or anus, but it's rectum-related and anus-adjacent because the prostate is the thing that makes anal sex pleasurable in "male" bodies (it gets poked when something is stuck into the rectum). Historically, it was believed that only "male" bodies had prostates. The lesser-known pussy prostate is called the periurethral glands. They are in a squishy tube, called the urethral sponge, which wraps around the urethra. It is the anatomy responsible for creating the G-spot. (See Chapter 4 for more about the pussy's prostate.)

Fifth-Favorite Anus Topic

The word *sphincter* may sound like it means "con artist" in Yiddish, but actually sphincters are muscular rings that keep tubes in your body closed. The anal sphincter keeps your butthole closed when you're not pooping. If your anus were a scrunchie, it would be the elastic inside. Part of it can be relaxed and tightened at will, and the other part is controlled by your autonomic nervous system, which you mostly don't have conscious control of.[3]

If something brushes the skin around your anus, the sphincter will automatically contract. This is, seriously, literally called the *anal wink*.[4] You're welcome.

Sixth-Favorite Anus Topic

I feel pretty neutral on ass play, but I think it's important to normalize and to educate about because it can be intensely pleasurable for some people with pussies, and I don't want anyone to miss out on a thing like sticking things in and around their butthole if that might just light up their lives. It's also a thing a lot of people do wrong and get hurt doing, so let's go over some things.

1. Anal sex is not immoral or weird or naughty or Bad. Depictions of butt sex can be found in Chinese and Japanese woodblock prints and handscrolls from the 16th to 19th centuries, in South American ceramics from 150 to 800 CE, and in French lithography and photography from the 19th and 20th centuries.[5] And not that something having happened historically makes it OK, but butt sex has been a Thing for forever, almost everywhere.

2. Ass play shouldn't hurt. If it hurts more than is pleasurable for you, stop. As Tristan Taormino, sex educator and author of *The Ultimate Guide to Anal Sex for Women*, explained in an interview on the podcast *Sexology*, anal sex is not painful by definition. "If it hurts, you have to listen to your body . . . not everyone loves it."[6] To find out if it's something for you, she suggests going slowly to warm up the anus (start with

something small!), combining it with genital stimulation, being gentle, and . . .

3. LUBE! Always use lube. Lots of lube. Like, a ton of lube. I like silicone-based lube the best because it's slipperier and doesn't leave a sticky residue, but check Chapter 16 for more on what kinds of lube can be used with what kinds of condoms and sex toys. Lubedy-lubedy lube. Never not lubing.

4. It's not just about penetration. Anuses are sensitive and pleasurable to stimulate in general. There's licking anus, rubbing anus, and putting a vibrator on your anus.[6] Butt remember, there's risk of STIs here as much as anywhere else!

5. It is incredibly easy to get something stuck in your butt, which is funny as long as it doesn't actually happen. That's why butt plugs have stoppers. If you're going to put something into your anus and that something is not attached to a person's body, make sure its back end is WAY wider than your anus. (See Chapter 16 for more info on how easy it is to get things stuck in your rectum.)

6. Use condoms. No, you cannot get pregnant from butt sex, but you can definitely still get STIs. So, yes, condoms are a good idea! In fact, because the tissues of the anus and rectum are delicate and can tear easily, infections are more easily transmitted during anal than during, say, regular ol' penis-in-vagina sex.[7]

7. Poop. That same horrible ex, The Waxer, was very funny (people can be many things), and one thing he used to say was: "Anal sex, always a crapshoot," by which he meant that there's always a possibility of some poop. Look, there might be some poop involved, but it's not going to be like a diarrhea geyser or anything, OK? If you've already taken a poop that day, you're probably in the clear. Poop only hangs out in the rectum right before it's about to come out; the rest of the time, it's higher up in your colon. You know when it's in the rectum because that's when you feel like you have to poop.[3] But all parties should be prepared for the possibility of some residue, and if some sneaks out, nobody should freak out and make the other person feel bad. Some people use enemas to clean their rectums

out before any ass play or anal sex but that's always seemed like a lot of work to me.

8. Anal play can be awesome and fun and feel amazing, but there's also a lot of coercion—unfair pressuring—that often goes on around it in heterosexual dynamics. The ass-crack-hair-positive dude I dated was the first person to introduce me to ass play. He started with his pinkie. He always used lube. He was gentle and went slow and always asked me, "Does that feel good?" He was patient. And it turned into something that I genuinely liked. That's how it should be.

The Waxer pressured me relentlessly to have anal sex. He never did enough to warm up my anus. When he was trying to work it in, he would bark, "Relax! You have to relax!" I often ended up in pain and pooping weird for days after.

One study found that "60% of heterosexual males report that they liked past experiences of anal sex 'very much,' while only 13% of heterosexual women [felt the same.]" It also found that "<10% of men disliked having anal sex with women while between 40% and 47% of women considered anal sex unpleasant and undesireable."[8] Another found that a lot of people end up having anal sex because they are submitting to the desires and dominance of their male sexual partners rather than because they want to.[9]

Anal play can be fun, but you don't owe it to anyone and should never be made to feel that you do. I know how complicated and convoluted and confusing it is to be on the receiving end of sexual coercion and all I can tell you is: *you are right*. That quiet little feeling in your stomach is right. If something doesn't feel good, it isn't good. (See Chapter 13 for more on being able to say what you do and don't want.)

9. If you're curious but nervous about anal, sex educator Melina Gaze recommends trying anal by yourself first. "If you're a beginner, it may feel strange or uncomfortable. Trying it alone first can take away the pressure of performing or having everything be perfect and great. You can start with a finger or beginner butt plug and a lot of lube. For some people it takes a few times to get used to the feeling. Go at your own pace

and learn about what you like so you can communicate with a partner. Talk about your concerns with your partner."

Least Favorite Anus Topic: Hemorrhoids and Fissures

Hemorrhoids are swollen blood vessels in and around the anus and bottom of the rectum. They can hurt, itch, and get irritated. Usually they are caused by pushing too hard while pooping (either because you are constipated or just overzealous) and are common during pregnancy. You don't have that many options for treating hemorrhoids but you can try ice, a hot bath, over-the-counter suppositories (little medicine capsules that go in your anus), or creams like Preparation H.[10]

Fissures are little tears in the anus. They can happen from one really giant, hard poop, a lot of diarrhea over time, anal sex, constipation, and/or pushing too hard.[11] To heal them, you need your butthole to relax. Again, a warm bath might help and, if things get desperate, doctors might recommend anal numbing creams or even butthole Botox.

Mostly, with both hemorrhoids and fissures, you just have to eat fiber and drink water to keep your poop soft, wait to heal, and try to keep your anus blissfully relaxed.[11]

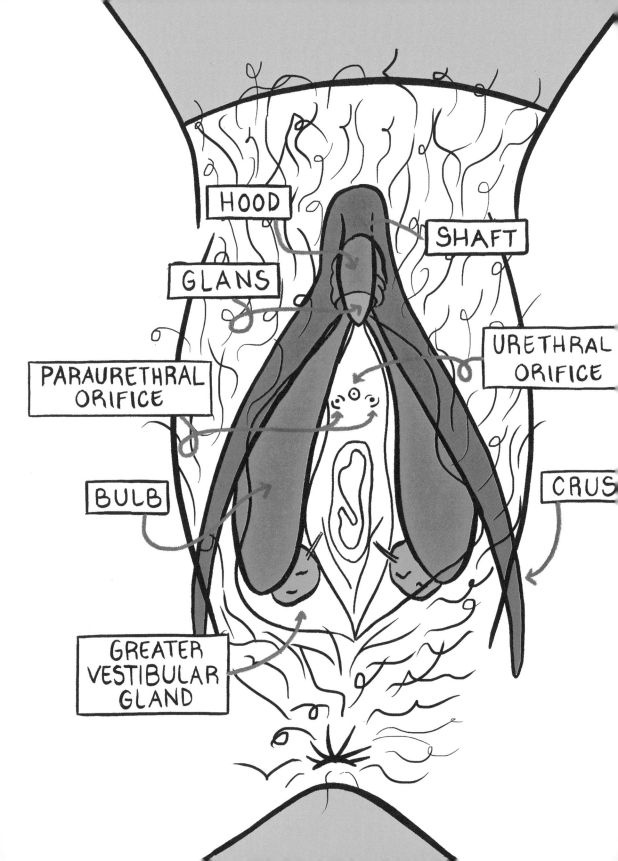

2
The Clitoris

As of November 2020, if you search PubMed—the most important and probably the biggest internet database of biomedical information—for "penis," you get 50,671 results. If you search for "clitoris," you get 2,444. The clitoris is the pussy's central pleasure organ and the anatomical equivalent to the penis (though I wish I didn't have to refer to the penis to make the point that the clitoris is relevant!), and most people could not draw one or tell you how it works, how big it really is, or where it is inside the body. (Of course, many . . . *cough* . . . *people* don't know where the part of the clitoris that sticks out of the body is, either.)

The clitoris doesn't get taught in school when we learn about "the reproductive system" (as if pussies are only for reproduction!). And even if you venture out to teach yourself about the clitoris, it's hard to find good information. As Dr. Helen O'Connell, the Australian urologist who formally mapped the internal structure of the clitoris in 1998, has said, "Typical textbook descriptions of the clitoris lack detail and include inaccuracies."[1]

Even the Oxford Languages dictionary definition of *clitoris* is inaccurate—"a small, sensitive, erectile part of the female genitals at the anterior end of the vulva"—as if most of its internal structure doesn't exist. Also, the clit is about the same size on average as a penis (nine centimeters, flaccid),[2,3] and yet *small* is strangely missing from the definition of *penis*. Huh.

The erasure of the clitoris is a problem. Clitoris champion and artist Sophia Wallace put it succinctly in her TEDx Talk, "A Case for Cliteracy": "We can't truly be free if our bodies are assailed. We can't truly enjoy democracy if half of the population can't speak about their own body, is censored when they say the words because these words are taboo, or are regularly having sex without orgasms."

But *why*? Why does the clit get so . . . shafted? Many people say it's because it's inside the body and therefore harder to observe than the penis. But most of the body is inside the body! And still, no other part of the body—internal or external—has been as historically invisible. So there has to be another reason. I think that reason is that the clitoris has always been a threat to The Patriarchy. Looking back on the ways the anatomy of the clitoris has been conceived through time illuminates how.

What It Actually Is: The Anatomy of the Clitoris

Let's start by establishing what I'm talking about when I talk about the clitoris. The little button of the clitoris that sticks out of the body is called the *glans*.[1] It's generally super sensitive. Many texts say that the glans of the clit has 6,000–8,000 nerve endings in it, and this is often stated as a way to say the clit is superior to the penis, which supposedly has fewer nerve endings. But it's really not a contest, y'all! (Also, I could not for the life of me find the origin of this "fact" about clitoral and penile nerve endings, and I think it may actually be based on one single study that was done on cows.) What's important is that the clit has many more nerve endings than the vagina and that it is the central engine of pussy pleasure. The skin that hangs over the glans is called the *hood*, or the *prepuce*.[4] Both glans and hoods can look very different from one body to another. Some hoods cover the glans. Others don't. But that's definitely not all of the clitoris.

The clitoris is kind of like those photo-op boards you find at tourist attractions, the ones you stand behind and stick your head through so that your face is on the body of a cartoon or a famous person. In this metaphor, most of the clit is behind the board (inside the body).

The neck of the clitoris (formally called the *shaft* or *body*) runs along the pubic bone, below the mons, then it splits into two.[1,2] The two arms (*crura*) are made of erectile tissue and are about five to nine centimeters long.[4,5,6] The two big bulbs (just *bulbs*) on the bottom, which hug the urethra and vagina, are made of spongy tissue that fills up with blood during arousal.[4] So, yes, people with pussies also get boners! If someone takes testosterone, their clit is likely to grow bigger, and to grow even more upon arousal, than before testosterone.[7]

A clitoris that has been constructed surgically from a penis will be made out of the head of the penis (also called the *glans*) and about 86% of the time, according to one study, still capable of orgasm.[8] It makes sense that the glans of the clit and the penis have the same name, and that one can be used to make the other, because they are basically the same thing.

For the first six-ish weeks of fetal development, all fetuses' genitals are the same.[4] Around the seven- to eight-week mark, the fetus and its genitals begin to differentiate by sex. The glans of any body is always the glans, from its beginning as a fetus, and it stays being the glans—it just grows to different sizes in slightly different locations on each person's genital package. We know now that every part of genital anatomy works the same way. Penises and pussies have the same parts; they're just kind of jumbled around into different configurations.

But it took, like, a really, *really* long time to get to this understanding of clitoral anatomy.

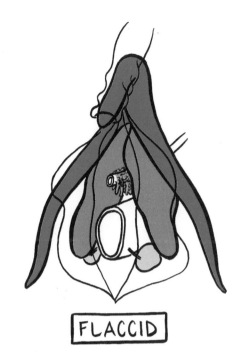

FLACCID

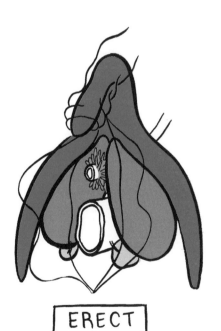

ERECT

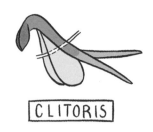

CLITORIS

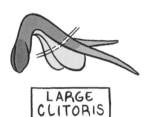

LARGE CLITORIS

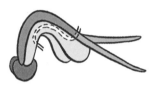

HYPOSPADIAS PENIS

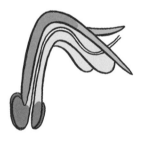

PENIS

HOOD

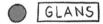

GLANS

SHAFT

CRUS

BULB

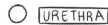

URETHRA

Centuries of Inching Toward Acknowledging the Aforementioned Anatomy of the Clitoris, Part 1: "Discovery" of a Thing Quite Perceptible to Sight and Touch and That Pokes Out of Half the Planet's Bodies

In ancient Rome there was a very influential doctor named Galen who basically said, *Women are like men except their bodies are kind of fucked up and worse. The vagina is an inside-out penis. And that clitoris thing some people have pointed out does not fit into that theory so stop asking about it.* So people basically stopped asking about it for like 1,400 years.[9] (The Middle Ages were a bad time for Science.)[4]

Fast-forward to 16th-century Italy. Andreas Vesalius, a prominent anatomist, agreed with Galen and was upholding his idea about vaginas being inside-out penises and clits not existing. Then, two of his students, Renaldus Columbus and Gabriel Fallopius (the one who would later pee on the fallopian tubes with his name), each said, "Yes, it is a thing!" around the same time and then promptly started arguing about who had "discovered" the clitoris.[4,6,10] Columbus (of course that's his name) wrote: "Since no one has discerned these projections and their workings, if it is permissible to give names to things discovered by me, it should be called the love or sweetness of Venus."[9] Wow.

Neither of them had "discovered" much more than the glans and shaft of the clit anyway, so they were really being super extra.[1,9] In response, Vesalius pooh-poohed his students' findings: "It is unreasonable to blame others for incompetence . . . you can hardly ascribe this new and useless part, as if it were an organ, to healthy women."[1] So first, he generously concedes that it's not Columbus and Fallopius's fault that they were incompetent, then says that the clitoris is not an organ that most "healthy women" have.

In the 17th century, Thomas Bartholin, who would later pee on the greater vestibular glands with his name, pointed out that Columbus and Fallopius were both "vainglorious" knuckleheads because the clitoris had been described as early as the 2nd century. (There are ancient Greek, Arab, and Persian records of observation of the clitoris.)[9,10] Beyond affirming the existence of the clit, Bartholin also challenged the idea that the vagina was an inside-out penis. This was important because it had been confusing people for way too long because if the vagina was an inside-out penis, what was the clit supposed to be? The inside-out penis idea had also been used as proof of an inherent imbalance between the sexes. Bartholin called it an "ideological plot hatched by those who accounted a Woman to be only an imperfect Man."[9]

A Not-Really-Tangential Tangent About Pee, Ejaculate, and Stories

I wonder if any of these be-penised scientists pondered the possibility that perhaps little kids with pussies had been discovering their own clitorises since the dawn of time. I mean, didn't, like, *everyone* with a clitoris, and probably a lot of people with penises, know about the clitoris?! In my mind, this whole "discovery" of the clit seems equivalent to: *Breaking news! Half of global population has dangly tubular organ-thingy hanging off their crotch!*

But I have to remind myself that we can't presume that people with pussies were aware of their own clitorises before scientific and linguistic recognition created a story about the clit that had become popularized public knowledge (which, like, we're still not there).

Here's a story that explains why the clit's existence may not have been as obvious as we would think. When I interviewed Dr. Beverly Whipple, the scientist who first formally established the existence of pussy ejaculation, I asked her, "Why do you think you had to do so many studies to prove that something happens if it happens to so many people?" She responded, "Well, women would come into my clinic saying they were urinating during sex." Dr. Whipple's patients, like so many people with pussies, didn't realize that "urinating during sex" was actually ejaculation because they thought people with pussies didn't ejaculate.

See? We use our stories to make our observations rather than using our observations to make our stories. As Thomas Laqueur, author of *Making Sex: Body and Gender from the Greeks to Freud*, wrote, "The history of anatomy during the Renaissance suggests that the anatomical representation of male and female is dependent on the cultural politics of representation and illusion, not on evidence about organs. . . . No image, verbal or visual, of the 'facts of sexual difference' exists independently of prior claims about the meanings of such distinctions."[9] Those prior claims and meanings—stories—were more important than the evidence in front of them, like whether or not their ejaculate smelled or looked anything like pee, which it probably didn't.

Centuries of Inching Toward Acknowledging the Aforementioned Anatomy of the Clitoris, Part 2: Things Briefly Look Up, Then Go to Shit

In 1672, Regnier de Graaf published what Dr. O'Connell called "the first comprehensive account of clitoral anatomy." It was actually pretty decent and even finally depicted the clitoral bulbs.[1,10] De Graaf wrote: "We are extremely surprised that some anatomists make no more mention of this part than if it did not exist at all in the universe of nature. In every cadaver we have so far dissected we have found it quite perceptible to sight and touch."[1]

Well, Regnier-boo, I can't say I share your extreme surprise. I think "some anatomists" were cis men who didn't want to acknowledge the clitoris because pussy pleasure scared them. As Rebecca Chalker notes in *The Clitoral Truth*, Jean-Jacques Rousseau, a prominent 18th-century philosopher, "believed, just as the Greeks did, that female reticence, discretion, and modesty really masked a fierce excess of passion that, if unleashed, would disrupt the male-centered social order."[4] And even if that passion weren't a fierce excess, many feminists have theorized that pussy pleasure became an ultimate taboo in The Patriarchy because *pleasure can set us free*. As The Great Audre Lorde wrote in *Uses of the Erotic: The Erotic as Power* in 1978:

> The erotic is a resource within each of us . . . firmly rooted in the power of our unexpressed or unrecognized feeling. In order to perpetuate itself, every oppression must corrupt or distort those various sources of power within the culture of the oppressed that can provide energy for change. For women, this has meant a suppression of the erotic as a considered source of power and information within our lives. We have been taught to suspect this resource, vilified, abused, and devalued within Western society.

I don't believe that any genital combination has more or less passion than another, but if people with pussies had known from the jump that they are biologically equal, they may have gotten pissed about their subjugated social position a lot earlier. And if they'd been enjoying the shit out of their clitorises, they may have had more power with which to do something about it. That's why what happened next makes so much sense: a few centuries during which Science minimized pussy sexuality and asserted that it was "weak, chaste, and passionless." [4]

In 1844, Georg Ludwig Kobelt published a huge study of the clitoris, even more detailed and accurate than De Graaf's, in which he set out to disprove the idea that had come into fashion: that the clitoris is small and insignificant and that people with pussies are less sexual than their counterparts.[4] He wrote: "I have made it my principal concern to show that the female possesses a structure that in all its separate parts is entirely analogous to the male."[1] And he was right! Remember the thing about fetal development and how the genitals are the same just rearranged? He also compared the nerves in the vagina to the nerves in the clitoris glans and concluded, "We can grant the vagina no part in the creation of the specific pleasurable sex feelings in the female body."[9] (He was onto something, but see Chapter 9 for why this might not be entirely true.) If only Kobelt's ideas had taken root. Alas.

In the ensuing years, Science began to consider the clitoris useless. In 1865, Dr. Isaac Baker Brown, president of the Medical Society of London, published *On the Curability of Certain Forms of Insanity, Epilepsy, Catalepsy, and Hysteria in Females*, which proposed cutting off the clitoris as a cure for all those problems, since their cause was—obviously—masturbation. The book was a huge success, and clitoridectomies, the surgical removal of the glans of the clitoris, became widespread in Europe and the US. A few years later, a group of doctors were like, *Wait, this is horrible,* and Baker Brown was forced to resign as head of his own hospital and expelled from the Obstetrical Society. His ideas unfortunately took much longer to go out of style. Cases of "therapeutic" clitoridectomies were reported until 1940.[10]

Meanwhile, where Kobelt's clit-power ideas were posited, they were mocked. One French author, Dr. Jules Guyot, wrote of the clitoris in 1852, "There exists an immense number of ignorant, egoistic, brutal men who do not bother to study the instrument that God has entrusted to them."[10] (I'm pretty sure God entrusted my clitoris to ME, but otherwise: YES, JULES!)

In response, the popular author Dr. Pierre Garnier wrote: "To claim that this miniscule apparatus, which is most often an insensitive little button so long as it has not been touched or artificially manipulated, is the most active erogenous centre, is to implicitly accuse all girls of once having resorted to masturbation or of one day becoming debauched."[10] *GASP* I find his central assumption extremely hilarious: if "girls" knew how erogenous their clits were, they would definitely play with them . . . I guess he was kind of right about that.

What's not funny is that Garnier's words demonstrate the serious taboo that existed around pussy pleasure. This 19th-century taboo facilitated a scientific and cultural erasure. It's simple: if something is considered foul and immoral, people will be less likely to talk about it, to write about it, or to consider it serious or important or worthy of study.

In 1905, Sigmund Freud wrote that the clitoris was an "infantile organ" and that clitoral pleasure was immature, secondary to the pleasure a mature, adult pussy should derive from vaginal penetration by a penis.[4,6] Thus he ushered in the era of people with pussies trying really hard to have vaginal orgasms and feeling inadequate when they couldn't, which is still happening. Freud further minimized the idea of the clitoris as the seat of pussy pleasure. (See Chapter 18 for more on the other horrible effects this idea had and why it actually *is* the seat of pussy pleasure.)

One study of anatomy textbooks from the 20th century found that, throughout the era, documentation of the clitoris waned. In 1948, the clitoris was taken out of *Gray's Anatomy*, perhaps the single most important anatomy textbook, and throughout the 1950s and 1960s, many texts followed suit.[11] As Dr. O'Connell put it, "The evolution of the female anatomy across the 20th century occurred as an act of active deletion rather than omission in the interests of brevity."[1]

Centuries of Inching Toward Acknowledging the Aforementioned Anatomy of the Clitoris, Part 3: The People with Pussies Who Dug the Clit Out of Obscurity, Sometimes by Watching One Another Masturbate

In 1966, psychiatrist Dr. Mary Jane Sherfey published *The Evolution and Nature of Female Sexuality in Relation to Psychoanalytic Theory*, in which she set out to reexamine Freud's theory in light of decades of evidence that seemed to contradict it—mainly that tons of people couldn't have vaginal orgasms, and that people wouldn't stop playing with their clits. She wrote:

> In fact, the whole problem of female sexuality . . . has received scant attention. This is most unfortunate, especially since . . . vaginal frigidity has not decreased with the increased freedom in the upbringing of girls (rather clitoral erotism and fixations seem to have increased) and . . . no form of psychotherapy or analysis has been singularly successful in the treatment of clitoral fixation.[12]

She goes on to ask: "Could the lack of psychiatric interest in the socio-psychological crisis of women today . . . and our serious therapeutic limitations and tragic failures stem, in part, from erroneous assumptions of vaginal and clitoral responsivity which form [Freud's] theory? Could much of the sexual neuroses which seem to be almost endemic in women today be, in part, iatrogenic?"[12]

Iatrogenic means an illness that is caused by medical treatment. She was suggesting that perhaps all the people going to their shrinks saying, "Something's wrong with me, I don't have vaginal orgasms," had nothing wrong at all except their idea that they were supposed to be able to have vaginal orgasms in the first place.

To support her hypothesis, she pointed out that the vaginal orgasm was the same as the clitoral orgasm, both by looking at fetal genital development (the same-parts-just-rearranged thing) and at the work of sexology pioneers Alfred Kinsey and William Masters and Virginia Johnson, who in the 1950s and 1960s had gone back to the idea that the clitoris was the seat of pussy pleasure. She concluded that "a large block of professional and public opinion . . . exists because people want the vaginal orgasm to exist."[12] (Weird right? Not sure why *cough* "people" would be so invested in the existence of the vaginal orgasm.)

Dr. Sherfey also studied why pussies can have multiple orgasms, and came to consider the pussy's capacity for pleasure and sexual intensity equal to, if not greater than, that of the penis. Yes, it was awesome and productive that Dr. Sherfey countered the superiority of the vaginal orgasm and the pussy-sexuality-as-less-passionate theories. But she also concluded, similarly to Rousseau, that people with pussies in fact have *such* a strong sexual drive that they have to be oppressed so that society won't come apart at the seams because who will take care of the babies if the moms are just out fucking everyone in sight?!? Dr. Sherfey believed that if the sexual revolution of the 1960s persisted, one outcome was certain: "A return to the rigid, enforced suppression will be inevitable and mandatory. Otherwise the biological family will disappear and what other patterns of infant care and adult relationships could adequately substitute cannot now be imagined."[12]

It is scary to think of a time when even such a smart and accomplished person with a pussy could not imagine a world in which people with pussies did not require external suppression to regulate their sexual urges and in which they might even be free to enjoy sexual pleasure responsibly while their partners shared in childcare duties.

In 1975, the Federation of Feminist Women's Health Centers (FFWHC)—which grew out of an underground abortion referral service that operated before *Roe v. Wade* and which opened aboveground clinics and health centers after it—decided to make a book about pussies and pussy health. To tell the story of FFWHC in *The Clitoral Truth*, Chalker interviewed Carol Downer, its founder and longtime CEO who was once arrested, tried, and acquitted on charges of practicing medicine without a license for showing other people how to use a speculum, mirror, and flashlight to give themselves cervical exams.[13] Downer recalled:

> Initially, we thought we would just review the popular and medical literature on sexuality, critique it, and write the chapter, but we were in for a big surprise. . . . Little of what we found in sex advice books or in medical texts seemed to correspond to our sexual experiences or to illuminate them in any useful way.[4]

So Downer and eight of her friends got together, talked about their experiences, took off their pants, compared their pussies to textbook illustrations, and took pictures and videos of one another masturbating, which they then studied carefully.[4] (I have imagined many times what it must have been like to be there in that room, masturbating for Science while my co-clit-conspirators looked on. I will never get over how brave and brilliant they were, how revolutionary it was of them to believe they could produce and improve knowledge despite every prevailing institutional narrative saying otherwise.) They dug out 18th- and 19th-century anatomy texts, and they also studied Sherfey's work. With this, they came up with their new definition of the clitoris, which included each part of the pussy that changes during orgasm. The FFWHC published it in *A New View of a Woman's Body: A Fully Illustrated Guide* in 1981.[4]

Just a year after the FFWHC had decided to create their book, Shere Hite published *The Hite Report: A Nationwide Study of Female Sexuality*, in which she conducted an open-ended survey, mostly about masturbation, of 3,000 people with pussies. She found that 82% of survey respondents said they masturbated and 95% of those respondents said they could orgasm easily.[14] She basically concluded: *Y'ALL. GUESS. WHAT. People with pussies aren't not coming because they're frigid. They're not coming because intercourse blows! And! In! Fact! We can actually get all of our pleasure from our clits and we don't need dicks at all. MUAHAHAHA.*

What she actually wrote was: "It is not female sexuality that has a problem ('dysfunction') but society that has a problem in its definition of sex and the subordinate role that definition gives women." And: "It is time we reclaimed our own bodies, and started to use them *ourselves* for our own pleasure."[14]

The book became an instant best seller and unsurprisingly made a lot of people Very Mad. *Playboy* magazine, in which Hite once posed topless (love her for being a serious academic who also did this—sex positivity, way ahead of its time), called it "The Hate Report." Still, *Ms.* magazine reported that it caused a "revolution in the bedroom." As Hite's obituary writer commented in the *New York Times*, the book "marked a sharp turning point after the 'sexual revolution' of the 1960s, which essentially had given women license to have no-strings sex with as many partners as men had always had, but which had done little to change the male-centric dynamic in bed."[15]

As it happens, many people had a vested interest in not changing the male-centric dynamic in bed. Hite was so hunted and harassed for her work that she ended up spending much of the rest of her life in exile in Europe.[15] (Please image-search Shere Hite. In every single photograph I've seen, she has obscenely much style. And, yes, if a man had *that* much style, I would also comment on it.)

In 1988, 27-year-old Helen O'Connell came across the FFWHC's *A New View of a Woman's Body*. She thought the book's methodology was amazing and

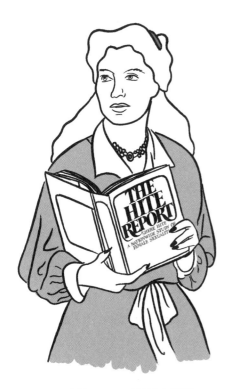

SHERE HITE

was especially excited about it after having been pissed off by the absence of the clitoris in other texts she studied.[16] Ten years later, she would take things into her own hands. Literally.

She and her team dissected 10 cadavers to look at their clitorises, urethras, and the relationship between those structures, and published their findings in a groundbreaking study in which she established that what were formerly called the vestibular bulbs are actually part of the clitoris. It was the first study to formally establish the clitoris's anatomy in the full penguin shape we know it today. In 2005, Dr. O'Connell published another study, "Anatomy of the Clitoris," using MRI scans to confirm her 1998 conclusions, which matched Kobelt's conclusions from 1844. Since Dr. O'Connell's work, there have been further studies using newer technologies to map the nerves, neurological pathways, and blood supply to the clitoris.

We've gotten to a level of considerable scientific documentation and detail of the clitoris, little of which is shown in most contemporary medical anatomy textbooks.[17] And yet there are still trolls trying to make the clit go away. Perhaps the most vocal is a dude named Vincenzo Puppo, whose Twitter bio says that he is a physician, sexologist, and "expert in the art of love making," and who seriously wrote in 2015 that "the internal/inner clitoris does not exist."[18] In my opinion, he has never managed to construct any basis for that argument. What he writes is (again, in my opinion) generally nonsensical. For example, in March 2021, he tweeted an accurate 3D model of the clitoris with the caption: "This 3D model is not the clitoris, it is useless for women, there are anatomical mistakes, there is no labia minora and clitoral prepuce . . . It is not the clitoris" (weird punctuation per original). That's like saying a drawing of a skull has anatomical mistakes because it's missing the nose and face skin.

Unfortunately, Puppo is very determined and manages to publish a lot of long, contentious responses to the work of people studying the clitoris. (One weakness that academia and journalism share is that it's easy to get published just by having a niche point. Saying no to the clitoris isn't new, but it is niche now that most of the conversation has thankfully taken a new direction.) The sad part is that he gets cited far too often by unsuspecting health sites and journalists. It's easy to imagine how this happens. Remember how few results there are when you search for "clitoris" on PubMed?

Unconquerable

Puppo is a nuisance, and I wouldn't mention him if I didn't think it was important. To me, he represents The Patriarchy's ongoing desire to erase the clitoris because the clitoris still represents a threat to The Patriarchy. Proving the existence of the clitoris is still a battle.

This is why I love the sculpture Ἀδάμας, which is pronounced *Adamas* and means "unconquerable" in Greek, by Sophia Wallace, aforementioned artist and creator of the CLITERACY movement. The sculpture is probably the first ever to portray the clitoris's full anatomy. It is a giant (43 × 72 × 11 inches), shiny, regal AF clitoris fashioned in a stance of strength and glory and bravado. Wallace's *CLITERACY*, a series of multimedia artworks, went viral starting in 2013 and a few times over the next few years. It catapulted the true shape of the clitoris into the mainstream zeitgeist. And, in fact, it is how I ended up seeing the true shape of the clitoris for the first time. (When I got to see the sculpture in person in Wallace's studio, I waited for her to go to the bathroom and literally took a selfie with it.)

"'Cliteracy' describes more than being able to sexually 'read' a clitoris, but more importantly the production of knowledge itself of the bodies of people with clits," Wallace, who's now a friend and teacher, told me. "To varying degrees, people with clits have historically been controlled, if not literally owned, by men. We have been trapped by the definitions, subordinations, and ignorance of those who colonized us. *CLITERACY* is about repossessing our bodies, our pleasure, and our authority over the knowledge of ourselves." (That's the goal of this book too!)

As *Making Sex* author Laqueur wrote, "The tale of the clitoris is a parable of culture, of how the body is forged into a shape valuable to civilization despite and not because of itself." I'm not sure why he says "valuable to civilization" when he means "upholding The Patriarchy," but he is right. The clitoris undermines The Patriarchy's narrative that the bodies of people with pussies are inherently passive receptacles. The full shape of the clitoris represents the idea that our bodies are equal, and that therefore we as people are equal.

The clit should be fully illustrated and labeled in every anatomy text. It should be a well-funded area of scientific research. It should be taught to kids at home and in school. It should be paid a great deal of attention to in bed. It should be an acceptable word to say out loud. It should be known. By everyone.

Because as another of Wallace's works states: "Democracy without cliteracy is a phallusy."[19]

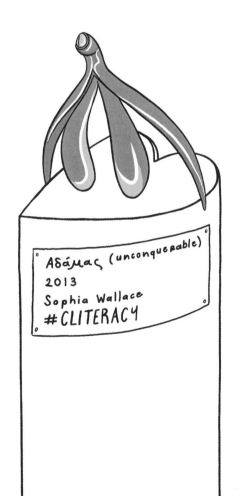

Αδάμας (unconquerable)
2013
Sophia Wallace
#CLITERACY

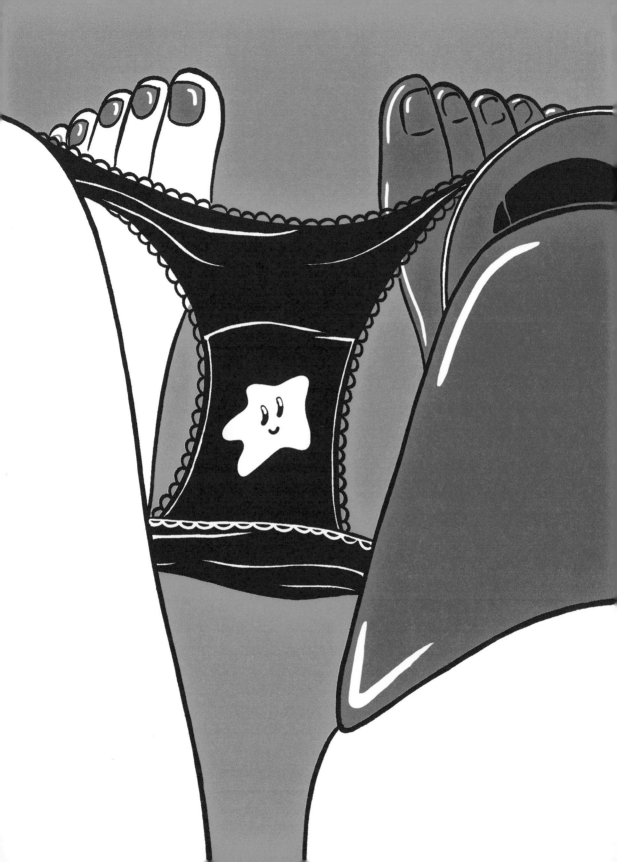

3
Liquids and Goops (Everything Except Pee and Blood)

What Is in My Panties?

Discharge has two main components: liquid secreted from your vaginal walls and mucus from your cervix. Cervical mucus is how pussies clean themselves. Mucus is a part of the immune system; it has antibodies that fight germs.[1] Cervical mucus traps germs and dead skin cells from the uterus and vagina.[2] (See Chapter 26 for more on how the vagina uses lactic acid and good bacteria to keep itself clean.)

The amount and texture of mucus produced by your cervix change throughout your menstrual cycle. Some people track their cycles based on physical signs from the body, including temperature, position of the cervix, and amount and texture of discharge (cervical mucus and vaginal liquids). It's a supercool thing because it teaches you how to read signs from your body and can be used as a form of birth control called *fertility awareness*. For example, during your more fertile periods, cervical mucus helps any sperm in your vagina get into your uterus.[3] But fertility awareness as a birth control method is only 76–88% as effective as hormonal methods.[4] Whether or not you're doing it to avoid getting pregnant, keeping track of the texture, smell, color, and amount of your

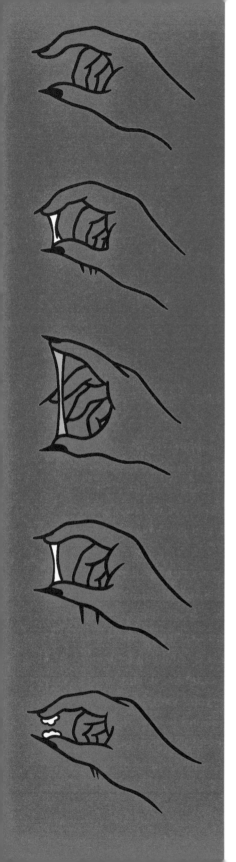

discharge is a good idea. It gives you a lot of clues as to what's going on in your body.

Before I try to describe what different kinds of discharge look like, I want to acknowledge that most of what's written about discharge, both in medical literature and in resources directed at the general pussy-having public, can be confusing.

If you've ever tried to look up information about your discharge, you've probably read something like this:

> If your discharge is, like, eggshell color but with a tint of egg white, you're fine. If it's more like ecru/bone/off-white-ish, or whipped egg whites, you might die. If it's meringue, then that's totally normal. Cottage cheese is maybe okay but if it's more like low fat than full fat, it might be a problem. If it's like cream cheese, go to the ER right now.

My point is that it's hard to look at your underwear and decide if the egg whites are whipped, if it's cottage or cream cheese. But the more you pay attention, the more you'll notice how your discharge is linked to your cycle, and you'll be able to recognize what you're looking at.

What is "normal" varies! Just try to have a solid idea of what *your* normal is so that you know when something is *not* normal for you and your body.

Generally, during menstruation, the cervix produces little to no mucus. Just after menstruation, it's nearly dry. Leading up to ovulation, around the ninth or tenth day of your cycle (day one is the first day of your period), there's more and more cervical mucus being produced, and it gets sticky, creamy, and less see-through, more of a solid color (whitish, yellowish). Right before and around ovulation, it gets slippery, stretchy, more see-through, and, yes, kind of like egg whites. After ovulation, in the luteal phase that leads up to your period, there's less cervical mucus being produced; it gets drier and stickier.[5]

If you're taking testosterone, the menstrual cycle might change or stop,[6] which could cause changes to the cervical mucus. If you've had a vaginoplasty, you probably don't have a cervix, in which case, you won't have cervical mucus. If you're taking hormonal birth control, depending on the type, you may or may not ovulate, which would change the consistency of your cervical mucus. Some kinds of birth control also make the mucus thicker so that it's harder for sperm to get through.[7]

When Your Discharge Gets Funky

If you notice the amount, smell, or color of your discharge is outside of *your normal*, you may have an infection. Again—trying to read about this and guess what's going on can be exasperating.

> If it's fishy and grayish or not gray or not fishy, it might be bacterial vaginosis. If it's thick and chunky or not chunky or smelly or possibly not smelly but slightly weird, it might be yeast. If it's green, you're probably dead right now and your ghost is reading this.

Good news: trying to self-diagnose is not your best option anyway. Different infections can manifest as different symptoms in different people, and different infections can often cause similar symptoms. One study (with a small sample size) showed that 66.3% of people who self-diagnose yeast infections and buy over-the-counter pussy creams have misdiagnosed themselves.[8] If something is off, just bring your cute, stanky self into the doctor if you can. For the love of God, don't be embarrassed. Ob-gyns are, like, bored of infected pussies.

Getting "Wet"

I can't even tell you how hot of a mess the scientific literature is on this topic. It's hard to get funding to study pussy pleasure and its anatomical structures (because in The Patriarchy, those are not considered important things). But it also just seems like pussy scientists are not reading one another's work. Anyway, here's what I've sussed out: when a pussy gets aroused, there are components to the wetness:

Greater vestibular glands (formerly called the *Bartholin's* glands) juice is made by tiny glands located on both sides of the mouth of the vagina. They produce fluid when your pussy gets aroused. This juice may serve as lubrication, may serve to deliver pheromones that say to your sexual partner(s) that you're healthy and fertile, or it may do both.[9]

Cervical fluid is not exactly an arousal fluid since mucus production does not increase during arousal but still it might be in there (texture and quantity based on where you are in your cycle) so I'm going to consider it a component of "wetness."[10]

Vaginal-wall juice comes out of the walls of your vagina and is called *transudate*. It's basically very, very filtered blood plasma. The vagina makes more of it during arousal.[11]

Periurethral glands (formerly called the *Skene's* glands) juice is made by glands that, like the Bartholin's glands, were named after men who, in the grand tradition of imperialist colonizers, "discovered" and then named them after themselves. These glands are located inside the urethral sponge, a.k.a. the G-spot. (See Chapter 4 for more on this structure.) They are sometimes called the "female prostate."

One purpose of the "male" prostate is to stop you from peeing when you have a boner. The periurethral glands do the same thing for people with pussies—if you've ever had a superhard time peeing right after an orgasm, these glands are why.[9]

Another function of the "male" prostate is to make a lot of the ingredients in male ejaculate. Again, periurethral glands do the same thing:[9] they can produce a small amount of milky liquid.[11] This is what is often called "female ejaculate" even though we don't say "female pee" or "female blood" or "male ejaculate" or "male prostate." Why assume the gender of the body in question? Let's just say "prostate" and "ejaculate."

Here are some of the things about the periurethral glands that seem to really confuse Science:

1. Whether the ejaculate they produce comes out during orgasm, like with the male prostate function, or just "during coitus." (Yes, the study I cite says "during coitus," meaning penis-in-vagina penetrative sex. Which, given that the height of arousal for people with pussies is often *not* during penetration, makes me wonder how many people with pussies are a part of this debate.)[12]

2. How many people have periurethral glands. Some studies say half of people with pussies do, others say six in seven, and still others say two-thirds.[11] It seems very unlikely that all people with pussies don't have them. It's almost as if The Patriarchy doesn't want to believe that people with pussies could have prostates because that would make us . . . biologically similar to men, which would . . . *shudder* undermine a lot of the theoretical framework of The Patriarchy.

3. What the periurethral glands' structure is. Maybe researchers can't figure out or agree on how many people even have periurethral glands because researchers are defining the structures differently and, therefore, counting differently. Some say that the glands empty fluid into the urethra. Others that it comes out of tiny single or multiple holes *next* to your pee hole.[11] This seems like it should be an easy question for Science to answer.

4. Whether or not this is where squirting comes from. Multiple studies have found periurethral gland juice *in* squirt juice,[12] and that they *might* both come out of your urethra,[11] but many studies conflate the two juices. This is despite that their chemical makeups have been shown to be very different.[13]

Can you imagine this kind of inconclusive science existing about the "male" prostate and ejaculation?!

Squirt juice: There are many silly and bad ideas out there about squirting. For example:

1. "Squirting is not real." Squirting is real. I have seen it. It is awesome.
2. "If you don't squirt, you're not reaching the heights of pleasure." You don't need to squirt to have a great time. Remember: porn is fiction.

3. "Squirt liquid is not ejaculate."[12] True, the periurethral liquid is more biologically parallel to "male" ejaculate, but who's to say squirting is not also a form of ejaculation? Here's a definition of *ejaculation* that I like, by sex educator Melina Gaze: "The release of fluid during sexual stimulation or at the moment of sexual climax." This leads us to . . .
4. "Squirt liquid is pee." As Dr. Rachel Levy, my friend and a very brilliant ob-gyn, says, "People are ON ONE about urine vs. squirt."

So is it pee or not? Hold on, I'm going to take an obnoxiously long time to get to the answer because I think we need to reflect on exactly why we are collectively ON ONE about this. I think it's because dudes don't want people with pussies to ejaculate because that's, like, their special thing. Like, men were ejaculating before it was *cool*, you know?

Scientists actually spent decades observing ejaculation (both periurethral liquid and squirt juice), unable to call it what it was. Alfred Kinsey, as well as William Masters and Virginia Johnson, all wrote that they observed liquids being expelled by pussies during arousal *and* orgasm, but all denied that it was ejaculation. Ancient Chinese, Indian, Greek, and even Renaissance-era European texts all describe female ejaculation, yet Masters and Johnson's take was, "The erroneous belief that women ejaculate probably stems from descriptions in erotic novels."[13]

As Rebecca Chalker put it in *The Clitoral Truth*, "Until the eighteenth century, when male and female sexuality began to be seen as radically different, there was no debate as to whether women 'ejaculated,' what caused it, or where the fluid came from. In the eighteenth and nineteenth centuries, the concept of female ejaculation was not discounted so much as obliterated due to the medical and social myopia through which women's sexuality was viewed."[13]

Basically, we can't see the ejaculation forest for the gender-narrative trees.

Squirt juice is clear, not yellow, and does not smell like pee, yet we look at squirt juice and say, "Pussies don't ejaculate, that's not a thing. This is pee." We are so attached to our gender narratives—to what we have been told are the radical physiological differences between "male" and "female" bodies—that it's easier to take something that *does not look or smell like pee and call it pee* than to look at a pussy gushing liquid upon arousal and/or orgasm and call it *ejaculation.*

OK, so, thank you for coming to my TED Talk, now here's the answer to "Is squirt juice pee?": A few studies have shown that it comes out of the bladder.[14,15,16] A few have shown that compounds in pee are also in squirt liquid.[14,15] A few have concluded that it's way more dilute than pee.[15,16] And a few have shown that it can also contain chemicals not found in pee that are likely periurethral liquid mixed in.[14,15,16]

There's no scientific consensus, but again, I would like to say, it's not fucking pee. If squirt juice is pee, then tomato juice is marinara sauce. Put that on your pasta, bitches.

Why Your Pussy Might Be into Freakier Porn Than You Are, or, Why Your Pussy Might Get Wet at Seemingly Weird Times

Many times I have scrolled through Pornhub looking for non-gross, or even just less-gross, porn for so long that I've ended up losing my boner. But something weird happens: I get wet anyway. This confused me for years until I read Dr. Emily Nagoski's book *Come as You Are* (essential reading, people!). In it, Dr. Nagoski explains a concept called *arousal nonconcordance.* It means that, for a person with a pussy, their genitals showing physical signs of arousal—that is, their pussy getting wet—does not predict whether the person would say they *feel* aroused.[9] In other words, it's very normal to get wet but not feel turned on. This is because your genitals may respond to anything they deem sexually "relevant." People with pussies report feeling turned on by approximately 10% of what their genitals find relevant.[9] I see porn featuring people in very ugly outfits, and my pussy thinks, *Hey, that's sex. That's sexually relevant.* And even though my brain is thinking, *Whyyyy,* I end up wet anyway. Totally normal. (Whatever kind of porn gets you going is fine, really. You do you. There's also a lot of cool feminist porn out there, and scrolling through Pornhub is not the best way to support the people that are making it anyway.)

PS: It's OK if you don't get that wet, and it's also OK if you get extremely wet. Everyone gets a different level of wet, and all of those levels are great as long as you're enjoying yourself. If you don't feel like you produce enough lube, use some lube from a bottle, or make sure you and your genitals are fully aroused before sexual play. A lot of people with pussies just take some time to get revved up. And even if you are revved up, it's very normal to still not get wet.[9] But also, lube is not a lesser second option. Using lube has been shown to increase pleasure significantly, so don't be lube shy![17]

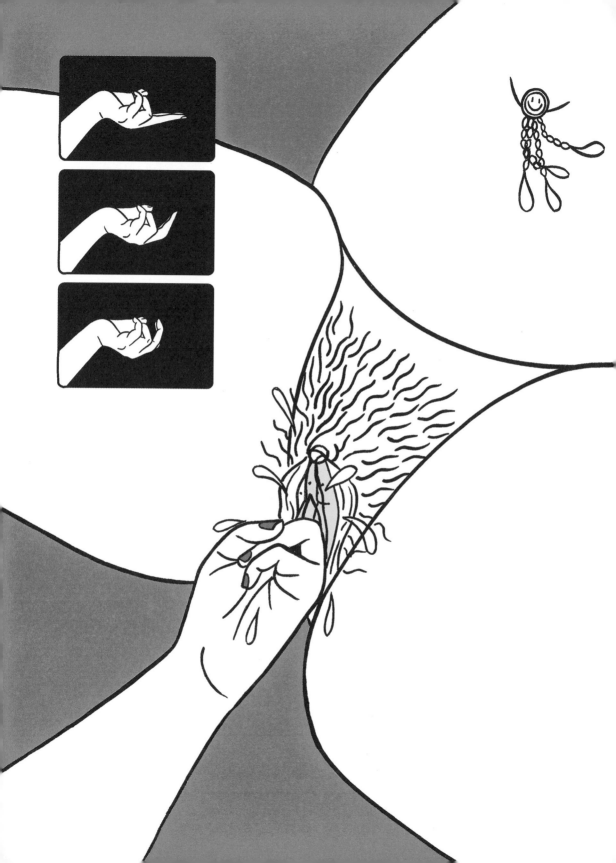

4
The G-Spot

THE G-SPOT, THE MYTHIC-BUT-ACTUALLY-REAL, SOMETIMES EXTRA-SENSITIVE PART of the inside of a vagina that, when properly stimulated, can, in some cases, produce vaginal orgasms definitely does exist. And yet, this year, *Cosmopolitan* ran an article about how it's a total sham and doesn't exist. Which is weird. Because we have basically known what the G-spot is and how the G-spot works for over 50 years.

The G-Spot Is Where Pleasure Parts Are Smooshed Together

The structures that explain the existence of the G-spot are the bulbs of the clitoris and the tube of erectile tissue that surrounds the urethra, called the *urethral sponge.* It's corpus spongiosum, the same kind of erectile tissue that surrounds the urethra in a penis. It contains the paraurethral glands, sometimes called the "female" prostate,* and is super connected to the clitoris, which is why it can feel good to stimulate.[1,2]

In 99% of anatomical descriptions and depictions that I've ever found, the vagina and urethra are parallel and separate structures. But a 1998 landmark study published in the *Journal of Urology* by Dr. Helen O'Connell, "Anatomical Relationship Between Urethra and Clitoris," established that the two are, in fact, attached. In the same study, Dr. O'Connell famously established the

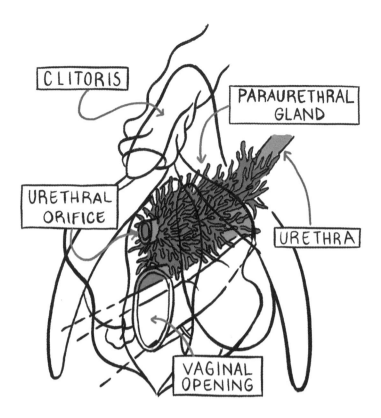

CLITORIS

PARAURETHRAL GLAND

URETHRAL ORIFICE

URETHRA

VAGINAL OPENING

internal structure of the clitoris. Dr. O'Connell concluded, based on cadaver dissections, that the urethra is actually embedded IN the vaginal wall on one side and surrounded by the urethral sponge on all other sides.[2]

During arousal, the urethral sponge fills with blood (it's a boner). The clitoral bulbs engorge, squeezing the also-engorged urethral sponge and the vagina together. Not only are they squeezed together, but the erectile tissue of the bulbs and the urethra share veins and nerves with the vagina. That's why the urethral sponge and the clitoral bulbs can get stimulated through the vagina: they're all smooshed and wired together. The urethral sponge, clitoris, and vagina function as one glorious, pleasure-producing, integrated system.[1]

This is why a vaginal orgasm is really still a clit orgasm. (But see Chapter 18 about why that distinction makes no sense.) Wherever your urethral sponge presses against your vaginal wall when you are aroused is your G-spot. You can think of the G-spot as the clit's back door.

So why are we still debating whether or not it exists?

The Mysteriously Persistent Non-Mystery of the G-Spot

One of the best, most thorough articles ever written about the anatomy of the G-spot, called "Beyond the G-Spot: Clitourethrovaginal Complex Anatomy in Female Orgasm" from 2014, begins like this: "Whether the [G-spot] is a discrete entity, a complex structure, or a gynaecological myth created for journalistic purposes, or with the aim of supporting surgical aesthetic manipulations of the female genitals, remains unclear."[1] . . . ?!?!

That's so funny because NO IT DOES NOT REMAIN UNCLEAR. Plenty of scientists and feminist health advocates actually had, by the year 2014, already explained the existence of the G-spot and described the structures behind it. Rebecca Chalker gives an amazingly detailed anatomical explanation and a historiography of the G-spot's disappearance from and denial by Science in *The Clitoral Truth*, which was published in 2002. In fact, "Beyond the G-Spot" itself goes on to very clearly describe the anatomy of the G-spot. But that wouldn't have been as fun if they hadn't first made it out to be a mystery, now would it?

Both scientific studies and clickbait headlines questioning the G-spot's existence abound. *Cosmopolitan*'s 2020 article called "The G-Spot Doesn't Exist" by Elizabeth Kiefer is a mea culpa for the way the G-spot has been misinterpreted and misrepresented, which has caused shame, sexual frustration, and unhealthy sexual dynamics.[3] People with penises are free to hump, come, and call it a day because if their partners *should* be able to orgasm vaginally with G-spot stimulation, penetration *should* be enough, right? This, in turn, can lead to people with vaginas feeling bad if they can't orgasm vaginally and also to them not getting the pleasure they deserve. That's not wrong. But the article attempts to remedy this by getting rid of the whole concept of the G-spot.[3] In doing so, Kiefer throws the Science-and-Anatomy babies out with the Bad-Sex bathwater.

Kiefer (barely) interviews Dr. Beverly Whipple, a neurophysiologist who helped to coin the term *Grafenberg spot*, which was later shortened by her publisher to G-spot (now in *Merriam-Webster's*) and to popularize the concept in 1982. She was also one of *Cosmopolitan*'s 10 Sexual Revolutionaries You Should Know in 2013. Once Kiefer lets Dr. Whipple briefly clarify that her team never meant that the G-spot was a literal spot but rather an area, Kiefer goes on to dump Whipple entirely and proclaim the G-spot a sham.[3]

To prove her point, Kiefer references studies that she does not actually cite. These silly studies looked for some discrete structure or nerve density *in the vagina*. And it's true: there's nothing inside the vagina to find. But Dr. Whipple and her team never said there was.

Kiefer closes the article by saying, "Whipple stands by her 'area.' Italian researchers have suggested renaming it the somewhat less sexy 'clitoral vaginal urethral complex.'"[3] The "Italians" are the authors of "Beyond the G-Spot." (Only one is actually Italian.) And while I made fun of their G-spot-as-gynecological-myth introduction, their research would have had a lot to offer Kiefer's article were she to have touched upon it at all.

Dr. Whipple never gets a chance in the article to explain what she *did* mean. Had the *Cosmo* reporter actually read Dr. Whipple's book about the G-spot, she would have found hundreds of pages of anatomic explanation, zero mentions of some invisible organ or structure hiding inside the vagina, and an entire prescient chapter about how the G-spot should not create pressure for women to orgasm vaginally.

When I reached out to Dr. Whipple for comment, she wasn't interested in refuting the article. "It just has so much inaccurate information, we could do that for a very long time," she said. To her, what matters is pleasure: "What I want to focus on is that I want women to feel good about what brings them sensual and sexual pleasure, and realize there's not just one way. There are many ways, and people should feel good about what they enjoy. They should be able to identify what brings them pleasure, and be able to communicate that to partners. That's what's important."

Dr. Whipple may have been extremely Zen about the *Cosmo* article, but I'm still hung up on why pussy science just doesn't seem to stick. (See my longer rant about this in Chapter 3 in the section about the periurethral glands.) I think one of the (false) gender narratives that makes G-spot science so slippery is *the "female" and the "female body" and sexuality are mysterious and unknowable.*

Maybe pussy scientists (and *Cosmopolitan* reporters) don't fully survey the work of those who've come before them because, deep down, they think, *But nobody* really *knows, so I'm safe if I don't do an exhaustive search because it's all speculation anyway.* I asked Dr. Whipple about this too: "I think you have a point there. But I've never studied it so I can't say." Spoken like a true scientist.

Whatever the reason, researchers the world over have gone looking for something that nobody ever said existed. The most mysterious thing about the G-spot is why (*God, why?!*) so many of these researchers did not, in their searches, read the original papers about it.

The "Italians," who have worked closely with Dr. Whipple, made a very good point in their article. The structures in question "have not been completely and unequivocally described, probably representing a unique case of remaining major uncertainty regarding human gross anatomy."[1] It's true, there are still disagreements and unknowns about pussy pleasure and anatomy. But there's a huge difference between not knowing everything and not knowing anything.

The Unambiguous Texts That Sent the World on a Goofy-Ass Quest for the Holy Vagina Grail

During World War II, Ernst Grafenberg was a German Jewish refugee and ob-gyn practicing in New York City with—by the account of one of his patients—a great deal of concern and sympathy for the emotional pain experienced by transgender and intersex people, groups that still seriously lack in health care today. He also had intense interest in the sexual well-being of people with pussies, which he developed during wartime while treating poor people whose bodies had been devastated by childbirths and botched abortions. "He told me how helpless he'd found himself when faced with the brutal reality of some women's existence," his patient recounts.[4] This led him to spend many years studying egg implantation and redesigning the IUD.[5]

In 1950, he published the article "The Role of the Urethra in Female Orgasm" in the *International Journal of Sexology*, in which what he actually fucking said was:

> An erotic zone always could be demonstrated on the anterior wall of the vagina along the course of the urethra. . . . Analogous to the male urethra, the female

urethra also seems to be surrounded by erectile tissues like the corpora cavernosa. In the course of sexual stimulation, the female urethra begins to enlarge and can be felt easily. It swells out greatly at the end of orgasm. The most stimulating part is located at the posterior urethra, where it arises from the neck of the bladder.[6]

All the answers are there! The urethra. It gets a boner. The boner can be felt through the vagina. It feels good. Yay.

Fast-forward to 1981, to a study called "Female Ejaculation: A Case Study" by a team including Beverly Whipple, which named the G-spot and aimed to confirm that yes, pussies ejaculate. What that article actually said was

At the April, 1979 testing session, the subject identified an erotically sensitive spot, palpable through the anterior wall of her vagina. We subsequently named this area the "Grafenberg spot," in recognition of the person who wrote of its existence and relationship to female ejaculation (Grafenberg, 1950). . . . [The area] coincided with a fairly firm area approximately 2 cm by 1.5 cm, with the long axis along the course of the urethra. . . . The area grew approximately 50% larger upon stimulation. . . . (The exact anatomical nature of this spot has not yet been determined.)[7]

So they had a patient who pointed out that the front wall of her vagina felt good to touch. And then they were like, *Grafenberg wrote about that! We shall call it his spot*. They measured it. They measured the boner. They confirmed that it's where the vaginal wall goes along the urethra. So they know where it is, they know that it aligns with Grafenberg's observations, and they know that it feels good to touch in at least some pussies. And, no, they didn't yet know everything about what was going on yet. But while the phrase *exact anatomical nature* could mean a lot of things, one thing it surely does not mean is *There's a magical mystery vagina grail waiting to be found.*

In 1982, Dr. Whipple, Alice Kahn Ladas, and John Perry published the smash-hit book that catapulted the G-spot into the zeitgeist, *The G Spot and Other Recent Discoveries About Human Sexuality*, in which they outlined even more anatomy:

In *A New View of a Woman's Body*, compiled by the Federation of Feminist Women's Health Centers, the area we call the *G spot* is called the "urethral sponge." The authors were unable to find this structure mentioned in medical textbooks, so they named it themselves. . . . The *G spot* is probably composed of a complex network of blood vessels, the paraurethral glands and ducts, nerve endings, and the tissue surrounding the bladder neck. The cellular structure of the *G spot* is, at this time, unknown. . . . In 1953, urologist Samuel Berkow, M.D. concluded that this tissue is erectile and can be viewed as a "corpus spongiosum" . . . But his interest was in urination and he felt that the function of this [tissue] was to . . . control urination. . . . Unfortunately, other urologists failed to find this [function], and quickly forgot that the "erectile tissue" might have other purposes outside the domain of their own discipline.[8]

"Other purposes" like *pleasure*! The authors already knew the G-spot was right on the other side of the vaginal wall as the urethral sponge. They knew that the urethral sponge did not exist solely for pee control. They knew erectile tissue produces pleasure. They were even right in their hypothesis about what the G-spot was composed of, although they didn't know its cellular structure, which, like, (again) would not equal the discovery of a holy vagina grail, anyway.

They were also correct in their hypothesis that the urethral sponge should be considered the "female" prostate,* which it now widely is:

Shall we refer to this cluster of tissue as the "female prostate gland"? There is no argument about its anatomical and embryological similarity; the question seems to be merely one of semantics. . . . It should not surprise us (although this has not yet been validated scientifically and remains at the time a hypothesis) that it may in some women . . . generate a fluid.[8]

We now know that it does (see Chapter 3 for more on the periurethral glands, ejaculate, squirting, and why it took so long for Science to accept the glands as a prostate).[9] We also know that the "male" prostate is a pleasure-producing organ. So it makes sense that the "female" prostate would be too. What they didn't know at the time—the missing puzzle piece—was that the urethra has such an intimate relationship with the clit.

Even More Important Than the Fact That the G-Spot Exists Is the Fact That It Doesn't Matter If Yours Doesn't

If yours is not that sensitive, you are normal; you are fine. The fact that some pussies have this characteristic does not mean that yours should. Either way, it certainly doesn't mean you should be able to orgasm vaginally or just from penetration. (See Chapter 18 for more on why vaginal-orgasm superiority is a lie from The Patriarchy that perpetuates unhealthy sexual dynamics.) Just do what feels good to you! Dr. Whipple couldn't stress this enough when we spoke:

> We shouldn't be setting up expectations that there's only one or two ways to experience sensual and sexual pleasure. We have documented pleasure in the brain from many different types of stimulation. What's important is to be pleasure-oriented rather than goal-oriented. When you're goal-oriented, if you don't reach your goal, you don't feel very good about the experience. Whereas if you're pleasure-oriented, any activity can be an end in itself.

As Whipple, Ladas, and Perry put it in the last chapter of *The G Spot*:

> Sexual activity should be a pleasurable experience and not a performance requiring some specified outcome. Pleasure, enjoyment, and the path of mutual exploration and sharing are more important than any end result. The subject of sex reaches deep into our most elemental feelings and touches us in the most sensitive areas of our being. New information about it must not add pressure.[8]

Amen! Really, we make a giant deal about the G-spot, but there are so many ways to enjoy our bodies, and if we fixate on one area as if it's a holy grail, like the G-spot, we could miss out on the fun of all the others. In Dr. Grafenberg's original paper, he also encourages exploration. He literally suggests sticking a dick in your ear[6]—or at least in the "external orifice" of it, which . . . I can't really imagine physically getting one any farther in . . . but, hey, best to specify lest someone get really, really determined, right? Anyway. Bottom line is have fun with it, y'all. The pleasure is the point.

*It's fairly common now that the periurethral glands and sometimes entire urethral sponge are referred to as the "female prostate." That assumes the gender of the owner. And, also, we don't call the other one the "male prostate" so, like, why? Let's just say *prostate*. Just like we say *liver, lungs, heart, pancreas, thumb*, and so on.

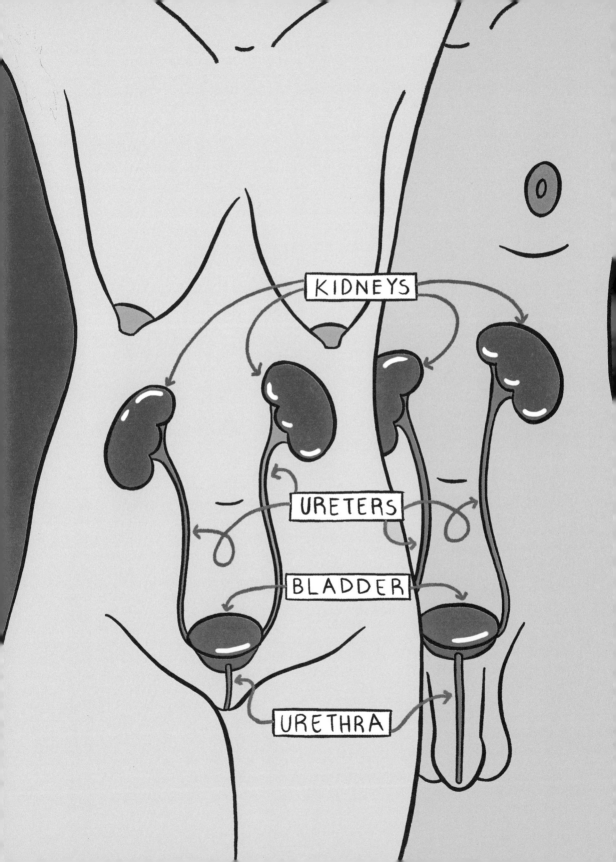

5
The Urinary Tract and Peeing

Your Plumbing

The urinary tract is all of the components that make, move, process, hold, and expel urine (pee) in your body: kidneys, ureters, bladder, and urethra. Your kidneys are badass bean-shaped organs that filter about 30–37 gallons of blood every day to remove stuff that shouldn't be in there. The reason we pee is to get rid of waste in our bodies and to balance the amount of fluids in us to levels that our bodies like. The ureters are two li'l tubes that move pee from the kidneys to the bladder. The bladder sits between the uterus and the vagina, and it's where your pee hangs out until it comes out of your body. The urethra is the tiny tube that goes from the bladder to the surface of your vulva, including the exit hole that pee comes out of.[1]

Urinary Tract Infections (UTIs)

UTIs are so fucking exasperating. They can make you feel like you have to pee all the time, then you try to but you can't or you only can a little bit, or you pee super often, and when you pee it hurts like hell and smells.[2] Insert a million crying emojis here. Almost one in three people with pussies will have at least one UTI that they need antibiotics for by age 24 and almost half will get a UTI in their lifetime.[3]

A UTI can mean any or multiple parts of the urinary tract are infected. If it's the bladder, then it is called a *bladder infection* or *cystitis*. UTIs are caused by bacteria—usually *E. coli*.[4] Since your butthole, along with the poop that comes out of it, and your vagina, which tends to have communities of bacteria living in it, are pretty physically close to your pee hole, it was long believed (and is still reported in tons of reputable health-information websites) that UTIs are caused mostly by poop bacteria and vagina bacteria getting into your pee hole. (See Chapter "Old, Rude as Hell Narratives About Pussies Being Dirty." JK, that's not a chapter. But it could be.)

But actually, for the last decade, it has been known that your pee hole is pretty good at getting poop germs out if and when they do get in there. The strains of *E. coli* that cause UTIs are special little fuckers that adapted to colonize the urinary tract. They can get in there from catheterization (getting a tube stuck up your urethra), sexytimes, or from just living your life.[4]

Many UTIs will resolve themselves without antibiotics. But if you have a UTI, it's best to go to the doctor, who will probably prescribe you antibiotics because UTIs can spread to your kidneys, which can be dangerous. Antibiotics for UTIs may be overprescribed, but researchers recommend that a doctor keep an eye on your healing process whether or not you take them.[4] There are a few things consistently recommended to help avoid UTIs if you are prone to getting them (and if you're not, just keep doing what you do!):

- Wipe front to back
- Pee after sex
- Drink lots of water
- Don't use tampons
- Don't go in hot tubs
- Don't wear tights
- Don't hold your pee for a really long time

Doing these things is unlikely to hurt you (unless you miss out on an extremely cool hot-tub party), but research does not show that these practices actually help very much. I'm saying this because if you get recurrent UTIs and you feel like you're trying really hard to do everything right, you shouldn't feel like it's your fault.[2] UTIs are just a curse from God. I'm kidding, that's not science. But it feels true sometimes.

Other things that have *some* but not, like, *amazing* evidence of helping are cranberries (better in pills than in juice) and probiotics (*Lactobacillus rhamnosus*, *reuteri*, or *crispatus* if you can get them, but see Chapter 26 for more info on probiotics before spending your money on them).[2]

Stress Urinary Incontinence (SUI)

SUI is when you pee a little when exerting force, like coughing, laughing, sneezing, or trying to lift something heavy. This happens usually because of a lack of strength in the pelvic floor muscles that (among a bazillion other very important activities) keep your pee inside your body when you're not ready to let it out. SUI is one of those things people don't talk about, probably because peeing in your pants can be embarrassing. But it is fairly common. There's no standard epidemiological definition of SUI, and thus, there is a huge range of estimates of exactly how common it is among people with pussies: 4–35%.[5] But one study put it this way: "It is exceedingly clear that SUI is a prevalent condition affecting a substantial segment of our society as a whole."[6]

Some factors can make SUI more likely. People experiencing obesity are about 1.3 times more likely to also experience SUI because extra weight in the abdominal area puts pressure on the bladder.[7,8] People with pussies who have never had a baby and who do high-impact sports like gymnastics and running are a lot more likely to have SUI.[6] Between 30% and 50% of pregnant people leak some pee.[9] And vaginal childbirth causes at least temporary pee leakage in about a third of people, but evidence is unclear about how often it turns into a long-term problem.[6,10]

One treatment for SUI is pelvic floor muscle training (PFMT), which you may have heard of by the name *kegels*. It's best if you can get PFMT from a physical therapist (which is usually pretty expensive), but according to Annemarie Everett, PT, DPT, WCS, a pelvic-floor physical therapist who specializes in treating SUI and anal incontinence, you can also learn PFMT at home. Here are a few of her tips for getting the hang of contracting your pelvic floor to strengthen it, just like we do strength training for other muscles:

First, do what you would do to stop yourself from farting, except don't contract the muscles with 100% effort. Stick a mirror or a phone camera between your legs so you can see the part of you between your vulva and your anus—the perineum—moving in real time. It's not easy for everyone to "find" their pelvic floor, so you might need to give it some time. You should see the perineum moving up with each contraction. Wash and lube up a finger and stick it up your vagina or anus. You should feel a squeeze and then a lift upward, in that order. Try starting to contract those muscles while inhaling and exhaling and while holding your breath. (The breathing is to make sure your abdomen is not tightened.) Once you get the hang of it, try three sets of 8–12 long contractions per day.

You'll need to have some patience. "Strength building takes time!" says Everett. "Most people require at least three to six months to reach their desired level of improvement. Once you have achieved your goals, you can determine whether a lower frequency is required to maintain your desired results."

In the meantime, once you get a hang of contracting your pelvic floor, you can help stop leaks by squeezing when you cough, sneeze, or laugh.[11]

Overactive Bladder Syndrome (OAB)

OAB is when you feel like you have to pee all the time, when you do have to pee all the time, when you get sudden urges to pee, or when you have to pee a lot at night. When it becomes a syndrome instead of just having to pee a lot is hard to say. According to one enormous international study, about 12.3% of people with pussies have OAB.[12]

If you're not happy about how often you have to pee or how intense sudden urges to pee can be, know that the "small bladder" trope is a myth. You can retrain your bladder as an adult. Like PFMT, this can be learned at home. The University of California San Francisco has great resources that I've included at the end of this chapter. If you want to see a health care professional about it, it may be helpful if you keep a bladder/pee diary for a few days beforehand. (There are apps that can help you do this—search for "bladder diaries" in your app store.)

Peeing in Public Bathrooms Is a Privilege You Can Help Others Have

Trans and gender-nonconforming people have a really hard time with public bathrooms. In a large-scale 2015 survey on trans health in the United States, nearly a quarter of respondents said that someone had questioned or challenged their presence in a restroom, nearly 60% had avoided using public bathrooms out of fear of that happening, and almost a third had limited their eating or drinking to avoid having to use a public bathroom in the previous year.[13]

My friend Dante Ureta, trans activist and writer, explains:

> Trans people are always subject to the scrutiny of the public eye. Our actions are questioned and our words are rarely believed. That's why, when I had a more androgynous presentation I got anxiety every time I had to go to the bathroom. People often tried to kick me out. Over time, I learned to go accompanied by someone, so that if it came in question, they could affirm that I was the gender assigned to that bathroom since it was easier for people to believe others than to believe me. So if you are with a trans or gender-nonconforming friend, it never hurts to casually ask them if they would like some company in the bathroom. Just try to do it with tact and empathy and without making it a big deal.

Piss Chills

When I was a kid, my brother told me that boys get this thing called *piss chills*, which is when you get a little chill and shiver when you pee. That has always happened to me too and I've always found it kinda pleasant, but I told my brother neither of those things because I was extremely alarmed that this thing that "only happened to boys" happened to me too.

Turns out, piss chills can happen to everyone. I found zero peer-reviewed studies on it, but it does have a cute fake-scientific name, *post-micturition convulsion syndrome*, which is not an institutionally recognized syndrome. One urologist interviewed by *Live Science* suggested that it happens because blood pressure drops when you pee, and your body's sympathetic nervous system kicks in to raise your blood pressure back up, causing shivers.[14] Still, no studies so . . . piss chills = official mystery!

Peeing in Your Partner's Mouth as a Sexual Act Might Save Your House from Getting Robbed

Once, two guys in black ski masks broke into my friend's yard, presumably to rob their house, but what they saw immediately upon entering was my friend's upstairs neighbor peeing into his boyfriend's mouth (a more or less harmless thing to do if you're into that).[15] The robbers screamed and ran away and never tried to break into the house ever again.

RESOURCES

- totalcontrolprogram.com
- ucsfhealth.org/education/bladder-training

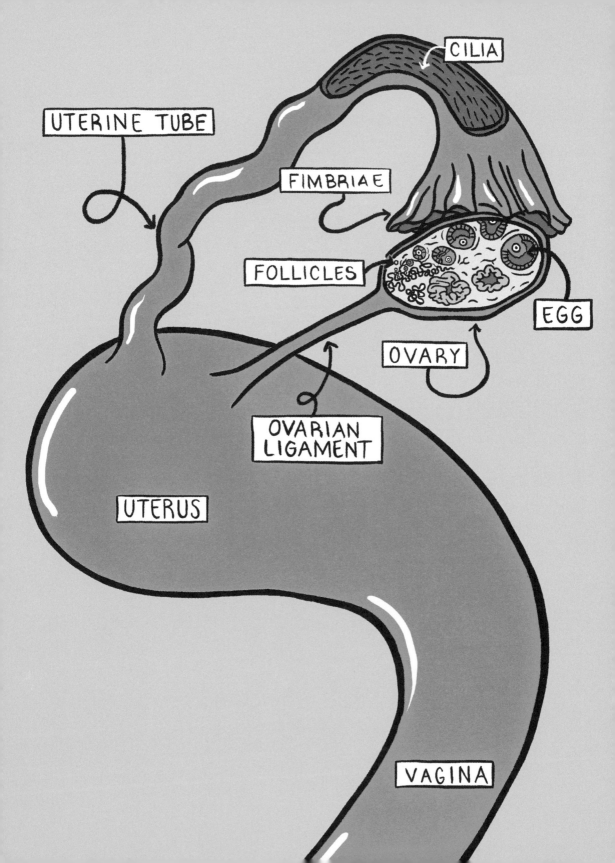

6
The Uterine Tubes and Ovaries

What Do the Ovaries Do?[1]

Ovaries are your gonads—your primary reproductive organs (in "male" bodies they are the testes). They are about the size of an almond. When you are born, your ovaries have about 2 million follicles in them, many of which will get absorbed by your body. When you reach puberty, you'll have around 400,000 but only 300–500 follicles will mature into eggs over the course of your life. Eggs develop and get released into the uterine tubes during ovulation as part of the menstrual cycle. Usually it's one egg per cycle, but it can be two or more sometimes too! Ovaries also produce hormones like estrogen, progesterone, and testosterone.

What Do the Uterine Tubes (Formerly Known as Fallopian Tubes) Do?[1]

These tubes are about four inches long, and they carry eggs from the ovaries into the uterus. Despite what too many illustrations out there show, they don't actually connect *to* the ovaries; the end of the uterine tube and the ovary are not attached. So an egg, once released from an ovary, floats out into the abdominal cavity. That's when the strange, long, fingery things on the end of the uterine tubes come into play. They swoosh around and try to get the egg to float into the opening of the tube. It's like a whole circle of those tall inflatable smiley guys dancing together, trying to lure the egg into the car wash that is the uterine tube.

The tubes are lined on the inside with tiny hairs called *cilia*. The cilia, along with the muscles of the tubes, undulate to move the egg toward the uterus, and if there are sperm around, to help the sperm move toward the egg.

When Ovaries Grow Blobs

Polycystic ovary syndrome (PCOS) is different depending on who you ask. Some definitions of it require that someone has three of three problems to have PCOS, and others are content with two of three for a diagnosis. The three problems are little cysts on your ovaries, too much androgen hormones (like testosterone), and irregular ovulation. So you can have PCOS and not have cysts on your ovaries. You can also have cysts on your ovaries and not have PCOS. Depending on whose definition you use to count, between 5% and 20% (that's a ton!) of people with pussies have PCOS.[2]

Common symptoms are irregular periods, bleeding between periods, tiredness, anxiety, extra hair growth in places you don't expect it to grow, thinning hair on the head, and acne. Because it is also associated with insulin

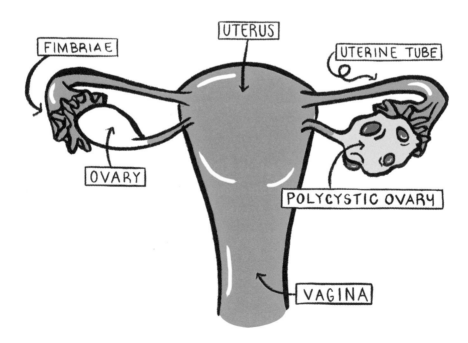

resistance, PCOS can increase your risk of endometrial cancer and type 2 diabetes, although there is some disagreement about whether insulin resistance is a cause or a symptom of PCOS.[1,2] (Anything called a *syndrome* is a collection of related symptoms without a known cause.)

PCOS can be awful and a lot to handle, and there's no cure for it, but there are a lot of treatments to mitigate the symptoms. Many people are treated for PCOS with hormonal birth control, which can regulate periods and help curb hair growth and loss.[1]

Trans men who have not started testosterone therapy may be at a higher risk for PCOS, but findings on the matter are inconsistent.[3,4] At least one study has shown that taking testosterone does not seem to worsen the symptoms, but at least one other found that it can worsen insulin resistance.[4,5]

Tarah Knaresboro, the fact-checker for this book, wrote the "PCOS" article for Pussypedia.net and had this to say:

> Especially if you're new to PCOS, getting used to having a lifelong condition and sorting through all the treatment options can be overwhelming. And if, like many people, it took a while for your symptoms to get diagnosed, you may be just plain exhausted with the health care system. This is normal and very understandable.
>
> But there is a good chance that, in time, you can find a way to treat symptoms that bother you. Go at a pace that feels right to you, and if you're talking with a doctor, stay in touch about what is or isn't working. You may need to try a few different things before you find a plan that works well for your life and needs. Although it may not always be easy, it is possible to live a full and happy life with PCOS.[6]

Ovarian cysts that are not from PCOS also exist. The most common ones are little fluid-filled blobs. They usually go away on their own within a few months. Because of this, it's hard to estimate how common they are. But they're thought to be very common. Most happen because something went awry when a follicle was trying to become an egg. If the follicle just keeps growing instead of eventually releasing the egg, it can become a cyst. Other times, fluid can accumulate in a follicle after it releases an egg. Most cysts are not dangerous but can be if they burst. If you ever have sudden, severe pain anywhere in your body—especially if it's accompanied by fever or vomiting—it's a good idea to go get some medical attention.[7]

What's in a Name?

The uterine tubes are usually called the *fallopian tubes*, but let's start calling them the *uterine tubes* because we could all really stand to stop calling our body parts by the names of the dudes who "discovered" them and then peed on them with their names. In the case of the uterine tubes, it was Gabriel Fallopius, the same douchebag from Chapter 2, the one who got in a fight with his douchebag friend Renaldus Columbus about who had "discovered" the clitoris. Fallopius may have added a lot to our collective knowledge of human anatomy, but body parts named after the men who "discovered" them is a legacy of colonialism, and as they say, fuck that noise.

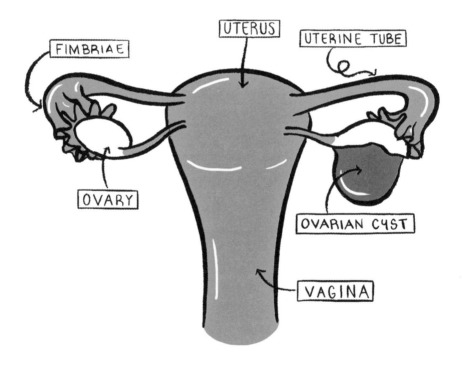

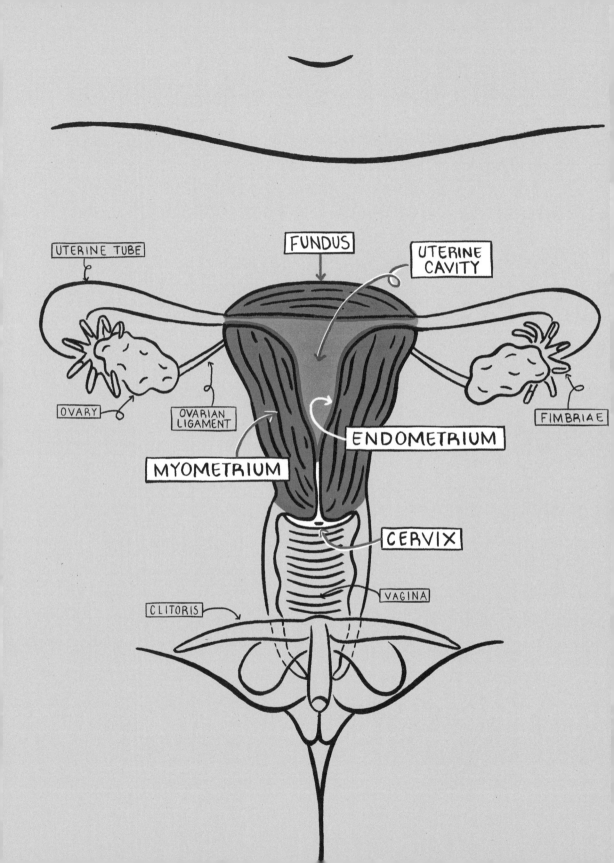

7
The Uterus

WE ALL MAY HAVE POPPED OUT OF ONE, BUT WE NEVER REALLY ESCAPE THE WOMB. The uterus is where menstruation happens, which, for most people who have one, means that you're actively dealing with your uterus's activities for a giant chunk of your life. Also, for more than 2,500 years, the uterus has been the focal point of all kinds of horrible ideas about people with uteruses being mentally ill. Those ideas continue to shape the way people think about people with pussies.

The uterus is made of thick, muscular walls that are lined with endometrium—what you see come out of the vagina, along with blood, during menstruation. Endometrium helps nourish a li'l fertilized egg that will live inside the uterus as it grows into a baby.[1] The uterus is often called a "sack," but that's a little misleading because it has solid walls and is not hollow with air inside. It's more of a solid structure with the walls mostly touching each other unless it happens to be growing a big fetus. The uterus is extremely strong because it has to be strong enough to push out a baby. That strength is why menstrual cramps can hurt so much; cramps happen when your uterus squeezes itself to get the old endometrium out. Sometimes it can squeeze so hard that it can't breathe. It literally cuts off its own oxygen supply, and then that hurts even more.[1]

I don't know it for a fact, but I think that happens to me. I would really fucking hate my uterus if it were a conscious being, but it's just a collection of cells receiving and reacting to electrical signals, and despite all evidence to the contrary, it is not actually trying to ruin my life for a few days every month. I have sat in meetings pretending that everything was fine and trying to participate in conversations while I felt like the bottom half of my body was being fed through a meat grinder, and I fantasized about throwing my uterus into one for real. I have spent hours at a time curled up in a ball on the bathroom floor waiting to puke from the pain. I have resorted to taking prescription muscle relaxers, which knock me out for the day, but at least I'm not screaming in pain and pooping a week's worth of future poops—like, OK, uterus, I get it, you're strong. But weird flex, dude. (Actually, researchers think you poop more on your period not because your contracting uterus squeezes the poop out but because a chemical that gets released to help make your uterus contract, called *prostaglandin*, also affects your bowels.)[2]

But back to the anatomy at hand. At the bottom of the uterus is its very narrow (basically closed most of the time) opening called the cervix. The cervix is the round protruding thing you feel at the back of the vagina. It kind of looks like the back side of a Bagel Bite. It produces mucus that changes texture over the course of the menstrual cycle (more on this mucus in Chapter 3), and it opens a tiny, tiny bit to let menstrual blood out and sperm in. It also opens a lot to let a baby out.

It's Not Hysterical, It's Historical

Wanna know why *hysteria* and *hysterectomy* (the surgery to take out the uterus) have the same root word? It's the same reason that people with pussies have been historically considered "hysterical."

It goes way back to ancient Egypt, when a doctor wrote down—warning, inexplicable logic ahead—that sometimes the uterus would up and start traveling around the body, causing people seizures and a "sense of imminent death."[3] Fast-forward to ancient Greece. Hippocrates, a famous doctor who would have enormous influence on Medicine forever on, coined the term *hysteria* from the Greek word *hystera*, for uterus.[4] Hysteria was a disease, he said, in which people with a uterus felt anxious or acted distressed because their uterus was wandering around their body. His reason for believing this happened was actually pretty predictable; he thought that uteruses, and therefore people with pussies, needed to get enough dick to be healthy and happy.[3] Literally, dudes have been telling upset people with pussies to "get fucked" since, like, 400 BCE.

In Rome in the 2nd century CE, the famous doctor Galen, who, like Hippocrates, had an outsize influence on modern Medicine, came along and was basically like, *Nah, the uterus isn't wandering around the body, it's just too full of orgasm juice that needs to get out.*[5] He talked about the "retention of female seed." Again, more dick and more orgasms were the solution. This nonsense was considered serious science for centuries and ended up informing gender narratives for millennia. This is how the sexuality of people with pussies got pathologized—made to be thought of as a form of illness.

In the late 19th century, Freud learned about hysteria, and it spurred him to write his hot-garbage theory that people with pussies are hysterical because we don't have penises. His Rx? You guessed it! *Catch a dick! Sex with penises.*[5]

Hysteria was considered by the medical establishment to be a real disease until it was taken out of the *Diagnostic and Statistical Manual of Mental Disorders* (a.k.a. the *DSM*, the book that is used by psychiatrists to diagnose mental disorders) in 1980![5] It was basically the medical establishment's catch-all diagnosis for people with pussies who didn't feel right and whose symptoms they couldn't figure out: they were "crazy," probably horny, and faking their symptoms.

In 1978, the *International Classification of Diseases*, ninth revision, published by the World Health Organization (WHO), defined hysteria as "a neurotic mental disorder in which motives, of which the patient seems unaware, produce either a restriction of the field of consciousness or disturbances of motor or sensory function which may seem to have psychological advantage or symbolic value."[6]

This definition could not be more disempowering if it tried. It means that the person doesn't realize it, but that they have "motives"—that, rather than wanting whatever's physically and/or physiologically wrong to be fixed, they're actually performing symptoms, and that that performance is somehow beneficial to them. (E.g., Person with a pussy: "I can't cook and clean the house today,

George. I'm super depressed and have a horrible headache." Doctor: "She's hysterical. She's not aware that she's doing this, but she's faking it so she doesn't have to do her housework.")

Some subtypes of hysteria included in their definitions were "selective amnesia," forgetting things on purpose; "sexual immaturity," which either meant not able to orgasm or "over-responsiveness to stimuli," which, wow, your guess is as good as mine as to how they measured and decided which pussies were responding "too much" to stimuli; mood swings; "dependence on others"; and, my favorites, "craving for appreciation and attention . . . and theatricality"[6] (i.e., "She's nuts, she's faking it, she wants attention, she's being dramatic").

Literally people with pussies have been gaslit by medical authorities for millennia! And just because hysteria left medical textbooks does not mean the destructive narratives that it created (i.e., the "hysterical woman," that people with pussies are dramatic and exaggerate their pain, that "horny chicks are crazy," and that "crazy chicks are just horny") left our culture or doctors' minds. This manifests as doctors not taking the pain of people with pussies as seriously as they do cis men's pain.[7,8] This is called *gender-biased diagnosing*, and it can be especially dangerous for people with pussies seeking treatment for severe pain that may indicate that something is urgently wrong. There exists a similar bias against Black people in the US, whose pain is also routinely downplayed and ignored by doctors, so Black people with pussies have an even higher risk of this kind of medical negligence.[9]

The Most Common Annoying and Bad Things That Can Go Wrong with Your Uterus, Absolutely None of Which Are Caused by Lack of Dick

Endometriosis is when tissue similar to endometrium grows outside of the uterus, often causing the formation of scar tissue.[10] About 1 in 10 to 1 in 15 people with pussies have it.[11] Endometriosis can make it painful to have sex, pee, and poop,[12] but its main symptom is extremely horrible, seemingly untreatable menstrual cramps.[10] Combine that invisible pain with gender-biased diagnosing, and you get a disease that's really hard to get diagnosed. On average, it takes between 6.7 and 7.5 years for a person with endometriosis to get diagnosed, often because doctors simply believe that someone is either too weak to tolerate "normal" cramping or exaggerating the severity of their cramps.[10,12] This is despite the fact that nearly 70% of adolescents with extreme, seemingly untreatable menstrual cramps will later get diagnosed with endometriosis.[10]

This medical gaslighting causes a whole second set of problems. As one doctoral thesis from a researcher at Queen Margaret University in Edinburgh found, people who waited and waited to get diagnosed with endometriosis experienced a plague of self-doubt. "They questioned their perception of the severity of the symptoms and ultimately their own sanity; mainly due to not being believed by medical practitioners and other[s]."[13] Meanwhile, without intervention, the disease progresses. The damage it does to the uterus is linked to infertility and bad pregnancy outcomes. Although it is considered a "benign" disease, it is estimated that people with endometriosis lose an average of 10.8 hours of work a week due to the disease's symptoms.[10,12]

Even though endometriosis is so common, there's very little known about the causes of the disease, and there's no sure-bet cure. More than 1 in 10 people with endometriosis will end up getting a hysterectomy as a treatment for their symptoms, but about 15% of those people will still have pain after.[10]

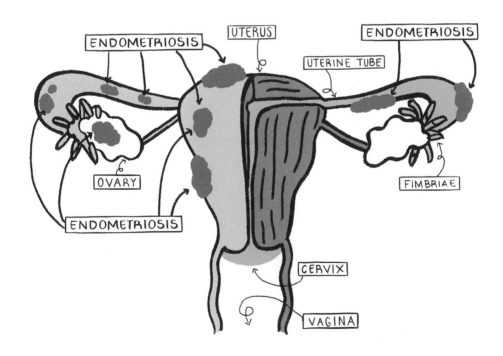

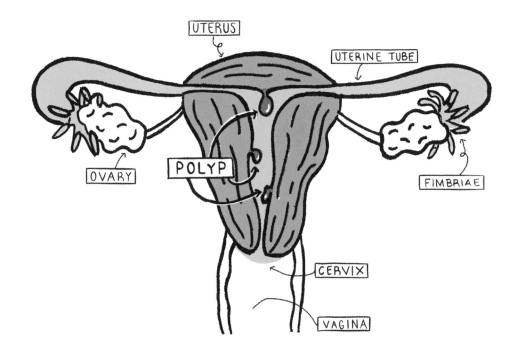

In recent years, there has been growing grassroots activism around endometriosis. There are many support groups on Facebook, like EndoMetropolis and Endo Warriors, and there are apps to help manage and track endometriosis, like Flutter, MyEndometriosisTeam, Phendo, Endometriosis Diary, and MyFLO.

Endometrial polyps, or **uterine polyps**, are buildups of the uterus's lining, which sometimes have no symptoms and sometimes cause heavy bleeding.[14,15] There is a small chance (about 3%) that they can lead to cancer.[14] Uterine polyps form in about 7–9% of uteruses, more commonly later in life and especially postmenopause.[16,17]

Abnormal uterine bleeding (AUB) just means bleeding a lot or bleeding when you're not supposed to be bleeding, and it can be incredibly annoying even if it's not painful or life-threatening. Besides causing anemia from losing too much blood, and therefore too much iron, you constantly have to worry about not bleeding onto your clothes, your bed, and public surfaces. Depending how old you are, there are a ton of reasons you might be bleeding a lot, so it can be

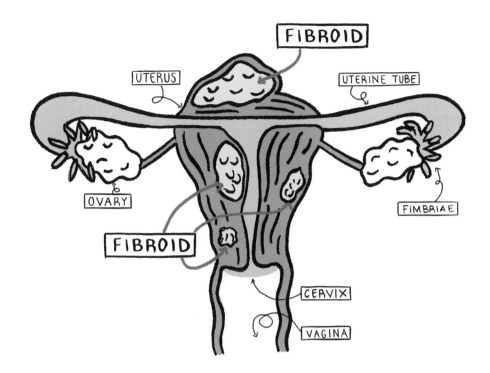

hard for doctors to pinpoint the cause. The combination of hard-to-diagnose and incredibly-annoying-to-live-with is kind of brutal, and I just want to acknowledge how seriously that sucks because doctors might tell you it's not a big deal even though it's a giant deal for you. If doctors can't figure it out at all and you've had other bleeding problems, ask to get screened for von Willebrand disease, a clotting disorder.[14]

Fibroids are noncancerous tumors that can grow on the inside or outside of the uterus *or* inside the wall of the uterus; they can be big or small and varying degrees of annoying. Many go away on their own. They are usually harmless and only require treatment about 20% of the time. Sometimes they can cause very painful periods and lots of bleeding; sometimes back pain, urinary problems, or constipation. In some cases, they can mess with pregnancy.[14] There are estimates of their prevalence ranging from 4.5% to 68.6% of people with uteruses.[18] *Our Bodies, Ourselves* says that about 30% of people with uteruses will get them by age 35 and about 80% by age 50.[14] Black people are both significantly more likely to have fibroids than other racial groups and significantly more likely to report severe or very severe symptoms.[14,19] They also report long delays in diagnosis (perhaps because their pain is not taken seriously), which can lead to having more sunk health care costs (i.e., spending lots of money while trying to get a diagnosis) and less of a chance to treat fibroids before a hysterectomy may become necessary.[19] Many doctors will recommend hysterectomies to anyone and everyone to deal with uterine fibroids, but it's worth getting a second opinion if someone wants to take your uterus out. Less-invasive treatment options, like uterine fibroid embolization (UFE), an outpatient procedure in which fibroids' blood supply is blocked, do exist.[20]

Hysterecto-Mania

In 2004, about a third of people with uteruses in the US had their uteruses taken out by age 60.[14] The US has the highest hysterectomy rate in the industrialized world, and my guess as to why is that, until recently,[14] hysterectomies were easy for doctors to bill insurance companies for. (And that The Patriarchy and Medicine have a long history of disregarding women's bodily autonomy. Throughout most of the 20th century in the US, hundreds of thousands of hysterectomies were forced on poor, disabled, and nonwhite people, as well as sex workers, for the sake of sterilization. See Chapter 21 to learn more about the history of forced sterilization in the US.)

There's huge disagreement about how necessary the operations really are. Studies range from saying that 10–90% of hysterectomies in the US have been unnecessary. Necessary or not, a hysterectomy is a major surgery with built-in risk during the surgery, like infection, hemorrhage, and damage to the bowel or urinary tract (though these complications are rare, it is important to acknowledge that they exist and are better avoided altogether if possible!), and after the surgery, like increased risk of heart attack and earlier menopause.[14]

Since the 1980s, there have been political movements and protests against the medical establishment's overzealousness for hysterectomies and underzealousness for their alternatives.[21] Even insurance companies have become aware of this problem and now often require a second opinion if a doctor recommends a hysterectomy.[14] The National Women's Health Network's official stance on the issue is

> Unnecessary hysterectomies have put women at risk needlessly . . . health care providers should recognize the value of a woman's reproductive organs beyond their reproductive capacity and search for hysterectomy alternatives before resorting to life-changing operations.[22]

If you get a hysterectomy, you don't have to feel any type of way about it, and whatever you do feel is valid. If you feel a sense of loss, let yourself feel sad. If it's no big deal to you, cool! If you feel super happy and relieved, well, great. Whatever you feel, reading about post-hysterectomy self-care is a good idea. Hersfoundation.org is a pretty great resource for information and has also been a force in political organizing around the issue.

Some people may get hysterectomies as part of gender affirmation. But trans men and other transmasculine and nonbinary people might also choose to keep their uteruses for a huge host of reasons, including that they might want to carry and have babies someday, which they absolutely can. Choosing to keep a uterus does not make anyone less masculine or less of a man, nor does still having a uterus that they would like to have taken out someday. However, it can be very distressing for someone to have a uterus they don't want. Hysterectomies are considered by the World Professional Association for Transgender Health to be a medically necessary part of gender-affirming surgical therapy, probably because Medicare is supposed to cover "medically necessary transition-related surgery."[23,24] Hysterectomies for gender-affirmation purposes are just beginning to be covered by some insurance plans, but there's a long way to go before they will be truly accessible for the majority of people who want them. (See resources on the next page for help with this.)[23]

The tragic irony is that so many people who didn't want and never needed hysterectomies have been forced to get them while they are denied to other people who desperately want them. It makes sense that The Patriarchy would be extra controlling over the uterus because the uterus is humanity's way of making more humans, which is something you need to man the nozzle

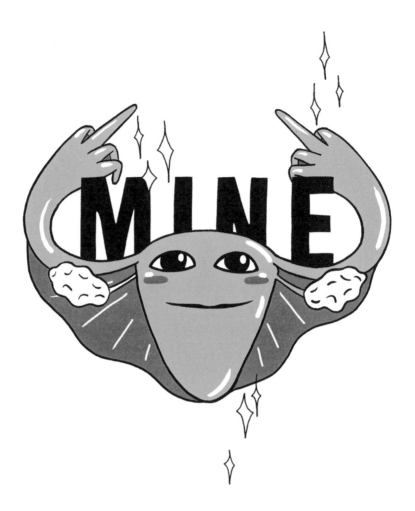

on if you want to control a society (i.e., to sustain The white-supremacist Patriarchy).

So even though I kind of hate my uterus, it's mine, damnit! And yours is yours. And we should all be able to do with them whatever we darn well please.

RESOURCES

For trans and nonbinary people who are looking for help getting a hyster-ectomy, Reddit may be a good place to start looking to connect with people who may have tips for the process. Also, the National Center for Transgender

Equality has a Trans Legal Services Network Directory of organizations that may be able to provide legal assistance in trying to get a hysterectomy or other surgeries covered by insurance:

- transequality.org/issues/resources/trans-legal-services-network-directory

For more information about and support for endometriosis:

- endometriosisassn.org
- endofound.org
- endometriosis.net

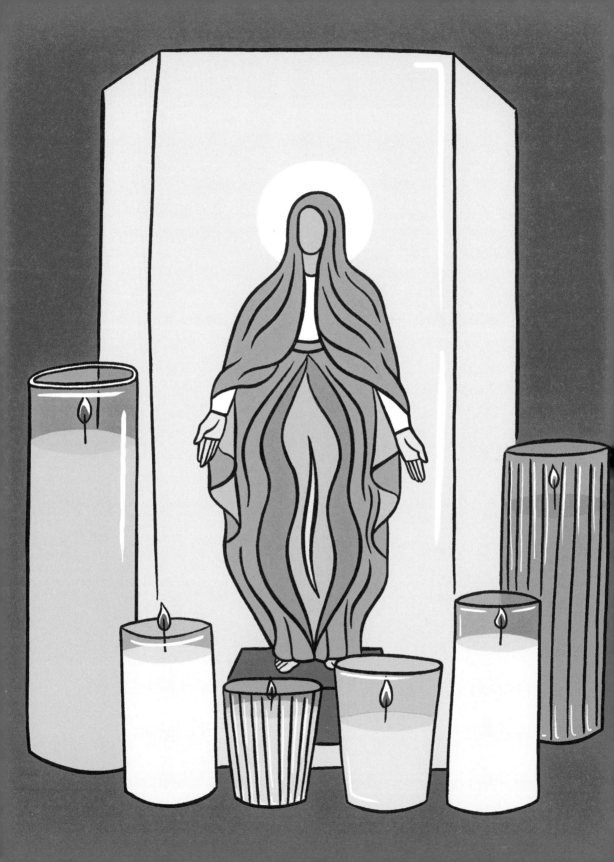

8

The Vaginal Corona, Formerly Known as the Hymen (and the Virginity Myth)

A HYMEN IS A LITTLE BIT OF ELASTIC MUCUS MEMBRANE TISSUE RIGHT AT THE EN-trance of the vagina, which gets stretchier during puberty and then often vanishes—entirely or almost entirely—later in life.[1,2,3] It exists for no reason. (Evolution sometimes leaves body parts hanging around. Like men's nipples, for example.)[1,2]

There are a bunch of kinds of hymens, and almost none seal the vagina. (The ones that do are rare—like, between one in 1,000 and one in 10,000.)[4] The most common shapes of a hymen are a ring of tissue around the vagina, a half-moon of tissue around part of the vagina, and a kinda messier version of a ring that kind of looks like an anus.[3,4,5,6] Less common shapes are a sleeve of tissue that's thick and might stick out of the opening a little, a ring but with a piece or two of tissue stretching across it, and a solid piece of tissue with a bunch of little holes.[3,4,5,6]

Many hymens do not break upon first being penetrated, and even if they do tear a little, they don't necessarily bleed and usually heal within 24 hours.[2,4,7] Only about half of people will bleed from their first vaginal penetration, al-though many of those instances may be bleeding from vaginal tearing due to

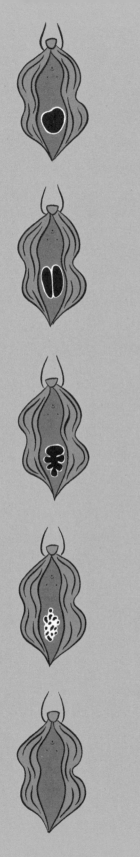

not enough wetness/lube, and not necessarily due to the hymen itself tearing.[1,2]

The notion that the hymen is a virginity seal that stretches across vaginas from birth 'til the moment a penis breaks it is a load of political bullshit. There is nothing accurate or scientific about it. Even the word *hymen* comes from the Greek god of marriage, Hymenaeus.[8] Our cultural hymen narrative comes straight from The Patriarchy's aching wish that the hymen were a mechanism to know—and therefore be able to control—what we do and don't stick up our vaginas. Sadly for The Patriarchy, it cannot because it is impossible to know what has or hasn't been in a vagina by looking at a hymen.[3,4]

In their 2017 TED Talk "The Virginity Fraud," Dr. Ellen Støkken Dahl and Dr. Nina Brochmann, authors of *The Wonder Down Under: The Insider's Guide to the Anatomy, Biology, and Reality of the Vagina*, explain:

> The truth [about hymens] has been known in medical communities for over a hundred years. Yet somehow, these [myths] continue to make life difficult for women around the world. . . . These myths have been used as a powerful tool in the effort to control women's sexuality in about every culture, religion, and historical decade. Women are still mistrusted, shamed, harmed, and, in the worst cases, subjected to honor killings if they don't bleed on their wedding night. Other women are forced into degrading virginity checks simply to get a job, defend their reputation, or to get married.[9]

Even in places where such extreme practices don't exist, the concept of "virginity" still enforces the damaging idea that a person's "purity" or value can be measured by what has been inside of their vagina, which . . . no it fucking can't. That idea also makes it hard for people with pussies to have a healthy relationship to their sexuality. This concept is often one of the voices in our heads singing, "You are bad for having sex, lalalalala, lala, la."

Also what does "virginity" even really mean if what counts as *sex* and *not sex* is an arbitrary distinction? A definition of "sex" limited to "penis in vagina" is heteronormative. There is no reason to draw a line in the sand of sexual activities to divide "real sex" from all the others. The only purpose that serves is to help The Patriarchy impose limits and control our activities. Like, is giving or receiving oral sex really less intimate or less of a big deal than vaginal penetration? I've had some make-out sessions that felt more important, intimate, profound, and vulnerable than some penis-in-vagina sessions.

The Swedish Association for Sexuality Education, which has been a leading organization in changing the global conversation about hymens, proposed that one thing we could all do to treat our collective ridiculitis around virginity and hymens is to rename the hymen the *vaginal corona*. The initiative has already had a pretty wide uptake among reproductive rights publications and organizations.

I like it because A) it doesn't have the cultural marriage and virginity baggage attached to it; B) a corona is a ring thing that goes around something, so this name gives a more accurate mental image; and C) it's a little crown for your royal vagina! That's cute! When we want to change the conversation (i.e., smash The Patriarchy), new words help.

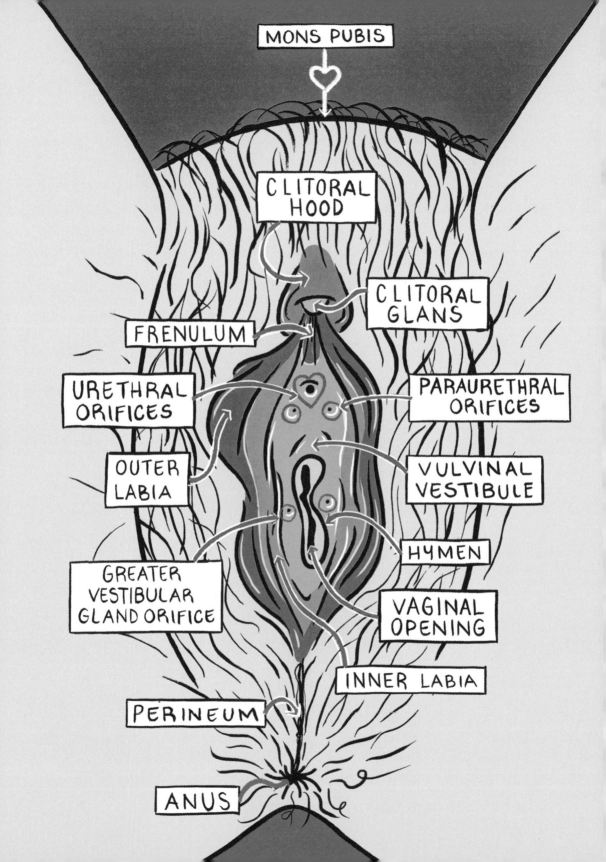

9
The Vulva and Vagina

Once upon a time there was a very unfair society (spoiler alert, it is this actual real one we live in!) where penises mattered more than vaginas. Like, a lot more. So they named vaginas "that thing that exists for a penis to go in." Literally, the word *vagina* comes from the Latin word for "sword holder."[1] That's why it's extra important to remember that the word *vagina* only actually refers to the vaginal canal—the little tube that connects the uterus to the outside world. The rest of what we often call the "vagina" is really the vulva.

Vulva Parts That Get Ignored When We Call the Whole Damn Thing "Vagina"

Which parts get included in the definition of the vulva depends on who you ask. I like to think of it as "everything you can see on the outside." First, ya got the mons pubis—the chubby, hairy triangle that sits above the top of the lips, in front. OK, maybe yours is neither chubby nor hairy, but mine is both. It's also sometimes called the *pubic mound* or the *mound of Venus*. It's a lump of fatty tissue covered by hairy skin that goes over the pubic bone.[2]

Pretend someone is lying on their back with their legs open and you're looking at their pussy (it's a great day). At the very top of the crack of the lips is the prepuce, or the clitoral hood—that thing that literally looks like your clit is wearing a sweatshirt hood. Under that is the glans of the clitoris. Below that, there's your teeny, tiny adorable little urethra—the pee hole that is the end of the tube that connects to your bladder. Under that, you have the opening of the vagina. Keep going down, and before the anus, you get to the perineum, or the "gooch," which is what my siblings and I have affectionately called our youngest brother since he was a toddler.

Around the center crack are the lips—the inner and outer labia. These used to be called the *labia majora* and *labia minora*, but the Federation of Feminist Women's Health Centers suggested the change since, in fact, the labia minora is often bigger than the labia majora on a lot of people's pussies, which is confusing. The outer labia are the hairy ones that extend inward from the inner thighs. The inner labia are the softer, usually hairless ones that are inside. They have lots of nerves in them and can be very sensitive. They also swell up with blood when you're aroused.[2]

Labia can look a million ways and still be normal. They can be super long and hangy-downy, really small and barely visible, red, purple, pink, brown, big and thick, small and thin, and everything in between. Vulvas in porn are just one kind of vulva and are often digitally edited to be smaller, less hangy-outy, and less detailed.[3] If your vulva doesn't look like that (mine certainly doesn't), good news: MOST DON'T! Vulvas really are like snowflakes, and if there are two just alike, there was probably plastic surgery involved. Check out Hilde Atalanta's project, @the.vulva.gallery, on Instagram to see a giant range of what they can look like, rendered in watercolor.

I spent many years being ashamed of my vulva—mostly of my hangy-downy labia. I don't know how I stopped. I think I just ran out of energy for that. If you are embarrassed about your labia, just stop. Your vulva is perfect, and you have so much else to do. These might literally be the Earth's last few habitable years. Please don't spend them letting The Patriarchy get you down on your perfect vulva. Also, anyone who shames you because you don't have a porn vulva is going to be bad at sex. That's not a fact, but it is a promise. I know it's not as easy as just stopping being embarrassed, but maybe if you can replace that mean voice in your head that says, "Your vulva is weird," with my mean (but loving!) voice saying, "Bro! You don't have time for this shit!" It might help. I hope it helps.

And let's not forget the pubes! Once when I was like fourteen, I was sitting on my toilet, looking down at my newly spawned pubes, thinking they looked very long. Then I noticed the hair scissors on the vanity. Then I got a Very Bad Idea. I took the scissors, pointed them into the toilet, quickly closed them across some curlies, and screamed. I had cut my also-newly-spawned labia. Very Badly. Now, I wouldn't think it was important to tell this story because I assume other people have better judgment and depth perception than I do. But I happen to know that it also happened to both a Very Smart friend and my own Very Smart mother. This makes me think we may not be the only three Otherwise Pretty Functional people to have had this Very Bad Idea.

So for the love of pussies everywhere, please be fucking careful if you trim your pubes with scissors. A few of my friends use short little scissors, which is probably a much better idea. These days, I don't do anything to my pubes except occasionally shave the bikini line if I'm going to the beach. I basically feel like I'm too busy to deal with my pubes, and also I think they're cute.

If your pube decision is going to come down to hygiene and safety, here are some things to consider. It used to be generally believed that pubic hair was dirty. That's why doctors used to shave pubic hair before childbirth. That is no longer considered true.[4] The two prominent theories about why pubes exist (for wafting pheromones and for minimizing chafing when there's rubbing going on) say nothing of cleanliness.[5] Shaving, waxing, or whatever you're doing probably poses a risk of some kind of injury. There are a few studies showing that people who remove their pubes get more STIs and at least one suggesting that's not the case.[6,7,8] Basically, it does not seem significantly safer or cleaner either way—to leave your pubes on or to take them off.

Pubes or no pubes is a personal decision. I'd say the only way to do pubes wrong is to do something that you don't want to do.

The Actual Vagina: A Lot Going On

The vagina is a tube, but the shape it actually sits in most of the time in your body is . . . not what it looks like in most illustrations and hilariously hard to explain. Here's how one study put it: "The overall shape of the vagina cannot be characterized by one single geometric shape, nor visualized in any one plane." Basically, it's collapsed most of the time (there are lots of parts around it, squishing it closed), and if you look at it in a cross section, it forms a soft W.[9]

And that amazing tubular soft W is so far from being a passive, inanimate recipient. Vaginas do a lot. They are active participants in sex. They grow an enormous amount to bring babies into the world. They transform when they are aroused. They change throughout the course of a life. They keep themselves clean. And they are host to an entire dynamic ecosystem (see Chapter 26).

Vaginas are made out of smooth muscle, which is the kind you can't intentionally move (like your intestines, and even your irises!). The inside layer of the muscle tube is stretchy connective tissue, and inside of that is the skin that you feel when you stick your fingers in there. This skin is called *vaginal mucosa*.[10] It is similar to the skin that lines your mouth except that it's very, very wrinkly. (The wrinkly-ness is what allows it to stretch enough to let a baby out.)[4]

The first, outermost layer of the mucosa is made up of dead skin cells and is called *stratum corneum*, from the Latin for "horny layer" (lol) apparently because the dead cells are harder than the suppler ones beneath. The horny layer cells store glycogen, a carbohydrate. Researchers estimate that the horny layer sheds cells every four hours. When the horny layer sheds, it feeds its glycogen to the *Lactobacillus* bacteria that live in your vagina, which make the lactic acid that keeps your vagina too acidic for most bad bacteria to survive.[11]

Another way the vagina keeps itself clean is with liquids. The skin below the horny layer filters blood to create a clear liquid called transudate which keeps the vagina moist.[12] There's usually also cervical mucus in the vagina. These two liquids constantly flush out the vagina, ridding it of bad bacteria and anything else undesirable.[13] That's why people say vaginas are self-cleaning ovens. (I wish we didn't compare vaginas to domestic appliances. Like, tigers also clean themselves. Just saying.) (See Chapter 3 for more on these liquids and Chapter 26 for more on how the ecosystem of bacteria plays a big role in keeping the vagina clean.)

Your vagina also has a huge array of different kinds of immune system cells in it. There are specialized receptors that keep a lookout for unwanted germs and tell immune-system fighter cells (one kind of which is literally named *natural killer cells*) when to launch an attack.[13]

The vagina's skin has another trick: it is good at bringing chemicals right into your bloodstream,[14] which is why in college I heard rumors about girls getting drunk by sticking vodka-soaked tampons up there, which is something that nobody should ever, ever, ever do. (I'm not sure anyone ever actually did this. I hope not. I imagine it would hurt like hell and probably kill all the good *Lactobacillus* bacteria that keep your vagina happy.) It's also why some medications can be administered vaginally, which can be helpful in getting more of the drug into your body since the digestive system and liver get rid of a bunch of medicine you take through your mouth before the medicine can help you.[14]

Bottom-Surgery Vaginas

Vaginas can be created surgically too, most commonly using the penis, scrotum, and sometimes other grafted skin that has been rearranged. It goes into the body between the rectum and the urethra.[15,16] The labia are made out of the scrotum, and the clitoris is made out of the head of the penis.[16] This is called *vaginoplasty*.

Surgically created vaginas don't produce their own natural mucus, lubrication, or *Lactobacillus*, so sometimes they can need more lube or even internal cleaning with douches, especially during the time after surgery when daily dilation of the newly formed vagina is needed.[16] But they are capable of feeling awesome! Seventy to 84% of people who have had vaginoplasties can orgasm.[4,15]

This is not so wildly surprising. Really, a vaginoplasty is just a rearranging of parts that are already made of the same tissues. A penis and pussy are the exact same thing when they're developing in the womb, until the sixth week of pregnancy when they start to evolve in different ways. After that, what's called the *genital tubercle* either becomes the head of the penis or the glans of the clit. Both are erectile tissue. The wrinkly, stretchy skin either becomes the outer labia or the scrotum. Really, "male" and "female" genitals are, as Dr. Emily Nagoski, author of *Come as You Are*, puts it, "All the same parts, organized in different ways."[3]

In bodies with intersex variations, the vagina and vulva might have characteristics that differ from what I've listed here and that do not fit into what is usually considered "male" or "female." For example, they might have a clitoris that is bigger than "normal," or a vagina that has an opening that is joined with the urethra. There are an unknown number of possibilities, none of which should necessarily be considered a deformity or even a problem that needs treatment! (For more on intersex variations, see Chapter 30.)

Changes Throughout Life

With major changes in levels of estrogen in the body, like during puberty, pregnancy, and menopause, the vagina and its microbiome change too.[17,18] During puberty, the vagina begins to take the form that it will have until menopause. As the vagina grows, its walls thicken, and its skin develops a horny layer and begins to contain more glycogen.[18,19]

Before puberty and after menopause, there is less estrogen in the body and therefore less glycogen stored in the horny layer. The vagina's skin is thinner, and the vagina has less *Lactobacillus* in it.[13,18] The same thing happens when taking testosterone: the vaginal walls thin and *Lactobacillus* decreases.[20]

People going through menopause, people experiencing the drop in estrogen that comes right after giving birth,[21,22] and people who take testosterone will also probably notice that their vaginas start to produce less lubricant, which can sometimes make penetration—or even just walking around—uncomfortable.[19,20] For folks taking testosterone, there are ways to treat this with estrogen rings, creams, and tablets that only give enough estrogen to the vagina to help without counteracting other effects of testosterone throughout the body (see Chapter 26 for more about changes to the vaginal microbiome when taking testosterone).[19]

Pregnancy and Post-Baby

During pregnancy, the vagina and vulva change in preparation for birth. Blood supply increases and sometimes the vagina and vulva change colors to something more blue or purplish.[19,23] The connective tissue under the skin of the vagina starts to relax, and the muscles under those start to beef up by building bigger fibers.[19] The cervix will also start to produce more mucus, which means there will be more discharge in the vagina (and your undies).[24] The extra estrogen in the body means more glucose in the vaginal skin, which helps the microbiome fill up with more lactobacilli than normal.[13] During pregnancy, vaginas are more prone to yeast infections, and it might be because the extra glycogen in the vaginal tissues, which normally feeds *Lactobacillus*, also feeds yeast fungus.[25]

After a baby . . . well, your vagina just pushed a baby out of it! So, yes, it's going to be somewhat different, though not totally different forever. There may be some injury to the vagina and the patch between the vagina and the anus, especially if an episiotomy (the cutting of the perineum) was performed. In one study, more than a third of people who had just had babies reported pain during penetrative sex for up to six months after giving birth for the first time.[22] The vagina's opening might be a bit bigger than its pre-birth size, but this usually goes back to normal over the next 6–12 weeks.[19] It's also normal to have some urinary incontinence, a.k.a. you pee yourself a little bit. One study showed that three months after vaginal delivery, over a third of people still had at least some pee leakage.[22] (This is treatable! See Chapter 5 for more on how.)

I felt unsatisfied with the research I was able to find about how people felt about their pussies after giving birth and about the recovery process, so I did an informal survey of 20 people (which is in no way a scientifically valid process or a representative sample, especially since they were all in my immediate or secondary social circles). I asked them how their pussies felt and how they felt about their pussies after giving birth. What I found was that everyone's physical recovery process was different, ranging from super quick and easy to years of pain and frustration. But there were a few consistencies:

1. Recovering from an episiotomy is pretty painful.
2. Almost everyone who didn't have an easy recovery suffered from anxiety about whether their recovery process was "normal" and whether they would return to "normal." As one friend put it, "When I asked the doctors about what was going on, they would say, 'That's normal.' But I hate the word *normal*. Just because it happens often doesn't mean it's OK."
3. The thing I heard most was, "I didn't want to look at it." People expressed feeling scared of seeing it, of knowing what had changed. They also expressed feeling disconnected from their bodies in a way that made them

not want to have sex. Sometimes this disconnection was just born of distraction—having an infant to keep alive, turns out, is a lot of work. Sometimes it stemmed from postpartum depression and sometimes from feeling that their new bodies were too foreign to them or just in too much pain.

When something is hurting and you want it to stop hurting, it's reasonable that not knowing how long it will take to heal could cause anxiety. But I suspect that much of this anxiety and avoidance stems from shame imposed by The Patriarchy—that false idea that we can "ruin" our pussies by having children, that vaginas get "loose," and that the state of our vaginas changes our overall desirability and value as people. And again, while my sample was not representative, I have a hunch that these experiences are pretty common. I hate that this bullshit comes to haunt us in the aftermath of one of the most difficult and amazing things a human can achieve, in a moment when I wish everyone could just feel proud as fuck of themselves.

If Your Vagina or Vulva Hurts, Like, a Lot

If your vulva or vagina tends to hurt, you might have vaginismus, vestibulodynia, vulvodynia, dyspareunia, or genito-pelvic pain/penetration disorder (GPPPD). GPPPD is a newish diagnosis, created in 2013 to encompass these many different kinds of pussy pain. GPPPD is when, for at least six months, your vulva or vagina hurts before, during, or after penetrative sex or just for no apparent reason.[26] GPPPD can make it very hard for people to have enjoyable sex lives.[27,28] And it can also be an emotionally shitty road to diagnosis because getting there will necessarily involve doctors searching for the source of the pain and not being able to find it. This is the kind of medical situation that often leaves people feeling gaslit and dismissed.

Because GPPPD includes a range of experiences, the data-based estimations of how many people have it vary a lot. But the broadest and most recent review of studies I found, which looked at 36 articles in 2018, says that 14–34% of premenopausal people with pussies and 6.5–45% of postmenopausal people with pussies have GPPPD.[27] About 8–10% of people with pussies experience pain in their vulvas specifically.[28]

Sometimes a vagina might hurt because pelvic muscles tense up and "close" the vagina when trying to get something in it.[26] Sometimes your vulva just hurts for no apparent reason.[28] Often anxiety is involved, though whether pain is caused by or causes the anxiety—or both—is not always clear.[29] Researchers think that, in many cases, fear of pain causes anxiety, which in turn causes pain.[27] GPPPD might be caused by physical problems in muscles, bones, or organs, might be caused by psychosocial problems like trauma or fear ("Affected women often come from families and cultures with strong beliefs about the dangers of penetrative sex," one study of vaginismus noted),[29] or might be caused by both.[28,30,31] It also might be causing both. Or neither.

As Dr. Ellen Støkken Dahl and Dr. Nina Brochmann point out in *The Wonder Down Under*, it's important to be cautious when pointing at psychological causes, even if they might turn out to be real: "It's easy to slap a 'psychological causes' label on conditions whose physical causes aren't immediately identifiable, but we should be very careful about doing this. . . . [I]t can lead to confusion and anger [and] create a misleading impression that a woman herself, or her personality, is responsible for the pain. This isn't constructive. Genital pains may well turn out to have psychological causes for some women, but that's no cause for shame."[32]

GPPPD may well have some psychological causes. God, there's so fucking much sexual trauma out there, it's easy to imagine. But I would add that we should stay vigilant about asking ourselves if, when, and to what extent we might be informed by the historical tendency to dismissively view people with pussies as "hysterical" when they have undiagnosable problems. (See Chapter 7 for more on the history of hysteria.) I worry that while the mind-body connection is a new and exciting field of research, both the people deciding what they want to research and the people who decide what research to fund could potentially favor that path over continuing to search for physiological causes because it rings the familiar hysteria bell in their brains that subconsciously causes us to emotionally, financially, or intellectually invest more. Or in other words, "Psychological causes? Hey now! That sounds about right!" This will matter most for the people deciding what research to fund; if we give up on looking for physiological causes and focus more on the psychological, we could end up delaying important discoveries.

Treatments for GPPPD include creams, medications, physical therapy, couples therapy, and behavioral therapy, putting gradually bigger thingies in your vagina, or even hypnosis . . . but it is often just a bitch of a problem to treat.[29,33,34,35,36] In worst-case scenarios, there's also surgery.[27] There's a long way to go in figuring out GPPPD. It's a fairly new area of research, but I was surprised to see just how much research is actually underway. So while we may have to wait a while to see GPPPD become a super-treatable problem, the picture is not totally bleak.

The most important thing is to seek out the specialists who work with these pain problems, who can try to help. Also, a few studies have shown that open conversations about pain and coping strategies with supportive sexual partners—especially partners who don't give up on figuring out how to have sexytime in a non-painful way—can help.[27,37,38,39,40]

The Vagina Can Still Sit with Me at Lunch

Vaginas do not get "loose" from having a lot of sex.[32,41] That is another gross patriarchal lie invented to shame people with pussies for having sex. And also, even if they are naturally bigger or wider than whatever your perception of "normal" is, that does not get in the way of having awesome sex.[41] And, yes, while the clitoris is amazing and long ignored, the vagina also still has a role in sexual function. OK, that might seem obvious, but I'm saying it specifically because there has been a feminist backlash against The Patriarchy's focus on the vagina at the expense of the clitoris. It's a backlash that has gone overboard, if you ask me.

For example, back in 1970, Anne Koedt published her wildly popular essay, "The Myth of the Vaginal Orgasm," in which she wrote that the vaginal orgasm "does not exist." In a way, she was right, but in a way she also was not. (See Chapter 9 to learn about why.) She clarifies, "It is the clitoris which is the center of sexual sensitivity and which is the female equivalent of the penis." It was cool and productive for Koedt to shift focus from the vagina to the clitoris . . . but then she went too far, saying that people who claim to have vaginal orgasms are merely confused or are lying.[42]

And then, in 2002, Rebecca Chalker wrote in *The Clitoral Truth*, "As heretical as it sounds, in terms of sexuality, the vagina is more useful to men than it is to women."[2] And while that's a subjective statement, I'd like to say: um, no.

The vagina does a lot. When the vagina gets aroused, it produces multiple different kinds of fluid (more on this in Chapter 3), the cervix lifts up, the vagina lengthens, and its upper portion expands outward. This is called *vaginal tenting* or *vaginal ballooning*, and researchers believe that it may be a mechanism that helps give sperm a chance to wriggle out of semen and mix with the fluids that help them glide into the cervix hole.[43]

On top of its active role in helping with conception, it also plays a role in sexual pleasure. The vagina appears to have what researchers call a *vaginal pacemaker*, cells that respond to rubbing by sending electric waves through the vagina, causing the vagina to contract and increase arousal.[44] Even if you never orgasm from vaginal penetration without direct clitoral stimulation, vaginal penetration might help the arousal process along. And some people absolutely do orgasm through vaginal penetration! Because the urethral sponge and therefore the clitoris are stimulated through the vaginal wall. (See Chapter 4 for more about how this works.)

So, yes, the vagina (again, which does not include the vulva) has the worst name ever and has definitely historically gotten way too much attention (and also, somehow, at the same time not enough attention). But we don't need to send it to the corner of the room to sit with a dunce cap on its head. In spite of all the shitty cultural narratives that surround it, the vagina does so much for us and deserves a seat at the Pussy Table IMFHO. The end.

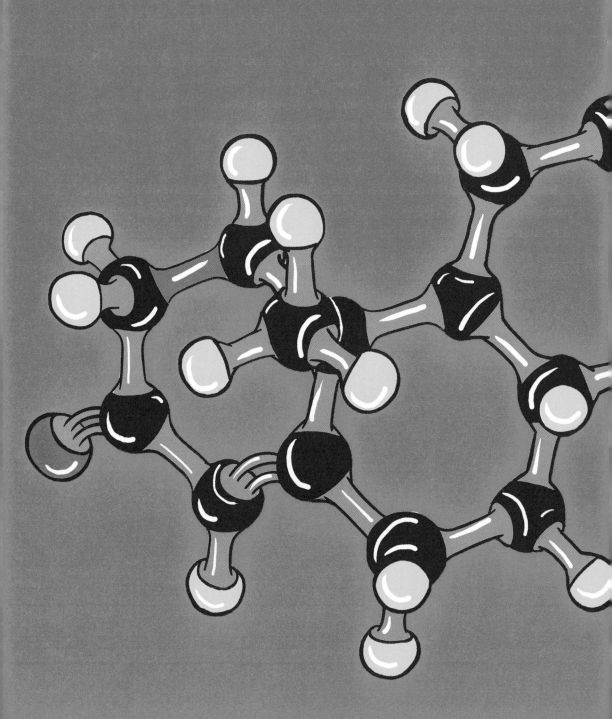

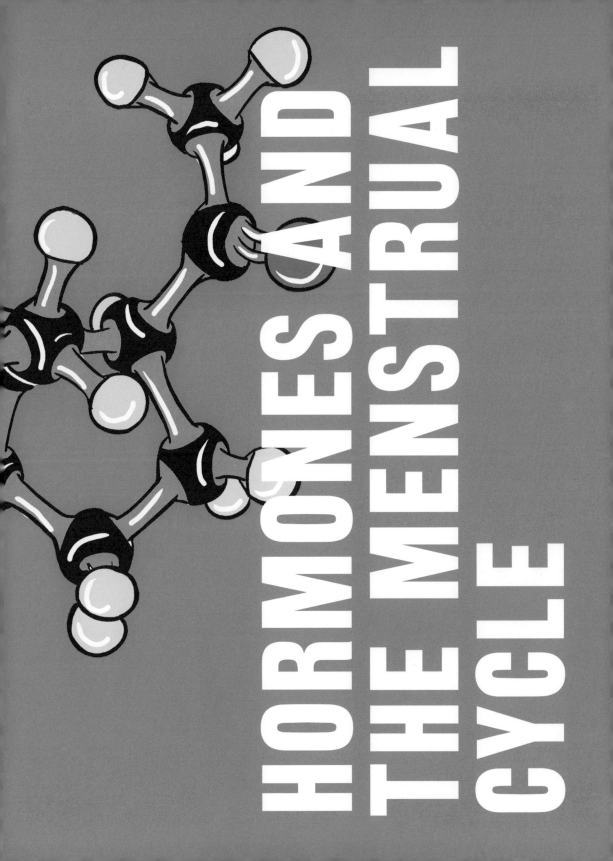

HORMONES AND THE MENSTRUAL CYCLE

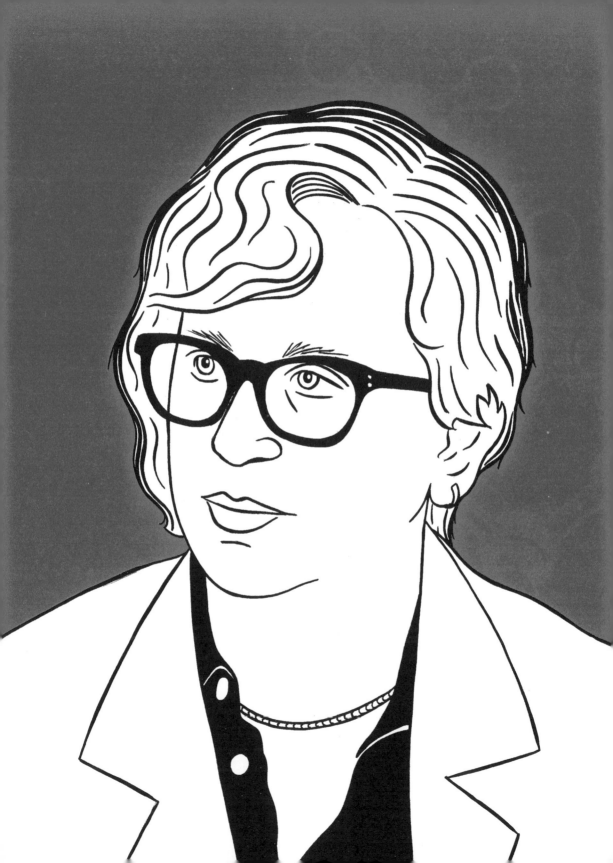

10
Gender-Affirming Hormone Therapy

Interview with Dr. Madeline Deutsch

You can't research trans health, especially hormone therapy, very long without coming across the work of Madeline Deutsch, MD, MPH. All transgender health research roads seem to lead back to her. So I was very surprised and excited when she agreed to an interview. When we connected over Zoom, Dr. Deutsch was both cooking dinner and talking to me with the facility of someone who is used to doing three to four jobs every day.

Dr. Deutsch is a physician who actually sees patients; is the medical director for UCSF Transgender Care, perhaps the most important transgender health program in the country; and is also an associate professor at the University of California San Francisco (UCSF). As I write this, she is also the president-elect of the World Professional Association for Transgender Health. She's trans and very proud to be able to work in her field.

In 2006, two years out of her medical residency, Dr. Deutsch was working in a high-volume urban trauma center in Los Angeles. She became disillusioned with emergency medicine: "I felt that I was continually plugging my finger into holes in a large, leaking dam and I didn't feel like I was actually making a big difference upstream." She began to contemplate a career change.

Around then, a colleague of hers started an in-home, preventative-medicine concierge service. The idea inspired her. "Being queer and trans, and understanding the limitations in access that my community has to these kinds of services, I said, 'Let me try to open a little private-practice office in LA, offering a range of LGBT preventative and primary care [services], and I'll do hormone therapy, and let's see what happens.'"

What happened was that she got very busy very quickly and, after a few years, ended up joining forces with UCSF, becoming a professor there in 2012 and, starting in 2013, growing her practice into a very important program that offers a huge range of trans health services and publishes some of the best—and only—extensive trans health content on the internet.

Dr. Deutsch also conducts and publishes what she twice referred to in our conversation as "just a little" research about hormone therapy and transgender health. But when I texted my public-health-researcher friend Dr. Jackie Jahn, asking if having your name on eight published articles in a year is a lot, she replied, "THAT IS A SHIT TON."

In Dr. Deutsch's picture on UCSF Transgender Care's website, she is wearing cute grandma glasses and an argyle sweater. But the argyle belies a very punk-rock mentality. She questions everything, the establishment and the antiestablishment alike. That bravery and instinct to question are probably what made her the trailblazer that she is. She seems to be constantly straining to see past the dam, to look upstream, to place everything in a broader context. Talking to her becomes an exercise in doing the same.

Sometimes people use the term *hormone replacement therapy* and sometimes *hormone therapy*. What is the difference between the two?
Terminology is important. I refer to it as "gender-affirming hormone therapy" because that's a descriptive term. *Hormone replacement therapy* is like, well, what are you replacing? It's typically been used in the context of managing menopause. Regardless of whether or not you agree with those semantics, if you also use it for people who are taking hormones for gender-affirming reasons, it's just not clear.

Gender-affirming hormone therapy is to allow someone to have physical changes to their body with the intent of affirming their gender. It can involve not only estrogen therapy but also other agents like testosterone-blocking medication and a full range of androgens—plus testosterone for masculinizing treatments.

How and when did hormone therapy for gender affirmation become a Thing?

It started in the 1950s, not very long after [researchers] figured out what sex hormones were. There was an endocrinologist at Johns Hopkins named Harry Benjamin, and he's identified as the—I don't like to say "father of" because it's a sexist term—but the parent of hormone therapy, in that he took it from an out-there premise and brought some technique and structure to the process. For a period of time in the '50s, '60s, and '70s, Hopkins and other heavy-hitter academic institutions like Stanford had some really active transgender-medicine programs that were researching hormone therapy and also prescribing hormones and doing surgery. By the '80s, there had been a couple of high-profile cases of some ethical lapses in the field. Also, the arc of culture in this country bends conservative. So, one by one, these programs closed. Insurance companies stopped paying for these services, universities got anxious, and things shut down.

Then we got into the Dark Ages in the '90s when hormone therapy moved away from university research and got pushed into the private-practice realm. It became the Wild West. Funding for the research dried up as the country tacked center and right. When I started doing this work in 2006, I could barely get anyone to rent me space when I told them what I wanted to do!

Then in the 2010s, we had eight years of Obama, who brought some cultural shifts, and there were a few high profile cases like Chaz Bono and Caitlyn Jenner. "Don't Ask, Don't Tell" [the US military's anti-LGBTQ policy] got repealed, marriage equality became the law of the land, and trans people were allowed to start serving openly in the military. Now [gender-affirming hormone therapy] has become a well-understood and a fairly mainstream line of medicine. It's still at the fringe and still kind of Wild West in regard to standards and training, but less in regard to general public acceptability. Even with the toxicity of this recent election cycle, nobody really got too involved with queer and trans stuff. It just wasn't front and center. In the 2004 midterms, queer people were going to be the end of the world. I think it's become baked into the culture of the country at this point.

Yeah, it does seem to be more baked into the culture, and it seems like kids are able to start coming out as trans much earlier in life because of that. What do you say to parents of young kids who are asking to go on hormones?

The first thing I would say to any parent who is anxious about their trans youth is: Check your own pulse. A little bit of mindfulness. Take a deep breath; it's not the end of the world.

Kids will tell you who they are. There is not an epidemic of trans kids suddenly waking up and saying, "I'm trans," and then waking up two years later and saying they're not. By the time a kid makes their way to their pediatrician's office and says, "I want to go on hormone therapy," that kid has been thinking about this for a long time. This is the end of a very long road for someone.

The data that we have on kids who desist in their gender goals is not soundly based data. There are a lot of confounders in it. The kids were generally taken to an institution where it was known that the institution was not particularly affirming. And they had to sit across from some stern-looking psychologist who stroked his chin while talking to them about their gender feelings and, surprise surprise, a lot of those kids—who were also taken there by parents who were not particularly into [the idea of their child being trans]—wind up stating that their gender has reverted to their birth-assigned sex. The real question is, How many of these kids in 20 years will be depressed alcoholics, or transition, or commit suicide?

Also, with kids, you don't start hormone therapy before puberty. If your nine-year-old comes up to you and says, "Mom, I'm a boy," you just say, "OK." My general recommendation is just to figure out how to best affirm their gender identity. So if you live in rural Louisiana, maybe going to school tomorrow with a totally changed gender presentation is not the smartest thing to do. Maybe be a bit more intentional. Maybe prepare an announcement, maybe wait a few months and change schools. You don't have to go lunging at someone with hormones the day that they tell you [they're trans], especially someone prepubertal. You have to wait for a certain pubertal stage to start someone on hormones. The fear memes of "Crazy doctors are putting eight-year-old boys on estrogen" are not actually what happens. So just, again, check your own pulse.

The data we have is that, when trans kids' families support their identity, their mental health outcomes are identical to those of non-trans kids. And when we don't support trans kids' identities, and when we don't allow them to affirm themselves, those are the kids that wind up with bad mental health outcomes.

What about from a physical health perspective? What do we know about the long-term health effects of hormone therapy?

We don't have a lot of data. There are some lower-quality, medium-term, and a couple of longer-term studies that are pretty reassuring. There are not huge signals in the data coming out saying that there are major problems. There might be some health risks in regard to cardiovascular considerations in some older transgender people. But we know that the harms of not giving somebody hormones are very high.

It's like the COVID vaccine: If someone came up to you and said, "There's a new vaccine against herpes and it was developed in 10 months and it's been tested on 30,000 people," there's no way you would take it. You would say, "Come back to me when you have a few million people and five years of data," like with every other vaccine. But with COVID, we know that people are going to die, and your likelihood of dying from COVID is much higher than the likelihood of dying from the vaccine. So you say, "OK, there are some unknowns associated with this vaccine, and it's new, we don't have enough data, but we know the alternative is death." That's how you can look at hormone therapy, in my opinion.

What else should people consider when they're considering starting hormones themselves? What do people who do their own research about it often get wrong?

I like to tell people, don't try to overengineer hormones. There's a lot of emphasis [from patients] on *my doctor gives me this many milligrams and I hear that if you take it rectally three times a day, it's gonna work better.* Most of this stuff is not true. Patients come to me and say, "Oh, I read a study that said that I should take my hormones *this* way . . ." Turns out, it wasn't a study, it was an article written by someone expressing their opinion.

It's particularly prevalent among trans women I see, but it is also prevalent among trans men. You have to remember that the forces of sexism that exist in society certainly apply to transgender people and potentially in a more intense fashion. One of the goals of sexist marketing, like the cover[s] of *Vogue*, is to send the message to women that, unless they achieve a certain standard, they're not worthy women. Then you market your product based on that desire. A cis woman might look at the cover of *Vogue* and internalize that she's not a valuable woman. Transgender people don't just get the message that they're not valuable but also that they're not even women. It creates ongoing trauma. Transfeminine people don't have the benefit of having been socialized from a young age as girls, when ideally they would have picked up some resilience and ability to tune out or push back against that kind of messaging. It's a shark tank of what it means to be accepted as a woman. And it can be really destabilizing for people.

So the connection back to not overengineering hormones is that the hormones can change your body but that they're not going to help with trauma?

That's a different issue, but also true. Hormones and surgery don't fix everything. They just give you a vagina or breasts or a beard. We have lots of data to support that taking hormone therapy brings objective improvement to a range of psychosocial measures. But they can't solve everything that is wrong with the world or with your life.

The issue I'm talking about though is that because of the current climate, and because there's an intense demand for *I want a lot of changes and I want them now*, there have unfortunately been a lot of predatory providers in the field, making drastic marketing claims: *You should take the hormones this way, and if you don't, then your doctor is underselling you and you should come to my cash-only hormone practice! What your doctor is giving you right now is total junk!* It's the same as *My weight loss program, my pill for five easy payments of $99.95.* Unfortunately, there has been a general decline in respect for science and professionals in the field. Look what's happening with COVID.

I was recently talking to an 18-year-old patient who is going to be starting hormones and they were asking me about some unorthodox and inappropriate approaches, and I was like, "Well, you know that's not—" and they said, "Well, I understand that's your opinion, but let me tell you what mine is." And I try not to be prescriptive and paternalistic in my care, but I was like, "Actually, I do want to tell you that I am the doctor here at the end of the day."

It's a microcosm of what's going on in this country where you see people saying, "I'm standing over here, and I believe that Black people are inferior. And when you don't allow me to share my beliefs, you're closed-minded and you're discriminating against me, and we just need to have discussions about all perspectives." It's not like you're saying you don't like the Beatles. You're frickin' racist. So obviously, we're getting off topic, but it's the same lack of critical thinking at play.

Yes. Identity politics are definitely being weaponized against us. And it's getting harder for people to understand what to believe. When it comes to research and critical thinking about [gender-affirming] hormone therapy, what are some things that Science just doesn't know yet that people shouldn't believe any claims they read about?

Methods of administration, dosing beyond getting the hormone levels into the female or male range, this component of the range versus that component of the range—we just don't have any evidence to support that one approach is better than the other. That's one big area. There's also a lot to be desired in the area of surgery and surgical techniques, differences between approaches. None of these things have been studied.

Only recently, there was a dark period of 20 years where this was almost all happening in private practice and there wasn't much going on in the academic community. I don't say "dark" because the care that's delivered in private practice is bad. In fact, it's often quite good, and actually, a strange side effect of the fact that we went 20 years without much academic output was that it was unencumbered by regulations. There was a great deal of innovation and movement toward a much less restrictive approach. We're way ahead of places like Europe that have maintained a tight grip on it through the scientific-academic government complex. But there does need to be some oversight. Unbridled free-market competition is what results in people selling dangerous consumer products that kill people. There's a balance that has to be found.

What would you like to see happen in the ecosystem not just of hormone therapy but of trans health care in general?

There needs to be evolution both vertically and horizontally. The program I run at UCSF is a university-based academic medical center. We have a multidisciplinary program. We have a range of specialties affiliated, from primary care and hormone therapy to different kinds of surgery, to hair removal, to voice therapy. And we're trying to make it a more integrated experience so people can one-stop shop as much as possible. Then, different specialists can talk to each other and coordinate care, like getting people two surgeries on the same day, or making sure that people with complicated medical problems can still get surgery.

Even though this care has been provided since the 1950s, there hasn't been a standardized approach to training providers in things like hormone management and surgery. It tends to be based on opinions. There just isn't a lot of solid, long-term research data because funding has significantly lagged. We need a standardized approach, and we need more funding opportunities for research and for training to develop those programs.

When you say, "funding has lagged," what does that look like? Do research proposals just get turned down?

A few things happen. Research proposals can get turned down, and research proposals can be not understood. I have been involved in reviewing research proposals for the National Institutes of Health, the primary government funder of big-ticket health care research in the US, and unfortunately, the people reviewing proposals often have no expertise in the area of research. It's like if you were designing a new car and then you send the proposal to a bunch of airplane engineers to review. They're qualified people, but they build airplanes; they don't build cars. That has been an issue. Also, in this ass-backwards country, at the end of the day, some of it is political. After the scientific gradings are made, there's some level of administrative review based on the policy priorities of the [NIH]. So there's always politics involved.

Let's zoom in to the patient-in-front-of-you aspect of what you do. What do you wish other health care professionals did better in treating trans patients?

The most important thing is that this is not rocket science. It's actually pretty easy to do this care. And the most important aspect of it is not even the medical care. It's calling people by the name they want to use, using the right pronoun, not being afraid to say, "I don't know exactly, but I'm going to look it up." Physicians do that every day in the course of their general practice. I look things up three times a day that have nothing to do with trans stuff. That's what we're taught to do in our training.

Doctors have hang-ups about this kind of care because of the combination of the social stigma and there's this *eughhhh*. It's the same as, *Ewww,* vagina, *ewwwwwwww*. It's a thing! People's brains turn off and go to jelly. Doctors need to realize that becoming comfortable with it is medically necessary.

Is there anything else you want to add before we go?

Yes. There needs to be more dialogue between cis communities and trans communities. You mentioned that you don't use the word *women* in the project. I have complicated feelings about this. There are cisgender women who have experienced a deep and wide range of sexism and maybe are survivors of abuse. There's gotta be a way to use inclusive language that is not excluding anyone but that still honors the perspectives of people who feel invested in their identities as women and that being linked to them having a pussy. I don't have the answers. But I'd like to see more dialogue. Otherwise, you have the trans community locked in battle with certain aspects of cis-feminist spaces, and white men win when we fight with each other.

The problem is that there is no empathetic dialogue going on around this issue. TERFs [trans-exclusionary radical feminists] aren't purely racist, hateful people. When I see stuff like a trans women saying, "How dare you remotely equate vaginas to women or anything, or reference anything related to cis women at all," that's horribly dismissive and unempathetic to the experiences of some cis women and what they're looking for in their life. You're never going to have any human progress on this issue until there's more dialogue around it. I hope the Biden administration will set the tone for more dialogue and will begin to heal some of our differences. We'll see what happens.

RESOURCES

- Dr. Deutsch's video "Introduction to Female-to-Male Hormone Therapy": https://youtu.be/GAJZ4fwTuyc
- Dr. Deutsch's video "Introduction to Hormone Therapy—Male to Female Transition": https://youtu.be/kRxkGCbAhC8
- For tons of awesome trans health information or to seek providers: transcare.ucsf.edu

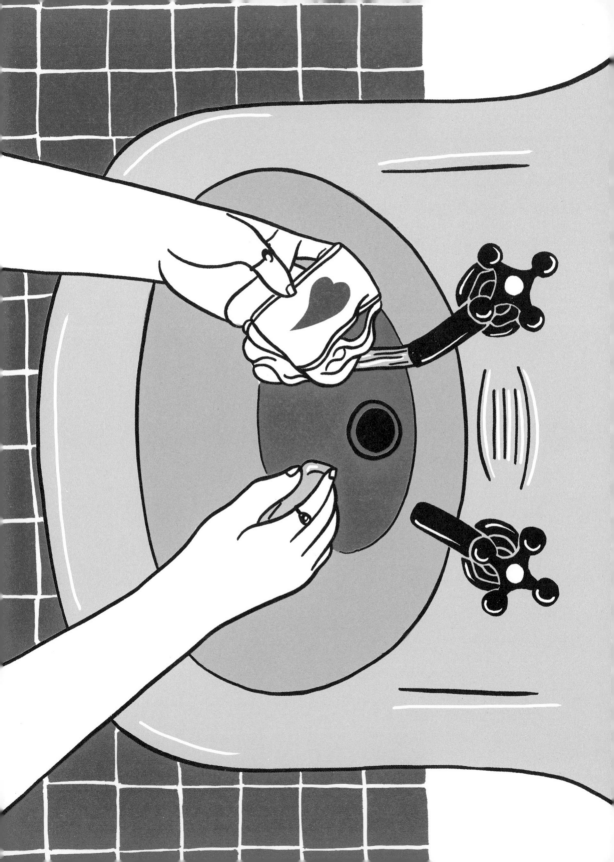

11
The Menstrual Cycle: Gender Narratives from Menarche to Menopause

MENSTRUATION IS PRETTY WELL COVERED IN SCHOOL SEX ED FOR MOST PEOPLE, which makes sense. So much information about our bodies is withheld from us except for reproduction-related things because it's in The Patriarchy's interest to teach little kids with pussies that their most relevant and important function is reproduction. Not that reproduction isn't cool. It's fucking mind-blowing to have the ability to grow a human inside of you. But our collective hyper-focus on it reinforces the idea that people with pussies should have a limited role in society. What if schools spent as much time teaching 12-year-old menstruators that they could do anything they want with their lives as we do teaching them about their periods and the ability to reproduce? Wouldn't that be nice? Here's a really wild idea: What if schools taught 12-year-olds about how our science, understanding, and experiences of menstruation are shaped by patriarchal gender narratives?

I won't hold my breath. But I will cover that in this chapter, as well as some of the basics.

Anyway, menarche, the menstrual cycles, and menopause comprise a trajectory that most "female" bodies will take over the course of a lifetime without significant intervention. In most cases, it goes like this: First, your body becomes able to reproduce and you start menstruating sometime during adolescence—this first menstruation is called *menarche*. Then you live out a few decades of menstrual cycles while your body waits for possible pregnancy. Then your body is like, *OK, that was enough of that*, and you go through menopause, in which you stop having a menstrual cycle and go through a long process of physiological and hormonal changes in your whole body.

(There are a lot of reasons why that process might not reflect yours. Like, for example, if your pussy was surgically constructed, if you had radiation, if you had surgery like a hysterectomy or oophorectomy that sends you into early menopause, if you take hormones for gender-affirming reasons, or even if you just take certain types of birth control.)

Menopause has two definitions. It refers both to the entire process and experience of going through menopause and to the exact moment that it has been 365 days since a person's last period because the ovaries have retired.[1] (In Chapters 9 and 26, I go over vaginal changes during menopause, to tissues and to the microbiome, respectively.) But contrary to popular narratives, menopause entails much more than vaginal changes and a decline in sex drive. It's a full-body process. Narratives about menopause need to expand or else when it happens, people are unprepared. Lucky for you, *What Fresh Hell Is This?: Perimenopause, Menopause, Other Indignities, and You* by Heather Corinna is an incredible book, packed densely with Everything Else about menopause.

Hormones: Bossy Little Molecules

Hormones like estrogen, progesterone, and testosterone are responsible for instituting the changes that happen in your body during this reproductive arc. Hormones are molecules that go around telling different parts of your body what to do. They have a huge range of jobs. For example, estrogen tells your ovary to release an egg, but it also plays a role in regulating your moods and behaviors, including your levels of horniness and stress.[2,3,4] And testosterone, which is not only a male hormone, helps the ovaries get ready to release an egg during the menstrual cycle.[5]

It's a pervasive idea, even among doctors, that testosterone makes people with pussies horny, but it's probably not very true.[3] Testosterone doesn't necessarily do the same things in a "female" body as in a "male" body. It's a common problem in Science that we study "male" bodies and then think we can apply what we learn about them to all bodies, which is often not true. Even though it is important to think about which sex chromosome–based differences between sexes are *not* real, or to what extent they're not real, it is also very important to think about which ones *are* real, and what implications they have for health.

That's important to note because in recent years it has become increasingly common that doctors are prescribing testosterone off-label (meaning taking a drug to treat something for which it was not approved by the FDA), for problems like low energy and low libido in postmenopausal people.[3,6] (This is not recommended, except in very specific cases, like for people who have undergone surgically induced menopause.)[7] In 2020, the American Association of Clinical Endocrinology and the American College of Endocrinology put out a joint statement explaining that the surge in off-label testosterone use is probably due to bullshit on the internet and reckless vendors who sell it for uses that have no research to back them up. The statement basically said, *Whoa, this is freaking us out. Y'all should really not do that.*[6]

There is some evidence that testosterone can help make people with pussies hornier, but there's more evidence that, in fact, it's estrogen that has the job of making us horny.[3]

Phases of the Menstrual Cycle

Physical, hormonal, immune system, and emotional changes take place throughout the cycle. For some people, their cycle is no big deal and they don't feel that different week to week. For others, their cycle has a huge effect on their lives. People's cycles vary from about 21 to 40 days, with an average of 28.[8] Some people's cycles are more regular than others.

Menstruation is your period. Your uterus squeezes itself to push out the endometrium—the stuff that lines your uterus and that comes out during your period along with blood. The squeezing is what causes cramps. (Hot tip that changed my life, from Dr. Ellen Støkken Dahl and Dr. Nina Brochmann, authors of *The Wonder Down Under*: take ibuprofen or another NSAID *before* the worst of your cramps would usually start, instead of after you're already in pain.)[9] If you're interested in suppressing your period altogether, there are a lot of hormonal birth control options that can do that (see Chapter 20 for more on those options).

Menstruation has been heavily stigmatized since the damn Bible, and still is, especially in the US. We are taught to hide it at all costs. How many tampon commercials sell their products not on the basis of their quality but on the basis of how *discreet* they are? This has been called the "culture of concealment" by menstruation scholars, and it reinforces the idea that our bodies are Bad and gross, which creates shame and stress, which just wastes time and energy and the ability to enjoy life for people who menstruate.[10] A thing we cannot stop our bodies from doing should not cause us shame. (Free the farts!)

Thanks to the work of a growing movement of activists and artists and actually—yes, I'm going to give them some credit—marketing people, this has started to change in the last 10 or so years. The menstruation-activism movement works to fight the period taboo.[11] Everyone can participate in this movement and help normalize menstruation just by publicly acknowledging it. If you don't feel good because you have cramps, say, "I don't feel good *because I have period cramps*." If someone says, "*Ew*," tell them (kindly) that *they* are being inappropriate. Instead of hiding a tampon to carry it to the bathroom, just hold the damn thing in your hand and walk past people and don't care if they see it.

Many trans, nonbinary, and gender-nonconforming people menstruate, which can be a source of stress, sadness, and logistical problems because it can be a reminder that a person has body parts they don't want.[12] Trans and nonbinary people can also feel totally neutral or positive about their periods.

But for those for whom it is difficult, part of that can be logistical problems with public bathrooms. Many men's bathrooms don't have garbage cans inside the stalls. The sound of unwrapping menstrual products in a bathroom stall has been awkward even for me, so I can imagine it could be scary for someone who doesn't want to arouse suspicion in a place they may already feel unsafe. And then there's the super-silly, pink, sparkly, ultra-heteronormative packaging on most "feminine" products, which can be yet another reminder for someone that a biological thing about their body is super culturally attached to traditional norms and expectations of "femininity."[12]

For people taking testosterone, periods can at first become lighter and/or shorter and start to arrive later. Some people will have heavier or longer periods at first. Then, for the majority of people, periods stop altogether within six months and for almost everyone within a year.[13,14] For people who take testosterone over a longer period of time, their ovaries may become less capable of releasing eggs.[13]

The follicular phase is during your period and the first week or so after your period is over when your body gets ready to release another egg. The name *follicular* refers to the follicles in your ovaries that form and release eggs every cycle (more on this in Chapter 6).[9] It's a great phase. Estrogen levels shoot up before ovulation.[2,9] Evidence suggests that this can make us less reactive to stress, more empathetic, more interested in social interaction, and hornier.[3,4,15] One 2018 study even suggests that people tend to have higher levels of antibodies during this phase, which strengthens your immune system.[16]

Ovulation is when the egg leaves its follicle, leaves the ovary, floats out into the abyss of your abdominal cavity, and then gets swooshed into the opening of the uterine tube by the tube's long, fingery things.[17] Some people feel a little twinge of pain on one side of their lower abdomen during ovulation. That is called *mittelschmerz*, which sounds like a kind of poetic cross-sensory onomatopoeia but actually comes from "middle pain" in German.[18,19] (Again, more on ovulation in Chapter 6.)

The luteal phase is when estrogen levels take a steep dive and progesterone begins to rise. Progesterone does its work of trying to get your body ready to conceive; it makes the inside of your uterus nice and cushy, and if an egg does get fertilized, progesterone keeps the egg comfortable and safe by keeping the endometrium thick.[18]

According to the findings of the 2018 study I mentioned previously, on the immune system and the menstrual cycle, progesterone turns your immune system down a notch during ovulation and keeps it down during the luteal phase, probably to stop immune cells from attacking a fertilized egg.[16] Interestingly, many studies have shown that symptoms of autoimmune disorders, like rheumatoid arthritis, can lessen during this phase. Other symptoms caused by non-autoimmune problems, like irritable bowel syndrome and diabetes, can worsen.[20]

If the egg is not fertilized by a sperm, it either disintegrates or gets flushed out of your vagina with discharge (depending on who you ask), progesterone levels fall, and your body gets ready to menstruate.[9,15] The luteal phase is also associated with premenstrual syndrome (PMS).

Premenstrual Syndrome (PMS): Is It a Thing? Goddamnit.

One day, my friend (and book agent) Elianna Kan told me that her mom, who grew up in the Soviet Union, basically thought that PMS was a hilarious, made-up thing for weak Americans who didn't have any better problems to keep busy with. She'd never heard of it in the Soviet Union and never experienced it. So I called her mom and she confirmed. No word for it, no concept for it, and no experience of it. Ever.* Or so she said. OK, weird. Also, exciting. I've always loved examples of how our words and narratives shape our reality and experiences. But this one turned out to be way more dramatic than I expected.

The dominant narrative about PMS is basically that, aside from the physical symptoms about which there is much more evidence, it makes you feel some combination of shitty, angry, irritable, and sad. But, actually, there's shockingly little evidence to back that up. Here, we're going to review what evidence there is(n't). The goal in doing that is not to prove that PMS is made up and does not exist.

I have terrible PMS, so I believe it exists. I am a firm believer in it and its power to make me a sad and cranky-ass bitch. There have been many a morning when I've woken up with my period, remembered the meltdown I had the day before, and felt acutely embarrassed. Even if I didn't believe in it, saying PMS doesn't exist when so many people say they experience it would be a form of gaslighting at worst and, at best, would be just not listening to people when they say what they know about their bodies, which is Bad.

But the evidence for PMS still merits exploration because there's a lot that doesn't add up. And what we think we know to be "true" informs our narratives about PMS. And our narratives about PMS inform our experiences of our bodies. And then those very real experiences reinforce narratives.

Many studies show that if you have to put your gender on a math test, and you identify as a girl/woman, and you write that on the test, you will do worse on that test, presumably because you have been subtly reminded of the stereotype that girls are worse at math than boys.[21,22,23] This is called *stereotype threat*, and it's been demonstrated with many different groups and different stereotypes. It's one of my favorite examples of how narratives—our stories and preconceived notions about things—influence our experiences in ways that turn around and make those narratives realer and truer. (Of course, the ultimate example of this is gender itself.)

So while it's important to listen to and honor people's experiences, it's also important to question what influences those experiences in the first place.

A History of PMS Research

Dr. Katharina Dalton is credited with establishing the concept of PMS in a very small-scale study she published in 1953 with Dr. Raymond Green. Before this study, PMS was called *premenstrual tension* and was thought of as a psychiatric disorder and described similarly to hysteria (i.e., with abundantly apparent contempt for people with pussies). Dalton cites, for example, the first description she could find about PMS as "a condition of indescribable tension and a desire to find relief by foolish actions difficult to restrain."[24]

In her study, Dalton drew data from emergency rooms and police reports—situations in which people were already having very negative experiences—and also counted any negative behavioral occurrences within two weeks before and one week after menstruation, which . . . *counts on fingers* is the whole month.[24] So it's kind of absurd that she took all those observations down and attributed anything bad to a "premenstrual" state.

She actually acknowledged this in the study herself: "We have preferred to use the term 'premenstrual syndrome,' but as our investigation has progressed it has become clear that this term also is unsatisfactory. Though the syndrome most commonly occurs in the premenstrual phase, similar symptoms occasionally occur at the time of ovulation, in the early part of the menstrual phase, and even, rarely, in the first day or two after the flow has ceased. . . . We [have] decided to retain the term 'premenstrual syndrome' in the full realization of its imperfection."[24] So she was saying, *We're looking at these negative symptoms happening all through the cycle, but we're still going to call it PMS.* That kind of breaks my brain. But OK.

Another problem with Dalton's study design was that she excluded data that did not fit her narrative of the existence of PMS. She wanted to narrow her subjects down to people who had experienced negative symptoms for three consecutive cycles and during the same phase of the cycle. So she excluded people who had negative symptoms but who had not experienced them in three consecutive cycles, or whose symptoms were not limited to a certain phase of their cycle.[24] So she only studied people who exhibited the thing that she was trying to show existed. That, my friend, is called *cherry-picking*. And it's a Bad way to do Science.

Another problem with the 1953 study is that Dalton told the subjects that she was studying their negative menstrual symptoms, which . . . well . . . if you were to be a test subject and they told you they were studying how much your palms sweat, wouldn't you be hyperaware of the sweat on your palms? This is called *priming* and it can bias the results of a study.

It wasn't just Dalton's study that had these problems. The way PMS symptoms were measured was, historically, a mess. Every researcher was using a different way to define and rate symptoms, so their results could not be compared. In 1968, to fix this problem, Rudolf Moos created an instrument for measuring PMS symptoms, called the Menstrual Distress Questionnaire (MDQ).[25]

The MDQ went on to become the most used way to study PMS symptoms for almost three decades. And that was Bad because the MDQ turned out to be a pretty shitty instrument. It asked people to choose from among 42 negative symptoms and only five possible positive symptoms that they could use to describe their experiences. Strange that studies kept finding that people had negative experiences, huh? Also, those 42 negative symptoms were not based on prior studies that had firmly established them as tied to the menstrual cycle, so the MDQ's very definition of the thing it was trying to measure was wrong. This did not go unnoticed; the MDQ was criticized for decades. It was not the only instrument developed for measuring PMS symptoms, but a bunch of the other ones sucked too, for similar reasons.[25]

Then came along Dr. Jessica Motherwell McFarlane and Dr. Tannis Mac-Beth Williams. They considered the design flaws in the MDQ, in Dalton's study, and in others that had similar problems, and they conducted experiments that tried to account for those flaws with new study designs. In their 1988 and 1994 studies, for example, they did not prime their subjects to think about menstruation symptoms. They even included men in the study so that their subjects wouldn't think it was about menstruation. They asked people to record how they felt—both positive and negative moods—every day and to remember how they felt, looking back over periods of time.[26,27]

Granted that these weren't huge-scale studies, they found almost no evidence at all for PMS. When looking at the day-to-day data people recorded, both "women's" *and* "men's" moods fluctuated more over the days of the week than "women's" moods fluctuated over the course of the menstrual cycle. "Women's" moods were no less stable than "men's." And it was more common for people to report feeling down during their period than during the week before. When people with pussies were asked to remember their moods, they reported feeling bad during their luteal phase (PMS time), even if at the time, they had recorded that they felt fine.[26,27] This is probably because when they looked back, they superimposed their narrative of PMS over their actual experience of it.

The 2003 study "Constructions of Femininity and Experiences of Menstrual Distress" by Dr. Lisa Cosgrove and Dr. Bethany Riddle looked at typical ideas of "femininity" and PMS symptoms. They found that the more stereotypically feminine someone was or wanted to be, the worse their reported PMS symptoms. The authors hypothesized that since The Patriarchy's idea of femininity requires people to avoid expressing any negative emotions, PMS served as a way that people who aspire to be "feminine" could express bad feelings without making themselves seem less "feminine."[28]

In 2012, a group of researchers designed a study of other studies that built on McFarlane and Williams's work. They sought out as many other studies about PMS as they could find that met a few important criteria that accounted for design flaws in how PMS had previously been studied. For example, a study had to look at people's symptoms every day over time, its subjects couldn't be already seeking treatment for a problem, and it had to look at people across their whole cycle and not just during the luteal phase (like many other studies did, which kind of meant the luteal-phase results couldn't be compared to anything and were therefore sorta meaningless). In the end, they compiled and analyzed 47 studies.[29]

Their results? Not looking good for PMS. "Clear evidence for a specific premenstrual phase related mood occurring in the general population is lacking." Of the studies they looked at, 18 found no association between mood and menstrual-cycle phase. The same number of studies found an association between negative mood and the premenstrual (luteal) phase, but with negative symptoms also happening during another phase. Only seven studies found an association of negative mood with the premenstrual phase. As the researchers noted, "This puzzlingly widespread belief needs challenging, as it perpetuates negative concepts linking female reproduction with negative emotionality."[29]

Indeed it does. The PMS narrative reinforces one of The Patriarchy's oldest, dearest narratives: that people with pussies are hysterical—that they are "pathologically emotional, and thus have a reduced capacity for reason, due to their reproductive biology,"[30] as Sally King puts it in "Premenstrual Syndrome (PMS) and the Myth of the Irrational Female."

And that narrative has concrete political consequences. In "Menstrual Taboos: Moving Beyond the Curse," Dr. Alma Gottlieb writes that the dismissive neologism *she's PMS-ing* "typically indexes just one symptom: the supposed tendency for a menstruating woman to lose control of her emotions in general, and to express annoyance, critique, or anger in particular." Gottlieb notes that people invoke this trope "to explain why they oppose women's holding top political positions, which they claim would imperil citizens, due to unpredictable decisions."[31]

We Do Know That Hormones Influence Our Moods

Still, none of this is to say that the negative mood elements of PMS don't exist at all. There is plenty of evidence that changing hormones can change our moods.[2,4,15,32] (See Chapter 20 for more on how.) One 2018 review of studies found that there is substantial evidence that during the follicular phase, we are better able to recognize the emotions of others and that when we have more progesterone, like during the luteal phase when PMS happens, we are less good at recognizing the emotions of others and we are more prone to think others are feeling negatively.[32] There is also evidence that during the luteal phase, we are more reactive, generally, to negative feelings inside. As I mentioned earlier, there's a lot of evidence that one of estrogen's jobs is to help you deal with stress.[4] So during the end of the luteal phase, during menstruation, and for a little while afterward, when we have less estrogen, it makes sense that we could respond more intensely to stress.

Real changes in our hormone levels likely combine with narratives about PMS to create our experiences.

After calling Elianna's mom, I talked to another friend's mother who also grew up in the Soviet Union. She confirmed to me as well: No word for it. No concept for it. But she *had* experienced it. She remembered experiencing it, specifically in medical school when she had to take her oral exams. She had learned about the hormonal changes of the menstrual cycle, so even if she didn't have a word for PMS, she at least had an idea that it could exist. She remembered being upset when her oral exams fell on the week before her period because she knew she often felt tired and less sharp during those premenstrual weeks. But also, she noted to me that she couldn't remember having noticed the same phenomenon during the summers when she wasn't in school. She summed it up: "I think it's overblown in the US, and was not talked about enough in the Soviet Union."*

Why is it overblown in the US? It couldn't be just because we have a word and concept for it. We have words and concepts for lots of things we don't overdo, and even for lots of things we don't do enough, like "justice," for example. I think it's overblown in the US because we tend to pathologize and medicalize people with pussies so that The Patriarchy can keep saying people with pussies are sick and defective, and so that Capitalism can make money off selling "cures."

And there's no better story about the pathologization of PMS than the story of PMDD.

Premenstrual Dysphoric Disorder (PMDD): A Real Thing. But Also, Wow, Drug Money.

Premenstrual dysphoric disorder (PMDD) is when your PMS is really, really, really bad, both emotionally and physically. Like, so bad that it's messing up your life. About 2–8% of people who menstruate have it.[33,34] Ashley Biggs wrote, from personal experience, in the "PMDD" article for Pussypedia.net:

For many, thoughts of the possibility of having PMDD arises when they notice extreme PMS symptoms and sometimes unbearable feelings of anger or irritability that aren't always there. For those affected, PMDD can feel like multiple personalities, or like living with an inner monster and waiting for it to strike every month. Once menstruation starts, the symptoms begin to subside quickly, giving a brief respite. Unfortunately this period of relief can be clouded by the thought of knowing the difficult time will return.[35]

The exact causes of PMDD are not known for sure, but there was recently a breakthrough on that front. A 2017 study found a specific set of genes that are messed up in people who have PMDD. These genes determine how people's cells respond to estrogen and progesterone, which explains why the changes in those hormone levels during the luteal phase make people with PMDD feel dramatically shittier during their luteal phase.[36] This study also goes a long way in suggesting that PMDD is a very real Thing.

Still, PMDD is a case study in the influence of the pharmaceutical industry on health care and the way it pathologizes normal human experiences to sell drugs. The pharmaceutical industry doesn't just sell drugs—it sells diseases.[37] And PMDD is a pharmaceutical company's wet dream: a worse version of something that tons of people already experience, with pretty subjective diagnostic criteria, that can be treated with prescription drugs.

The company Eli Lilly, which made Sarafem (repackaged pink-and-purple Prozac marketed for PMDD), had to take a commercial off the air in 2001 after the FDA recognized that the company was blurring the line between PMS and PMDD.[38] When a more pharmaceutical-sympathetic head of the FDA was installed by the Bush administration, more pathologizing commercials came out. One Paxil (also an antidepressant) commercial went: "I always thought it was just PMS. Now I know otherwise. Grouchy? Emotional? Irritable? It may be PMDD."[37] This is the equivalent to a commercial saying, *I always thought it was just normal to be sleepy at night. Tired at the end of your day? Tend to pass out during boring movies after you've had a beer or two? It may be narcolepsy.*

PMDD became an official disorder in 2013, when it was included by the American Psychiatric Association in its *Diagnostic and Statistical Manual of Mental Disorders, Fifth Edition* (a.k.a. the *DSM-5*), the book that is used by psychiatrists to diagnose mental disorders. A panel of experts decides what gets into the *DSM*. More than half of the experts decided that what went into the *DSM-IV*, and 100% of the experts on the panel for mood disorders had ties to the pharmaceutical industry.[39] That caused a controversy, so the American Psychiatric Association introduced transparency protocols for reporting potential conflicts of interest among *DSM-5* panel members.[40] But transparency, not fewer conflicts of interest, was apparently their endgame because for the *DSM-5* panel, the percentage of experts with financial pharmaceutical ties went up to 70%.[40] This is a problem. As the authors of one study put it, "Pharmaceutical companies provide substantial funding for conventions, journals, and research related to what is included in the DSM, because what is considered diagnosable directly impacts the sale of their drugs."[39]

Having conflicts of interest really is just the norm in a lot of medical research. A common refrain is that pharmaceutical money is the only source of funding for large-scale studies.[41] But even if that's true, it is still probably causing bias in research. One 2005 study that looked at 397 clinical-psychiatry drug trials found that, even among double-blind, placebo-controlled studies (i.e., super rigorous and more likely to be accurate), pharmaceutical-industry-funded studies were 4.9 times as likely to report positive results.[42] A 2004 study looked at all the studies published in 2001 in the *New England Journal of Medicine* and in *JAMA*—two very prestigious medical journals—and found that, among those studies, researchers who had conflicts of interest were 10 to 20 times less likely to present negative findings, especially in drug studies.[43]

I found one hilarious study in which only 7% of researchers believed that their conflicts of interest influenced their own recommendations about prescribing medications, but 19% thought that conflicts of interest influenced their colleagues' recommendations.[44] So basically, the researchers interviewed thought that getting money from pharmaceutical companies wouldn't change *their* behavior but that it *would* change their colleagues'.

Pharmaceutical companies also pay doctors to prescribe name-brand drugs. In 2016 and 2019, ProPublica investigations found that the more money doctors receive from a company, the more name-brand drugs they tend to prescribe in general, and that doctors will prescribe more of a drug if they receive money from the pharmaceutical company tied to it.[45,46] This makes me worry that if a doctor is getting money from any of the companies that prescribe drugs to treat PMDD, and I go see that doctor and say that my PMS has been really bad, they might be extra likely to diagnose me with PMDD and prescribe me drugs that I would then buy and take even though I might not need them.

One of the most prominent PMDD researchers is Dr. Cynthia Neill Epperson. It's hard to find recent research on PMDD that doesn't have her name on it or cite her work. As of 2020, she had received research funding from and consulted for Shire Pharmaceuticals and Sage Therapeutics (biopharmaceutical companies), had been a consultant for Forest Laboratories (a now-defunct pharmaceutical company), and had reported personal and/or family investments in Pfizer, Bristol Myers Squibb, Johnson & Johnson, Merck, Abbott, and AbbVie (all pharmaceutical companies).[47,48] Now, that doesn't mean she's a dishonest researcher or even that her work is biased. But this whole system in which researchers are this closely tied to pharmaceutical companies is definitely not ideal.

Sorry

I'm not going to wrap this up neatly for you. Or tell you how to feel or think. The point is that we *don't* have answers. PMS isn't not "real," but it isn't exactly "real" either. PMDD isn't a conspiracy, but that doesn't mean there's not a lot to be suspicious about. The point is that when we try to make up answers because we feel uncomfortable without them, we create narratives that only lead us away from the truth. Uncertainty is annoying, but it's better than oversimplification. We just have to sit in the messiness and let the messiness sit in us. Everything together. I think that's how you get closest to knowing.

*A third friend's mom who also grew up in the Soviet Union *did* know a word for PMS and absolutely *did* know it was a concept and couldn't imagine why anyone else wouldn't have known that. I could not get to the bottom of this discrepancy.

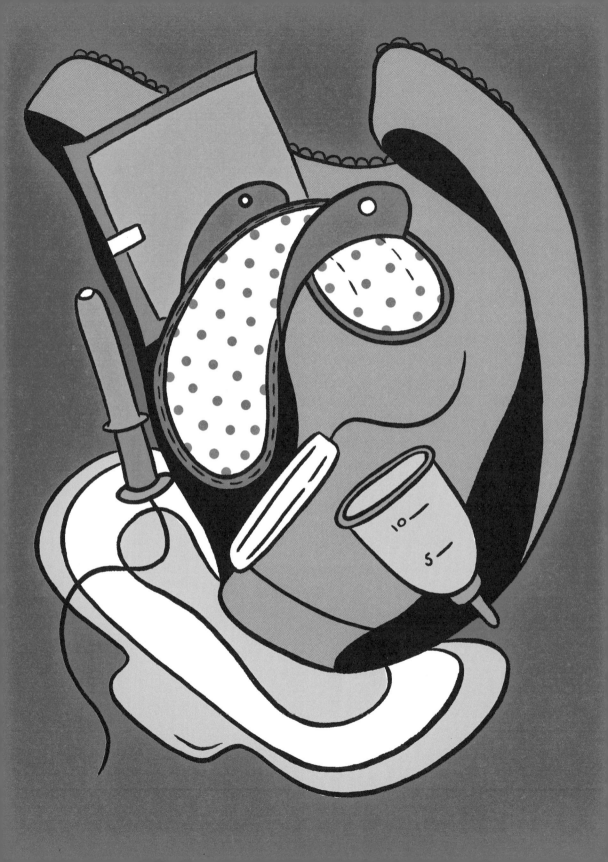

12
Period Products and the Earth

MENSTRUAL PRODUCTS ARE A FEMINISM ISSUE AND THEY ARE ALSO AN ENVIRON-mentalism issue, and guess what? Environmentalism is also a racism issue and a feminism issue and feminism and racism are also environmentalism issues. Everything is everything! (And I'm not even stoned!)

Here's how it goes: People with pussies bear the brunt of climate change more than cis men, since we are generally poorer. (One World Bank study found that, among people ages 25–34 worldwide, 122 "women" live in poor households for every 100 "men" who do.)[1] The poorer you are, the more fucked you are when it comes to things like hurricanes, droughts, or floods.[2,3] And even more if you're not white. For example, Black people in the US are much more likely than white people to live in polluted areas and, consequently, have a much higher rate of asthma.[4]

I saw climate change disproportionately burden people with pussies during some research I did about water in Mexico City for the *New York Times* in 2016. It is almost always the moms and the daughters who are charged with pro-curing water for their families/households, which can easily take up an entire day of the week. The less water there is, the more time-consuming it is to get, and the less time people with pussies have to do anything that might help them get ahead, increase their earning potential, or attend to their own health. It's

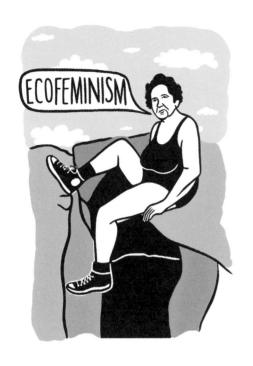

ECOFEMINISM

common globally for people with pussies to be the ones tasked with producing food, collecting water, and sourcing fuel for heat, which all become more difficult and time-consuming when the climate is increasingly extreme.[2,3] (Also, people with pussies, particularly those who menstruate, rely more on water for personal hygiene.)[5]

On top of that, because of sexism, people with pussies are excluded from the decision-making processes regarding climate-change-related public policies EVEN THOUGH they are potentially a huge resource for designing solutions, since they are so often the people who are interfacing most directly with the environment.[2,3]

People with pussies = huge untapped resource in helping to stop climate change.

See? Environmental destruction compounds sexism, and sexism compounds environmental destruction. It's a (melting) snowball effect. People have used the word *ecofeminism*, coined by Françoise d'Eaubonne (pictured above being a badass), as shorthand for a way of thinking about this connection since the 1970s.

A small, newish contingent of ecofeminism sees people with pussies as somehow inherently more connected to the earth because . . . of their menstrual cycles? Because they give birth? I'm not exactly sure, but I (and many other people who have written about it) find that kind of rhetoric, at best, to be magic-laden and woo-woo and, at worst, to be gender essentialist (i.e., generalizing about "all 'men'" and "all 'women'" inherently being one way or another). But this line of thinking represents only a small contingent of ecofeminist thinkers.

Speaking of people I disagree with, it comes as no surprise that people who are against environmentalism are also people who tend toward misogyny. As Martin Gelin reported in a 2019 article for the *New Republic*, "Male reactionaries motivated by right-wing nationalism, anti-feminism, and climate denialism increasingly overlap, the three reactions feeding off of one another."[6]

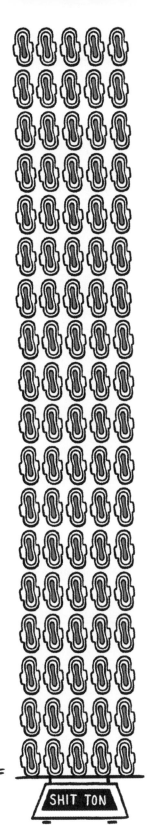

SHIT TON

But, Anyway, Menstrual Products

It's been estimated that the "average woman" will dispose of "250–300 pounds of pads, plugs, and applicators" in a lifetime.[7] This fact has been repeated all over the internet, but its origins are dubious. As Alejandra Borunda wrote for *National Geographic* in 2019, "Getting a handle on how much plastic waste comes from menstrual products is tough, in part because it's labeled as medical waste and does not need to be tracked, and in part because so little research has even looked at the scope of the problem."[8]

Still, we can make our own estimate. Let's make it a conservative one. Say each menstruator has a five-day period and uses three tampons and two pads per day. And let's take the average cycle length of 28 days to calculate 13 periods in a 365-day year. That would mean that, in a year, a given menstruating person would use about 325 individual products. According to the consumer data company Statista, in 2019 the "female" population of the United States between the ages of 15 and 49 was 74.63 million.[9] (People younger and older menstruate too, but we're guessing low here! Also, not all "females" in this age range menstruate, but we're going to pretend they do for a second.) So we can estimate that, every year in the United States, over 24.5 billion (325 products × 74+ million menstruators) menstrual products are used and thrown away. That's a fucking lot of garbage, and the real amount is likely much higher than this estimate.

Some of what goes into these products and then into landfills and the ocean is cotton, but a bunch

121

of it is plastic. Plastic is bad for basically everything and there is already way too much of it everywhere. Plastic tampon applicators (not really a thing outside of the US, by the way),[10,11] have earned the nickname "Jersey Beach whistles" because they wash up so often on the beaches in New Jersey, where children occasionally pick them up, mistaking them for toys.[12] And it's not even the over-whelming garbage factor that's the biggest problem with plastic.

One group of researchers at the Royal Institute of Technology in Stockholm in 2006 conducted a "cradle-to-grave assessment" of tampons and pads. They looked at raw material extraction, transportation, production, use, waste stages of these products, human health, ecosystem quality, and resource use, and they found that the biggest environmental impact that menstrual pads have is, sur-prisingly, in their production process, not in their long afterlives.[13] Pads have a type of plastic called low-density polyethylene in them. It's made with fossil fuel and takes a ton of energy to create. (The study looked at tampons too, but only those without plastic applicators, so there was no analysis of how much of an impact the production of US-style plastic-applicator tampons has. But it's prob-ably a lot.)

Sorry I'm a Bad Period Person

Before I launch into how we should all use alternative and sustainable op-tions, I must first admit that I, myself, do not. A few years ago, my best friend taught me the joys of ginormous pads and I never went back. Ya stick 'em in and *bam*—no worrying about leaking at all. I hate buying new clothes, so I really hate staining my pants. (Try soaking them in hydrogen peroxide, then rinsing in cold water if and when you do, though!) And I'm an anxious person, so with any other period gear I'm trying to surreptitiously touch or look at my crotch every five minutes to see if I've leaked. And my heart sinks every time I'm about to get up from sitting down on anything—like, *OK, here goes nothing, I've definitely bled all over this surface.*

I love giant-ass plastic, polluting diaper pads so much for the peace of mind they give me.

Pads are just easy, which is why I suspect most US consumers don't want to stop using most plastic products in general. As Anna Davidson aptly wrote in her 2012 article "Narratives of Menstrual Product Consumption," "It is clear that our current consumptive lifestyles need to change, and for the most part, it is clear what concrete actions need to be taken. The most problematic to shift appear to be the individual and societal narratives we tell ourselves to justify behaviors and prioritization we make."[14]

She's right. I'm a '90s suburban kid. Consumerism was the closest thing to a religion that I had growing up. (I mean, I'm a Jew, but as a kid, I definitely worshipped Abercrombie & Fitch more than I worshipped God.) This is probably why I feel so comfortable prioritizing my comfort over my health and my future children's future.

WTH Is in These Products?

Another reason I love pads: organic tampons are generally expensive and regular tampons freak me out because we don't really know what's in them. I figure I get enough toxins just breathing in the Mexico City air every day and don't need to also be sticking Mystery Flavor Dum Dums up my hoo-ha. Since the FDA considers tampons, pads, and menstrual cups to be "medical devices," manufacturers are not required to disclose product components, materials, and ingredients.[15]

Women's Voices for the Earth is a nonprofit that, for almost three decades, has worked to raise awareness and accountability around toxic chemicals, mostly in products that go in and around pussies. The organization did a round of independent testing of tampons in 2018 and found some nasty shit in them. They tested organic, mainstream, and dollar-store brands and found that all the tampons that contained rayon, which is most of them besides the 100% cotton varieties, also contained carbon disulfide, which is a reproductive toxin (a chemical that can hurt fertility/offspring). Some of the tampons tested contained reproductive toxins *and* carcinogens like toluene, xylene, and methylene chloride.[15] These tests were not published in a peer-reviewed journal, which is the gold-standard in Science as far as what information we can trust, but they are for sure enough to give me the heebie-jeebies.

Not that pads don't have their own mystery toxins. In 2014, Women's Voices for the Earth tested Always-brand scented and unscented pads and found that both had carcinogens and reproductive and developmental toxins that were (obviously) not on any public list of ingredients.[16] But the vagina is a mucus membrane that is very good at bringing chemicals into your bloodstream so—with no science to back me up—I make the loose, personal calculation that it's better to have toxins on my vulva than inside my vagina.

An important counterpoint to mention is that "toxins" are only "toxic" in certain amounts. There was a huge hoopla about dioxins in menstrual products a few years ago, but one study found that exposure to dioxins from tampons was approximately 13,000–240,000 times less than exposure from food.[17] Companies that make menstrual products say that the toxin levels in their products are below safe exposure limits (but, again, this is not peer-reviewed information).[18] Exposure limits are created by government agencies and may be totally legitimate, but it would still be awesome if these chemicals just weren't in these products at all.

So, yeah, there's reason not to feel totally safe about using pads and tampons, but there's not enough evidence to justify panic. Women's Voices for the Earth even says that their testing results "confirm neither a known level of danger, nor do they establish a threshold of safety for these exposures."[19] We don't know how safe or dangerous these products are. The only thing that's clear to me is that we should keep demanding information on labels and peer-reviewed and public testing and results.

And while we're talking about toxic things in tampons, I'd like to clarify that toxic shock syndrome, or TSS, is unrelated. It is a bacterial infection—not from chemicals. You can get it from leaving a tampon in too long, but it's very rare. There used to be some kinds of tampons more associated with causing TSS, but they are no longer on the market. To avoid TSS, change your tampon at least every four to eight hours.[20]

Sustainable / Less Toxic Options (Don't Be Like Me):
- Menstrual Cups: These look like precious little vagina chalices—like a wineglass without the foot. You fold its flexible rim and put it into your vagina and let it unfold, where it creates a kind of seal. You leave it there for up to 12 hours, then empty your chunky homemade cabernet into the toilet. Cups come in a variety of materials, but try to get one that's high-quality silicone. The better the quality, the more sanitary (see Chapter 16 on why different materials are more and less sanitary) and

the more years you can use it. They need to be cleaned between uses and boiled for 20 minutes before and after each cycle. Lots of people are very enthusiastic about cups, though some say they don't like the way they feel.

I bought a cup to try for the purpose of writing this and at first I didn't like it because it was annoying to get in and leaked while I was sleeping. I didn't think I would keep using it. But then something happened: When my next cycle started, the cup was already in my house. So I used it. And the same thing the next month and on and on. I still don't *love* it, but it can save me a trip to the store. Getting it in right got easier, but I still find it annoying how much blood I get all over my hands putting it in and taking it out. Not that it's gross—just kind of a mess. I'm not ready to give up my beloved giant diaper pads entirely. I mean, I don't buy fast fashion and I have a farm share and a rescue dog, OK?! Sue me.

Still, I have to say, an overwhelming majority of my friends at this point use menstrual cups and love them. Tarah Knaresboro, my dear friend and the fact-checker for this book, is very enthusiastic about the menstrual cup for the following reasons:

- The connection to my body of being able to check how much blood is in there and what it looks like is cooler to me (and more informative about volume) with a cup than with a pad/tampon.
- Honestly, they're the best for exercise, especially contact sports. If you have the right fit, you can move your legs around everywhere, and it stays right there.
- It's the most I've felt like I'm not even aware of my period, just grooving around 'til I empty it. Twelve hours is a long time!
- I think it's awesome when my hands are bloody. I feel cool and subversive.
- I love not having to buy as many products. It saves me money but it also saves me from having to remember to go out and buy stuff because it's just one thing that's already there.
- Reusable Pads: These are pads that you can wash and reuse. I bought and tried these and, well, they were OK. I didn't get the fancy kinds with absorption technology. Still, even with plain old cotton, it's useful for when

you have a lighter flow or as a backup for a tampon or menstrual cup. They're easy to wash at home in the shower . . . but I also wondered what would happen if I was out and wanted to change one. (You'd have to carry the bloody one around with you in a plastic bag?).

- Period Undies: These are underwear that can absorb your period flow. They've gotten very popular in the last few years. I've never used a pair because I definitely want the option of taking the thing that is holding my period blood in my undies *out* of my undies easily and often. So I don't really understand the concept. I've never used them and frankly was unwilling to buy them even for this chapter because I just can't make the idea seem at all appealing to myself. That said, multiple friends who use them are very enthusiastic about them and say they don't stink, don't feel bulky, and don't feel too moist. A few said they don't use it as a replacement for a tampon or a cup but rather as a backup to have peace of mind about leaking. Others said it was enough to contain their flow on its own. Some find the rinsing and washing routine easy and others find it impractical.

  In 2020, Sierra Club magazine journalist Jessian Choy commissioned independent testing of a few brands of period underwear. The results showed that Thinx-brand (but not Lunapads-brand, which is now called Aisle) underwear contained per- and polyfluoroalkyl substances (PFAS), particularly in the crotch area.[21] (PFAS has been called a reproductive toxin, but a literature review on studies that looked at PFAS and reproductive health did not find super-consistent results.)[22] The company responded by basically saying, *Well,* our *tests say there aren't any.*[23] They do have third-party testing results published on their site that say as much.[24] Again, neither sets of tests were peer-reviewed. ¯_(ツ)_/¯

- Free Bleeding: Free bleeding is a movement to just bleed without trying to stop the blood. To me, it seems more like a political statement than a practical solution. I think it's cool because it's a fun way to combat menstrual stigma—I love anything that freaks people out about things they shouldn't be freaked out about in the first place (hence the title of this book)—but I don't think it's cool to get your blood on public surfaces because that's not nice to others. It's one thing for people to have to look at your blood (cool) and another for them to have to touch it (not safe).

Not-Great Options

- Sea Sponges: Sea sponges are really cute and would be such an awesome natural alternative if they weren't prone to harboring bacteria.[25] They are considered by the FDA to be "significant risk devices."[26]
- Homemade Reusable Tampons: People are crocheting and sewing tampons and honestly it's cute—like they look like tampon puppets that should be characters in a Christmas claymation special—but there's no way to know what they're really made of or if they're sanitary or safe.

Individual Consumer Choices Are Not the Solution to Climate Change

Yes, we should try to take care of the earth in order to try to take care of one another. Feminism should include environmental consciousness.

That said, even if every menstruator on the planet started exclusively using sustainable menstrual products, we'd still have a long way to go to stop climate change. And stressing personal decisions as the answer to a global problem can obfuscate other important culprits. In 1953, the American Can Company, Coca-Cola, the Dixie Cup company, and others formed a plan called Keep America Beautiful, which was an anti-litter propaganda campaign specifically designed to shift national focus from their massive-scale polluting to individual "litterbugs."[27] In 2017, the Climate Accountability Institute's report *Carbon Majors* found that just 100 mega-polluting companies are responsible for 70% of the world's carbon emissions.[28] So yes, we should hold ourselves accountable as consumers, but we shouldn't lose sight of the big-polluter picture.

Also, in promoting the use of sustainable products, we should remember that they're not for everyone, so we don't end up shaming people who can't use them. These products are more expensive and not readily available everywhere. A menstrual cup might help you save money over time, but its up-front cost can be prohibitive to a lot of people. Also, for people with disabilities, these products are sometimes not viable options. As Alice Wong, activist and founder of the Disability Visibility Project, told A. K. Whitney in the 2019 *Dame* article "Is the 'Green' Menstrual Movement Ableist?":

> Each person knows what they need and what works for them and there has to be less shaming of people who may not follow the shift toward reusable items for legitimate reasons. It only drives people further away from overall engagement with environmentalism and sustainability.[29]

RESOURCES

- flexfits.com sells menstrual cups that are designed with input from people with disabilities.

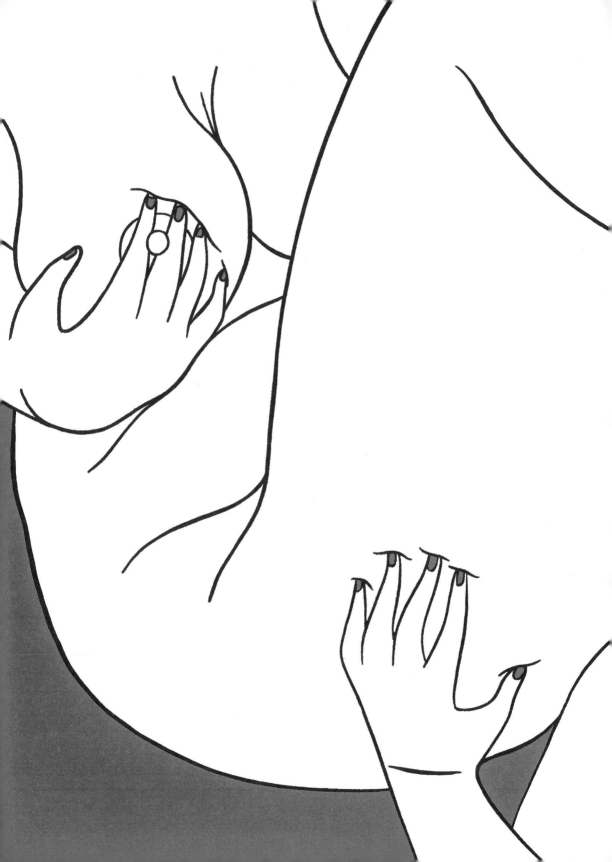

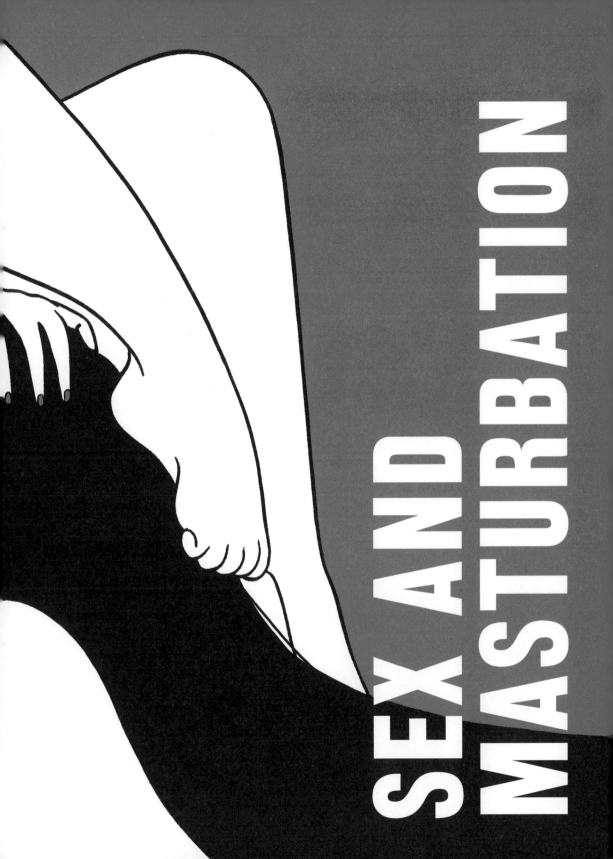

SEX AND MASTURBATION

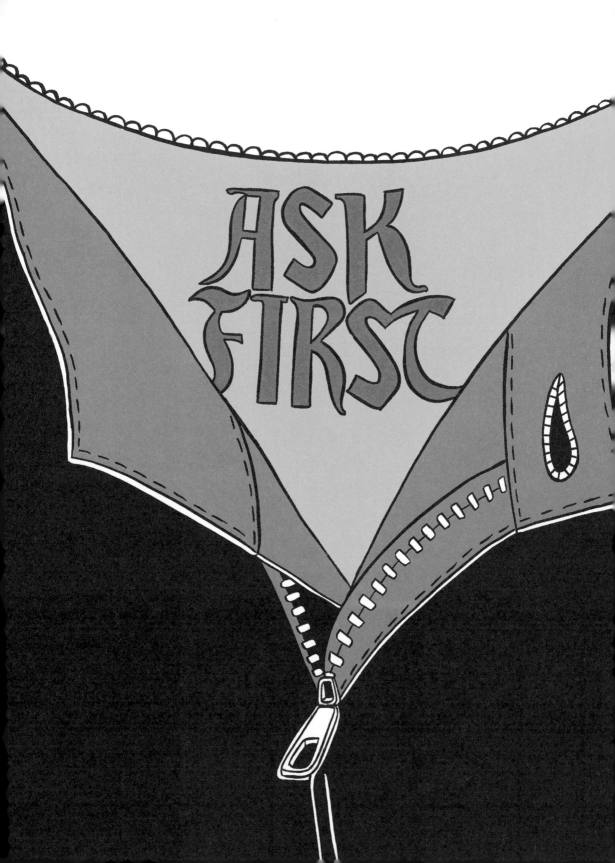

13
Consent

What Is Consent?

I wish I could give you a cute, brief definition of consent to kick us off here but I can't. If you ask the law, you'll get a different answer from each state. Ask a range of feminists and you'll get a range of answers. The dictionary defines general "consent" as "permission," but we're talking about it in the specific context of sexual acts because, while they hold potential for great joy and awesomeness, they also hold potential for great *ugh* and awfulness. Consent is evolving all the time as many people with different beliefs try to get as close as they can to a definition of sexual consent that maximizes awesomeness and minimizes *ugh*.

Here's my personal definition, though: nobody is allowed to do anything to you that you don't want them to do and you are not allowed to do anything to anyone else that they don't want you to do and, because it's hard to know what people want, everyone should ask each other and talk to each other a lot about what they want and don't want and then everybody should respect each other's wishes.

When There's No Consent

Trigger warning: sexual assault. If you don't want to read an account of sexual assault, skip the first paragraph below. The rest of this chapter mentions assault but does not describe it.

Here's how my rape went. I had just broken up and was sad. I texted a guy I worked with who I had a crush on and said, "I just broke up, I'm sad, take me out." I was 22. He was in his late 30s. When we met up at a subway stop in my neighborhood, he suggested we pick up beer instead of going out. Back at my apartment, he walked straight into my room, put the six-pack of Tecate down on the windowsill, and started kissing me aggressively. Then he pushed me down on the bed and started to take off my pants. I definitely said, "Wait, hold on, stop." In a quick move, he pulled his dick out and stuck it in me with no condom and no warning. I said, "No," and then I froze. I did not fight him or scream or, as far as I remember, say anything else until he was done. I watched it happen from above. Afterward, he casually cracked a beer and wanted to hang out. I was coursing with adrenaline, rage, and disgust but pretended everything was normal. It was obvious that he saw nothing out of the ordinary about what had happened.

After a few weeks of him asking if I wanted to "hang out" again, I decided to confront him. I asked him to get a coffee with me after work, and I told him I had not wanted the sex he'd forced, that I had said *no* and *stop,* and that I considered it rape. I will never forget the look of horror in his eyes. He was a handsome douchebag who had probably spent his life getting whatever he wanted, but I don't think he was a terrible person. He burst out crying and sobbed for a while outside of a fancy Brooklyn café. And then, when he could finally muster words, he said, "But, Zoe, you are young, you don't know. *No* doesn't mean no in the bedroom. That's not how it works."

Why This Dude Seriously Thought That *No* Doesn't Mean No in the Bedroom

If The Patriarchy were your sex ed teacher, this is what day one of class would be:

Your pussy is gross, so you are gross and unlovable. If you want sex, you are even grosser and a slut. If you're a slut, you're worthless and unlovable. Sexual acts are bargaining chips with which to procure love and marriage. So play coy! Don't ever make a first move, and don't even accept a first move too readily or you will seem like a slut and will have nothing to bargain with. When you are engaging in sexual acts, your pleasure is irrelevant. In fact, your pleasure is slutty. Listen, ladies, prioritize the man's pleasure, make them feel amazing about themselves, and avoid any kind of conflict at all costs or else you're a bitch. If you don't like men, what the hell is wrong with you? And if you say you are one, you are mentally ill. If any of this upsets you, you're hysterical.

Unfortunately, The Patriarchy actually *is* everyone's sex ed teacher. People who have internalized this message *do* play coy, even when we do want sex, which can lead to saying *no* when we mean yes. I wasn't one of the women who had said *no* when they meant yes to the man who raped me. But I *had* said *no* when I meant yes to countless men before him. And that's *my* end of the deal. These learned behaviors reinforce the idea that no means "try again in three minutes," or that "*no* doesn't mean no in the bedroom."

That said, I want to make a few clarifications:

1. When I say, "my end of the deal," I mean in contributing to the reinforcement of rape *culture*, not in contributing to my own rape.
2. Nobody has an "end of the deal" in their own rape.
3. That doesn't mean people don't have agency in their sexual encounters.
4. Levels of agency often depend on privilege.
5. Nobody gets to say how much agency anybody else has.
6. Plenty of people rape knowing full well in the moment that the other person does not consent, and those people are entirely responsible for their actions.

The presumable fix is to #unsubscribe from The Patriarchy, unlearn Patriarchy sex ed, and start saying *yes* when we mean yes and *no* when we mean no. And *not right now but maybe later* when we mean "not right now but maybe later." But that's not an option for everyone, whether because of a lack of privilege and/or sexual agency or because of past traumas. Also, sometimes these learned behaviors are a protection mechanism against harm—physical, emotional, professional, social. It's impossible to know when saying no to sex is even safe because we can't know who is going to harm us for refusing them. I once lost a job for saying no to sex. Other people have gotten murdered for saying no to sex. And for those with past traumas, it can be hard to ever feel safe, even when we know we are.

And yet, far too often, the reasons people don't say yes and no are way, way, way more trivial than that. No more "not wanting to ruin the mood" by communicating that you don't want sex. You know what ruins the mood? Unwanted sex. Talking about consent and pleasure and boundaries does not somehow make sex less spontaneous and fun. Sex is not supposed to be like sex in the movies. (It's better than that!) Say what you like and don't like without fear of hurting the other person's feelings or seeming slutty or freaky. What should upset a sexual partner more than not psychically knowing what you like or don't like is knowing you're not actually having a good time.

Saying what you want and don't want during (and before and after!) sex, and asking the other person the same, is hard because it requires #unsubscribing from The Patriarchy. But if you're up for it, it's an opportunity to heal yourself and our gross rapey culture. It's a twofer, y'all!

Now, I'd like to add another clarification to the previous list:

7. A lot of people have more agency than they think they do. Awkwardness is not an actual barrier to great, communicative sex.

If you at all can, be brave and start to practice consent. If you can't do it for yourself, do it for the people who really, actually do not have the privilege, agency, or ability to say *no*. Privilege is a moral obligation to help those with less agency than you, which you can act on by normalizing sexual consent every time you practice it.

Yes, More Consent!

The basic model of consent was explained beautifully by some anonymous genius who went by Rockstar Dinosaur Pirate Princess when they released a video with Blue Seat Studios called "Tea Consent" on YouTube in 2015. It goes:

You're making [a potential sexual partner] a cup of tea. [If] you say, "Hey, would you like a cup of tea?" and they go, "OMG, fuck yes, I would fucking love a cup of tea," then you know they want a cup of tea. If . . . they're like, "Um, you know, I'm not really sure," then you can make them a cup of tea, or not, but be aware that they might not drink it. And if they don't drink it . . . don't make them drink it. Just because you made it does not mean you're entitled to watch them drink it. And if they say, "No, thank you," then don't make them tea. . . . They might say, "Yes, please, that's kind of you," and then when the tea arrives they actually don't want the tea. . . . They remain under no obligation to drink the tea. . . . It's OK for people to change their mind[s]. And if they're unconscious, don't make them tea.[1]

Informed consent goes a step further. It means that the person offering a cup of tea has to disclose anything relevant about the tea when offering it, like whether the tea has any infections or is married. (For more on disclosing infections in the tea, see Chapter 22.)

Enthusiastic consent was popularized by the book *Yes Means Yes!* by Jaclyn Friedman and Jessica Valenti. "Real consent requires us to really be present when we're having sex with someone," wrote Friedman in a 2018 article for Refinery29. "It requires us to see our sex partners . . . not simply as instrumental to our own pleasure but as co-equal collaborators, equally human and important, equally harmable, equally free and equally sovereign."[2]

This model shifts from "*no* means no" to "*yes* means yes." If the person you've offered tea *says* they want tea but *looks* horrified or is just silent while they're drinking it, that's not enthusiastic consent because the person is not enthusiastic about the activity you're sharing. Consent shouldn't be just an absence of a no at the beginning, but rather the presence of enthusiasm and explicit affirmation throughout. This model requires checking in with your partners and clear affirmation or denial with each new action—the kind of communication that Patriarchy Sex Ed makes very difficult. It can sound awkward, or like a lot of work. But is it really more work than the emotional labor of pretending to enjoy things you're actually not enjoying? And is awkwardness really a reason to risk hurting someone?

Enthusiastic consent gets called radical, which is kind of hilarious. Because if you look at my story, you have to consider that, *even if* the guy thought that I had wanted the sex based on my "Wait, hold on, stop," I then went utterly silent and he still kept fucking me. A lack of enthusiasm should be an enormous red flag. Who the hell wants to have sex with someone who does not want to have sex with them? Correct: a rapist.

The world of BDSM has provided some other amazing frameworks for sexual communication and consent, especially around risk management.

SSC: Safe, Sane, Consensual means that all actors are safe from real harm, are sane (this rejects the pathologizing of BDSMsters, which is common to outsiders' views on BDSM), and are not exploited—that all decisions are made together by all participants.[3] But the SSC model did not accommodate people who were looking to take more extreme risks, and so was birthed . . .

RACK: Risk-Aware Consensual Kink.[3] In this model, safety is replaced with risk awareness. In reality, there is risk of harm implied in all sex, not just in kinky sex, which is why people are starting to use the term *safer sex* rather than *safe sex*. RACK was invented by Gary Switch, who wrote, "Negotiation cannot be valid without foreknowledge of the possible risks involved in the activity being negotiated. 'Risk-aware' means that both parties to a negotiation have studied the proposed activities, are informed about the risks involved, and agree on how they intend to handle them. Hence 'risk-aware' instead of 'safe.'"[4]

The Yes/No/Maybe List is a tool for negotiating proposed activities. You go through the list together and both say yes, no, or maybe to each activity. There are lists on the internet; Autostraddle and Scarleteen both have great ones. Or make your own. This may not make sense for a onetime hookup, but even in that situation it can be adapted from an exhaustive list to a simple conversation.

The 4Cs: Consent, Communication, Caring, Caution has three tiers: 1) surface consent—*no* means no, *yes* means yes; 2) scene consent—agreement on a planned activity; and 3) deep consent—awareness that, in the moment, a person may not be in a mental state to give or revoke consent and that it therefore should be discussed not just before and during but after the fact too. Caring is about honoring the other person's unique desires and concerns as much as your own. Caution is about risk awareness in activities and around each person's identities and past experiences.[3] Communication is the tool for all this.

Whether or not you use these specific models, consent should be given every step of the way when new things are going to happen. If someone's worn you down by asking so many times, or by guilting you, that you finally say yes, that's coercion, not consent. That person is being an asshole and doesn't deserve your bomb-ass pussy. If they say, "But you're wet," stop, get this book out, and make them read the section in Chapter 3 about arousal nonconcordance.

Complicating Consent

In his 2019 book, *Screw Consent*, Joseph Fischel, associate professor of women's, gender, and sexuality studies at Yale University, acknowledges that consent is an absolutely necessary legal tool, but points to its inability to address why we have so much bad, unwanted, consensual sex.[5] If we're using a limited definition of consent as simple "permission," I agree.

Some critics say that consent models reinforce traditional gender roles, in which "the man" asks permission and "the woman" accepts or rejects. The RACK, 4Cs, and enthusiastic models of consent all address this (thank you, queer communities, for rethinking gender roles and making better consensual-sex models for everyone!), but I imagine that, in the real world, the dynamics of consent pretty often play out in a traditionally gendered way anyway—for sure in heterosexual contexts, but in queer contexts too.

Fischel's argument and the gender-role criticism both lead me to think that #unsubscribing from The Patriarchy should be part of the definition of consent, or at least a permanent fixture in the conversation about what makes for authentic, non-coerced consent. Until everyone has the option to #unsubscribe from The Patriarchy, though, it's on whoever has more power within The Patriarchy—namely, cis men who have sex with people with pussies—to take a proactive role in making sure that consent happens.

Fuck Yes, Fuck No, Fuck Me

I'm not going to prescribe you cute, sexy ways to ask permission or to say yes or no. There are lists on the internet. My advice is this: Just make words come out of your mouth. Stumble around until you find some that feel natural to you. It might feel awkward at first. You'll live. Notice how else it feels, beyond the awkwardness. Notice how others react. Notice your reactions to their reactions.

It's not the words you use that make it sexy, anyway. The sexy part comes with the self-respect you get from expressing your autonomy and actively respecting yourself and others! It comes with feeling powerful and unashamed and in control and alive. And from actually liking what's going on rather than having to pretend to like it.

I can't tell you I'm some kind of enlightened sexual monk now, or that I've broken free of the shackles of The Patriarchy's imposed awkwardness when it comes to communicating what I do and don't want. The first time I hooked up with my now husband, he straight up asked me to teach him how to make me come. That was a first for me and I thought it was the most feminist thing I'd ever seen from a man. But it was also a daunting prospect. Sometimes I still have trouble telling him, "Not like that," even when he's just massaging me. But I'm learning to respect my own pleasure, to feel like I equally deserve it. I'm learning to communicate. And it's made everything feel so much better.

As The Great Audre Lorde put it: "For the erotic is not a question only of what we do; it is a question of how acutely and fully we can feel in the doing."[6] It's not about making consent hot. Consent is already so fucking hot.

If you have been sexually assaulted or want to talk to someone about sexual assault:

- Rape, Abuse and Incest National Hotline
    1.800.656.HOPE (4673) | www.rainn.org
- Planned Parenthood
    1.800.230.7526 | www.plannedparenthood.org
- National Domestic Violence Hotline
    1.800.799.SAFE (7233) or 1.800.787.3224 | www.thehotline.org

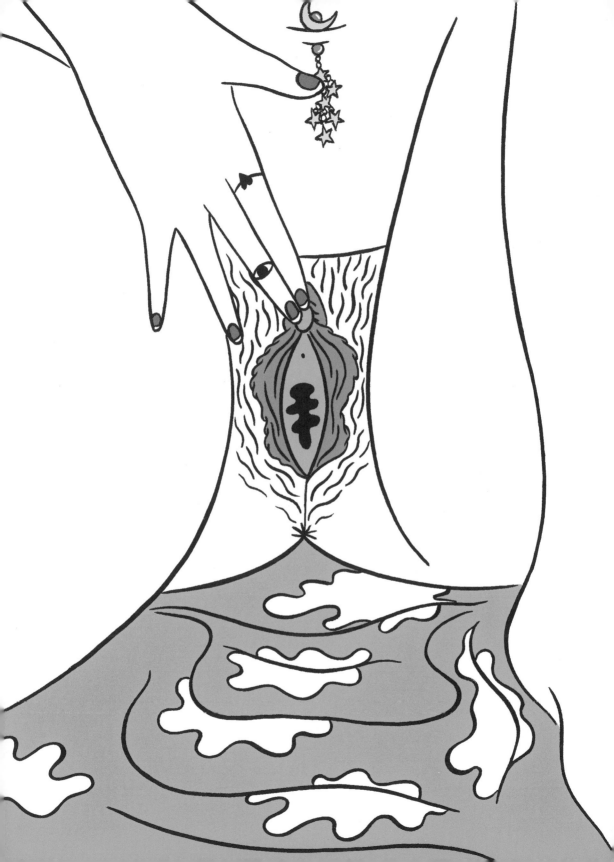

14
Masturbation: Yes

You know what's awesome? Masturbating. You know what I think when I see people who look like they spent an hour-plus getting ready in the morning before they left the house? "You could have been masturbating." You know what I do when I feel like I'm about to explode into human anxiety confetti? (Smoke weed and) masturbate. You know why? Because it fucking makes me feel better. Just like it makes a lot of other people feel better.[1,2,3] And that is why it is awesome.

Proving That Masturbation Is Awesome

Masturbation makes people feel better not just because of the direct physical pleasure but because when you are very aroused and when you orgasm, your brain serves you a cocktail of chemicals—dopamine, oxytocin, endorphins—that makes you feel euphoric and relieves stress and pain.[4,5,6]

Masturbating by yourself can help you build a foundation for your pleasure in partnered sex because if you know what feels good to you, it's much easier to communicate that to someone else, to do it to yourself when you are with others, or both. One study showed that the more people with pussies masturbated with their sexual partners, the more likely they were to "overcome orgasmic difficulty, to experience orgasm, and to enhance their orgasmic pleasure."[7]

There have been many other claims about what masturbation can do for you—that it helps everything from the immune system, to self-esteem, to abdominal bloating, to UTIs—but the research behind these claims leaves a lot to be desired. I am over health benefits being a major talking point. Yes, people who masturbate more have higher emotional intelligence, but that doesn't mean masturbating *makes* you more emotionally intelligent.[8] There's very little research on masturbation for people with pussies, and what research does exist is mostly studies with tiny sample sizes.

Perhaps, if we could prove more benefits of masturbation, it would be easier to convince policy makers that masturbation should be taught as part of sex education. (In 1994, President Clinton fired the extreme badass surgeon general Dr. Joycelyn Elders—who grew up too poor to ever see a doctor until she was 16, was the first Black US surgeon general, and, undeterred in her 80s, now campaigns for insurance companies to cover vibrators—for suggesting that masturbation should be part of sex ed.)[9,10,11] Also, it would be great to know about the benefits of masturbation just for the sake of knowing them. That's why we do Science.

But I also want to make something clear: The positive effects of masturbation are cool, but we do not and should not need health benefits to justify our pleasure. Pleasure is a right! So perhaps health benefits are beside the point. It feels good. That should be enough.

And Yet, Pussy Masturbation Is Still Super Taboo

The taboo on masturbation is at least as old as the Bible. As Sami Ross (my bestie since I was five) wrote in the "Masturbation as Self-Care" article on Pussypedia.net:

> Possibly the oldest condemnation of masturbation can be found in Genesis 1:28: "Be fruitful and multiply." In other words, this was pleasure with strings attached. Sure, have sex often, but only with the intention of making babies. . . . Historically, masturbation has been depicted as a sinful act because it's all pleasure and no procreation. The word comes from the Latin words *manus*, *tubare*, and *stupare*, which respectively translate to "hand," "to unsettle," and "to throw into disorder."[12]

I'm skipping over a bunch of civilizations and movements that condemned masturbation here, but in the 1850s, a bunch of pious haters in the United States (including Sylvester Graham, inventor of the graham cracker) waged a humongous public war on masturbation.[13] The medical establishment (which has never been very pro-pussy) got on board. In his article "The Antimasturbation Crusade in Antebellum American Medicine," Dr. Frederick M. Hodges wrote:

> American doctors, using the most modern "scientific" methods at their disposal, convinced themselves that masturbation was the underlying cause of nearly all social problems and diseases, ranging from rape, divorce, "pederasty," poverty, and criminal activity, to paralysis, epilepsy, venereal disease, nervousness, heart disease, fever, tuberculosis, apoplexy, insanity, idiocy, and even death . . . The medical condemnation of masturbation endured well into the middle of the 20th century.[13]

Yeah! It was all fucking weird! None of it was true, and Science no longer believes this. But the cultural taboo has shape-shifted and stuck. Masturbation went from being seen as immoral to being seen as unhealthy to being seen now as . . . I don't know, just kind of gross? (Remember that time in 2019 when the MTA stations in New York City were plastered with huge flaccid cactus ads for boner pills but wouldn't let a vibrator company advertise?)[14]

One thing hasn't changed: The Patriarchy uses the masturbation taboo as a tool to keep people with pussies down. Masturbation was once taboo for all, so why has the taboo against penis masturbation receded while the taboo against pussy masturbation remains? I mean, I don't believe that The Patriarchy is a conference table full of old white men plotting how to subjugate people with pussies, but sometimes I'm amazed that it's not. Because suppressing our pleasure is a really brilliant way of suppressing us. If you want to know why, go back and read the epigraph in the introduction because there's no way I'll be able to explain it better than The Great Audre Lorde.

While we may know that negative attitudes toward pussy masturbation are not valid, it can still be hard to keep the little black-hatted, sex-hating Puritan off your shoulder. Many people with pussies experience shame and guilt around masturbation.[1,2,3,15] It seems like the way we all collectively think and talk about masturbation has gotten less conservative, but that doesn't mean it's all of a sudden going to feel OK for everyone.

I totally get how hang-ups can stick around, despite your ability to refute their logic in your brain. (I'll talk about how that happens to me with sex toys in Chapter 16.) It makes me sad. I wish everyone in the world guilt-free masturbation and mind-blowing, self-induced orgasms. I really do. But also, if you don't have hang-ups about masturbating and you just feel awesome about it, well, that's awesome.

Orgasm or not, masturbating just feels good, beyond the physical pleasure. For me, it's about taking some time to be by myself, to be with myself, to tend to my body, to indulge my imagination. I love to fantasize. My imagination is so strange and funny, sometimes I make myself laugh out loud. Sometimes I really have to stop and marvel at the beautiful abstract forms and human scenes my mind can generate. Honestly, my mindporn rules, even if sometimes I occasionally get very hung up on and distracted by logistics like, "Wait, but if I'm on the table, he would have to be standing on a stool to . . ." I love that it doesn't matter how long I take, what sounds I make, or how my boobs are hanging. I relish that it feels like a small act of rebellion. It *is* an act of rebellion!

As adrienne maree brown wrote in *Pleasure Activism*:

Pleasure is a feeling of happy satisfaction and enjoyment. Activism consists of efforts to promote, impede, or direct social, political, economic, or environmental reform or stasis with the desire to make improvements in society. Pleasure activism is the work we do to reclaim our whole, happy, and satisfiable selves from the impacts, delusions, and limitations of oppression and/or supremacy.[16]

Clarifications on Some Masturbation Things

Masturbation is not only touching your genitals until you orgasm. Masturbation can be any combination of touching genitals, touching other erotic zones, tensing muscles, fantasizing, humping a stuffed animal, or any other activity on an infinite list of activities that might get you off, or not even get you totally off but that just feel good (including using sex toys, which is covered in Chapter

16). There's no wrong way or wrong amount to masturbate. It's normal not to masturbate at all. It's normal to masturbate a few times a day. You're not masturbating too much unless it causes problems in your life.

Even if you have a partner, you should still masturbate exactly as much as you want. It's not true that if your partner sexually satisfies you, you won't also maybe want to masturbate. Even during sex! Masturbation is not a secondary backup option to your partner being able to make you come. It does not reflect badly on a partner if you want to touch yourself in any way while hooking up. Nobody should ever have a problem with you masturbating, whether or not you're in a relationship with them.

If Your Masturbation Is Not Yet Fully Awesome and You're Not Sure Why but Want It to Be

If you feel weird or awkward about masturbating, maybe it would help for you to tell someone you love and trust with sex stuff (or even who you've never talked about sex stuff before with but you think you might be able to! People generally love talking about sex stuff!) that you're having trouble in this department and need some encouragement. Also, in the 2015 National Survey of Sexual Health and Behavior, over 60% of cis women between the ages of 18 and 50 in the United States reported that they masturbate.[17] So you're in good company.

If you masturbate and it's painful, that might mean something (perhaps vulvodynia) is wrong and you should go see a doctor if you can. If the pain is because of dryness and rubbing, use lube! Lube is awesome. If you don't know what to actually do when you masturbate, read on. If you just feel kind of distracted and can't get yourself that excited, that's because you're a human being!

Everyone and their mom should read *Come as You Are* by Dr. Emily Nagoski. It explains a dual-control model of sexuality. There are accelerators, and there are brakes. Accelerators turn us on (porn, fantasies, pineapples, whatever does it for ya). Brakes turn us off (feeling guilty, cold feet in the literal sense, fear that someone's gonna walk in). Your brakes can stop you from getting aroused even if you're flooring the accelerator with things that should hypothetically turn you on.[18]

So your environment and your mood really has to be right to let your accelerators do their thing. Do whatever you can to make that happen. Obviously, some of your brakes might be things that are hard to work through or not preventable. But do what you can. Lock your door. Put socks on. (I literally put socks on for both sex and masturbating 100% of the time. Cold feet distract me!) Try to identify what your accelerators and brakes are. Give yourself what you can to help yourself feel horny and safe and comfortable.

Here is a list of some of the ways people masturbate, compiled by sex educator Melina Gaze:

- Touching the clit in circles, rubbing, or flicking motions
- Massaging the glans of the clit through the hood of the clit
- Massaging the clit through underwear
- Humping a pillow or other object while facedown
- Tightening and releasing the pelvic floor muscles (as if you were holding your pee)
- Using the head of a shower or water jets in a pool*
- Tugging your own hair
- Talking dirty to yourself
- Putting stuff in your pussy, like fingers, toys, or washed and condomed vegetables
- Sticking stuff in your butt, if whatever you use has a stopper on it (see Chapter 16 for more insistence that it must have a stopper, and a hefty one at that)
- Lathering up with different kinds of lube and touching any parts that feel good!
- Caressing parts of the body, like the nipples, inner thighs, neck, and so on
- Watching porn, reading erotic literature, fantasizing, or listening to sexy podcasts

Melina's main message is "If it feels good, go there!" Also, if the way you masturbate is not on this list, that does not mean it's wrong. It's still awesome, and how cool that you are so creative! You do you, OK? Whatever that is. But do it fully, without being determined for it to end in orgasm. (If it does end in orgasm, great; if it doesn't, great, too.) As brown puts it, "The deepest pleasure comes from riding the line between commitment and detachment. Commit yourself fully to the process, the journey, to bringing the best you can bring. Detach yourself from ego and outcomes."[16] Enjoy a moment of self lovin'. The process and the pleasure are the point!

*When I was seven, my sister, my friend Jessie, and I got caught by Jessie's mom while we were all pressing our crotches into the jets in her hot tub. She told us, "Don't do that, you'll scramble your eggs." I believed her that it was possible, which did scare me. But we kept up the practice for years, calling it the Scrambled Eggs Game.

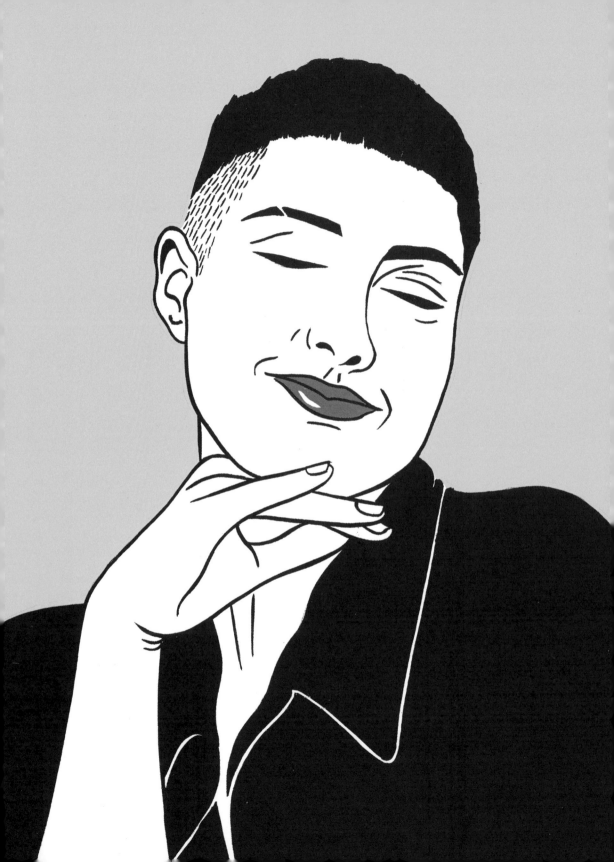

15
Pleasure

Interview with Melina Gaze

When I first laid eyes on Melina Gaze in 2015, they were basically naked, danc-ing, and singing cumbia into a microphone at a clothing-optional party in their apartment in Mexico City. Melina is an Ecuadorian American sexuality educa-tor and performance artist, raised in Miami and based in Mexico City. In one of their gender and sexuality-themed cabaret acts, they put a clear, five-pound bag of Totis (kind of like Funyuns) over their head, tell jokes, dance, and sing to the point you forget you're watching a person with snacks as a face until the performance sputters out of control and they're gagging on the Totis and writhing around onstage (like all good performance art ends).

Melina has also led pleasure- and social-justice-focused workshops and events for thousands of people, mostly adults but also young people, all over the world. In 2012, in collaboration with queer feminist collectives in New York, they started organizing discussion groups around pleasure. In 2018, together with queer anthropologist Sucia Urrea, they founded Vulgar.mx, a Mexico City–based sexuality-education collective that works to create pedagogical tools and offers training to educators and activists. Melina currently serves on the Diver-sity, Equity, and Inclusion Committee of the American Association of Sexuality Educators, Counselors and Therapists.

In 2016, when María and I were starting to put together Pussypedia.net, I had no experience working in sexuality education, so I knew I would need help. I was super excited to have an excuse to propose a collaboration to Melina. They ended up running a trans, nonbinary, and intersex-inclusion focus group alongside collaborators Alexandra Rodriguez de Ruiz, a trans activist and community organizer, and Kani Lapuerta, a trans activist and filmmaker, and created a set of guidelines that shaped both the website and this book. Melina taught me how to make my language more inclusive and sex positive. Hell, they taught me what *sex positive* means! Melina also put together detailed outlines for many of the chapters in this book, making sure that I covered many crucial bases that I didn't even know existed.

But maybe the most important thing Melina has done for Pussypedia is to have had countless long and patient conversations with me, which have given me a much better grasp on why we do Pussypedia and what Pussypedia should aim to do. So much comes down to pleasure and its diametric opposite: shame. Here is Melina explaining why.

How and why did you get into sexuality education?

Well, growing up, we just didn't talk about sex in my family—it was super taboo. And I went to public school in the '90s and early 2000s when the primary policy of the US government was abstinence only education, so that's mainly what I got. But I was also being educated by the culture around me: porn, the *really cool* eighth-grade boys at the back of the bus, MTV, whatever.

When I started having sex, I was having very unsatisfactory, often coercive experiences. I became kind of obsessed with the idea that I would never be able to have an equitable relationship because I didn't feel the same amount of pleasure as my partners did. I couldn't come; I felt weird in my body. I really thought I was broken and that I was doomed to be the vessel for someone else's pleasure for the rest of my life.

Then, I had a conversation with my friend Red Samaniego, who is an amazing trans, Mexican American writer, and they said, "Actually, you know what? I don't think it's just you. I think there are social factors at play that taught you that you're not supposed to touch your body, that you don't have a voice in sex, and that your role is to please your partners." That really blew my mind because I'd always thought of myself as "strong," like, I wouldn't be able to be influenced by that cultural garbage.

That's when we got some friends together and started organizing pleasure-oriented discussion groups for women [and] trans and nonbinary people to talk about sexual pleasure. When we started, I didn't have enough information or understanding to think of them as educational spaces. I was just trying to dig myself out of some really deep confusion, a lot of myths, and a lot of misinformation. But it's evolved into a more formal way of addressing the social and political dimensions of sexuality.

In connecting with others, it was enraging to realize how common experiences of assault and harassment were. It also became super evident how many people had versions of the *I'm broken or weird* narrative. I've been doing this work independently and with collectives since 2012. And, yeah, I love it. It's transformative for me to talk about pleasure, and I think it is for others who come to the spaces as well.

Why is it so important and helpful to talk about pleasure?

We have a right to information about our pleasure, to accurate and complete information about our anatomy, sexual and gender identities, sexual and reproductive rights, and consent.

And that applies to young people as well. So often there's a line drawn about *Don't teach anyone under 18 about their bodies because then they will have sex!* Actually, we have a human right to experience our sexuality, and part of that is pleasure. And you can do it in a gradual, age-appropriate way over time. But it's totally legitimate for teenagers to be learning about pleasure because a lot of them are sexually active, and these are skills we should be developing sooner.

The trajectory of sex ed in the US has been STI-risk prevention with a lot of abstinence only tossed in and maybe, if you were lucky, some relationship and consent education. But in general, it's a negative orientation. And, yes, we need to talk about things that can go wrong, so people can learn to protect themselves. But we need to balance that with the positive things about sexuality.

[As sex educators], when we talk about pleasure, we're more likely to be heard. And lot of people have sex *for* pleasure, so leaving it out just . . . doesn't make sense. There's also been some research showing how public health interventions that address pleasure help people to negotiate better for safer sex or the use of contraception and to have more satisfying, equitable experiences.

It's also important to talk about pleasure because certain groups of people have been denied access to bodily safety, autonomy, and information about their bodies, which impacts how they experience their bodies and their pleasure.

So it's not even just important for us individually. It's a social justice issue too.

Right! Queer and trans people have been pathologized for their gender and sexual identities. People of color have been criminalized for expressing their sexuality and literally just existing. Women throughout history have been denied access to information about their bodies and have been brutally repressed. People with disabilities have been forcibly sterilized or told they are not and cannot be sexual. Of course, this is not an exhaustive list, and oppression is not monolithic. There have been communities that celebrate sexuality and have rich histories of resistance that we can learn a lot from. But many people have been disenfranchised from their bodies. And I think pleasure education can help address those historical injustices.

It can certainly start with individuals expressing their pleasure. The simple act of masturbating can be political. To carve out that space, to reject the cultural shame and stigma—that is subversive. But we need to expand beyond individual action. We need conversations about sexuality-education policy, the health care system, economic inequality, racism, and government-sponsored violence. We have to address those structural problems so that everyone can access their right to pleasure.

Now I have to make a caveat: It's really easy for this rights argument to be co-opted by jerks—like if you ask someone to use a condom and they're like, *Oh, no, but I have a right to pleasure.* That is the absolute worst employment of these ideas. Part of a right to pleasure is the right to safe and consensual sexual experiences. It's not about exploiting someone else's well-being for your own gain.

Yeah. I think if I had thought of sex as something that was supposed to be pleasurable for me, it would have made it more obvious to me how many normalized behaviors are coercive and unacceptable.

Exactly. There's a lot of public conversation happening about sexual misconduct. People are starting to recognize that coercive behaviors are not just from a few "bad apples" but that it's actually a systemic, cultural issue. However, those conversations are rarely complemented with proactive tools to change sexual culture.

Historically, we've only talked about sex as a penis penetrating a vagina. We've talked about sex either as giving something away or as taking something away—*She's gonna say no, and you still have to press on and get it*. No. That's coercion. This is what we want to change.

Pleasure-informed education is an opportunity to do that because, for there to be pleasure, people have to feel happy and respected. So pleasure-informed education necessarily includes enthusiastic and informed consent. It also offers a more holistic framework of sexuality, where we talk about the entire interaction. Ideally, the whole [experience of sex] would be pleasurable from before sexual engagement, to during it, to after. So let's think about the tools to make it that way. Sex should be an act of co-creation in which each partner's pleasure and well-being is equally important.

And that doesn't mean we're going to eliminate all awkward or unsatisfying experiences. That's not gonna happen; we're human. But we do want to eliminate coercion and assault, and I think this broader understanding of sexuality education can help us work towards that.

What about people who are just starting to come into these ideas much later in life and have lived lifetimes of internalized shame around these things?

These are definitely ideas we can integrate into our lives at any point, and for some of us, it's a messy thing that we're continuously processing. I know it can be overwhelming for some people. So often sex positivity is communicated to us—especially on social media—through imperatives and directives. Like, *To be an empowered woman, you have to do* this! But if we want to advocate for bodily autonomy, we also have to respect that people are at different places in their processes.

Let's avoid creating yet another system that constantly tells us we have to be a certain way. We don't have to feel feminist guilt on top of the shittiness we feel from living in a patriarchal society. It's easy to get so caught up in a frenzy of individualistic, self-improvement consumerism through ideologies that are supposed to liberate us but actually make us feel inadequate. Like, it's not a contest to see who's the most sex positive. We can be gentle with ourselves. Maybe I feel ugly today and that's OK. If I'm not having "good-enough" orgasms, I don't need to beat myself up about it. It's also totally normal not to want to feel sexual pleasure at all, or not in the way I talk about it here.

OK, but if you're not having good-enough orgasms, or any orgasms at all, and you want to make them better, what should you do? What are some concrete strategies for seeking and expanding pleasure?
First of all, if sex hurts, if we feel our body doesn't represent us in a way that feels right, or we have experienced trauma that is getting in the way of our pleasure, it's totally our right to seek out professional attention.

Otherwise, from listening to a lot of people talk about their sexuality and about pleasure, I can say that masturbation is a really, really big one. A lot of people don't know what turns them on. That's common and normal. So do some exploration. Whether it's alone or with someone else, don't make it overly goal-oriented where it HAS TO END IN ORGASM. If we reframe sex so that we're guided by pleasure and not the need to orgasm, we may actually be more likely to come.

I know it can be awkward. It might not be a streamlined process. It might take longer than we expect, but that's OK! We're never taking "too long," every body is just different. If you're having trouble getting going, remember that some people experience spontaneous arousal—like just all of a sudden feeling horny—but a lot of us don't. So you might just need some stimulus to get excited. That could be porn, or lighting candles, or maybe just whippin' out some lube and starting to touch yourself. [See Chapter 14 for a longer list of masturbation techniques, provided by Melina.]

For some people, it's helpful to cultivate different tools for getting turned on. Both for solo and partnered sex, it's a lot about identifying your turn-ons and turnoffs so you can create contexts that are more conducive to your pleasure. [See the resources section at the end of this interview for tools and information.] These things change through time. If you fixate on one thing [that gets you off] and then that doesn't work anymore, don't think you're broken. That applies to sexual identity too. Like, what or *who* we like is allowed to change. For people going through gender-affirming treatment or surgery, what turns you on or feels good may change significantly.

And then, once you identify what feels good, it's easier to communicate that to partners. I know a lot of people feel awkward talking during sex—we don't give positive feedback when something great is happening, we don't say when something doesn't feel right, so our partner keeps going. I want to encourage all of us to be more communicative about what works and doesn't work for us. If it feels too awkward [to try it during sex], try a debrief after.

Like, we can work on being able to say, *One finger on the clit, two inside, come-hither motion, silicone lube, please!*—whatever it is. Tolerating something because we don't want to hurt our partner's feelings can feel pretty crummy. Let's practice our *yes*es and our *no*s. That's a skill we can apply outside of sex, in so many areas of our lives.

We don't have to feel bad about our needs. And we certainly don't have to feel bad because we *want* to feel pleasure. We can ask for what we want. We have a right to pleasure, however we define that for ourselves.

RESOURCES

These resources are recommended by Melina Gaze:

- **Vulgar.mx (@Vulgar.mx)**—This is the sexuality education group led by Melina Gaze and Sucia Urrea. They offer workshops on pleasure and social justice in Spanish and English.
- *Come as You Are*—The book by Dr. Emily Nagoski has great information to understand the pleasure response; she also has some turn-on and -off worksheets available for free on her website: emilynagoski.com /come-as-you-are-worksheets.
- *Trans Bodies, Trans Selves*—This book has valuable information on an array of topics, including sexual pleasure and relationships. It was printed in 2014, and there are now a wealth of bloggers and vloggers online

providing updated information about trans pleasure and different gender-affirming options.

- **Afrosexology**—Dalychia Saah and Rafaella Fiallo offer workshops on topics ranging from masturbation to self-love: afrosexology.com/workshops.
- **AnteUp!**—Bianca Laureano [from Chapter 17] offers radical sex ed resources, including curricula and workshops on intersectionality and pleasure anatomy: anteuppd.com.
- **O.School**—This website, by sexuality-education pioneer Andrea Barrica, has helpful articles and videos about sexual health, wellness, pleasure, and masturbation: O.school.

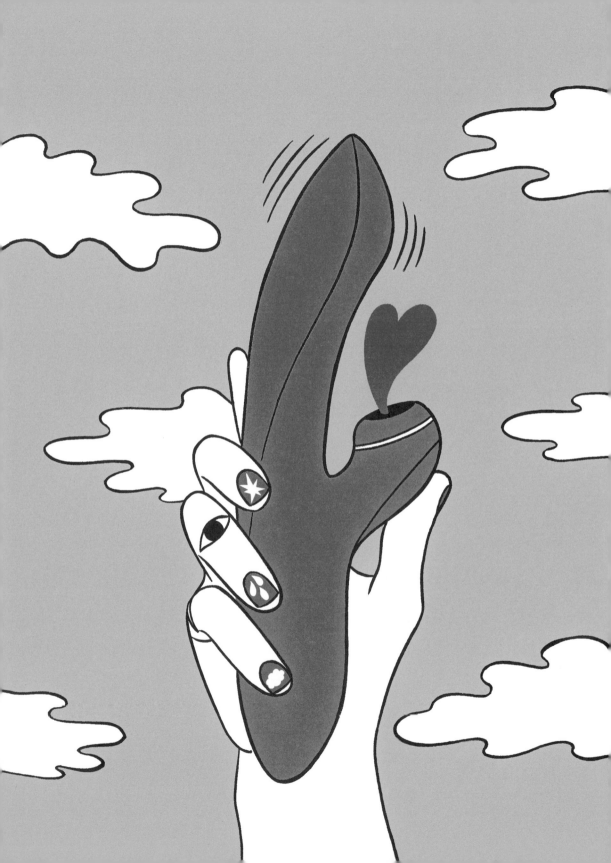

16
Sex Toys

I Have a Weird Hang-Up About Sex Toys

Once when I was eight, my friend Jessie and I were playing in her mom's closet and we found a giant, vibrating dildo. When we brought it to her mom (the same mom who'd told us that masturbating on hot tub jets would "scramble our eggs") to ask what it was, her mortified face and swift recovery of the object tipped me off to the fact that the dildo was both very important to her and very embarrassing. I recognized that it was a fake penis, and I knew what sex was, so I was able to put two and two together. When I was 12 or 13, I would look for dildos in other people's houses—those of friends, and even a bunny I was pet-sitting. When my search was successful, I almost never took the dildos out of their drawers or boxes, or even touched them. I just wanted to stare at them. They were intriguing in the way that moon rocks are. They felt like portals to some unreachable, mysterious, and very exciting realm.

Fast-forward to the summer before my first year of college. My mom generously offered to buy me my first vibrator, but when we went into the shop to actually buy one, the salesperson assumed my mom and I were partners, and I immediately no longer wanted the vibrator. During my second year of college, a woman I was having sex with pulled out her vibrator while we were in bed.

I didn't like the sensation—too intense. It also freaked me out. In recalling the incident to me recently, she said I was so embarrassed by the object that my shame alienated her.

I'd never owned a dildo or a vibrator until recently, which embarrasses me to admit. My curiosity about the pleasure potential of sex toys had not surpassed my weird shame about them until a few weeks ago when I put a condom on the back of my husband's hair clippers (the guard was on!) just to see how the vibration felt. (Outside, not inside! And don't try this. It was a Very Bad Idea.) It was . . . a little much for me? Later, I bought a real vibrator that I tried to use for a few days but just didn't really like. I could come with it but not as intensely as without it. Maybe it was the color, which is this terrible Microsoft blue that kind of makes me cringe. (The saleslady swore I would not be bothered by the color once I started using it. She may have been wrong.) Maybe I just don't love the sensation of vibration. Maybe I don't need a vibrator in my life. I've been perfectly happy without one. Or maybe this is a Thing caused by Patriarchy BS that I should try to get over. I'm not sure.

It's easy to be able to articulate a sex-positive logic all day yet still have weird patriarchal and puritanical voices deep in your conscience preventing you from enjoying otherwise good and harmless things. I want people who have hangups they can't seem to shake to know that even the girl who is willing to tell the world she tried masturbating with hair clippers has hang-ups too.

Why I Still Think It's Important for Everyone to Have Accurate Information About Sex Toys

Sex toys can include vibrators, dildos, vibrating dildos, anal plugs, anal beads, clit suckers, strap-ons, or even oblong vegetables washed and dressed in a condom. Then there's all the fun BDSM toys like leashes and collars, whips, and gags, which are awesome too but which I don't get into in this book. Sex toys can be used all over the body in many creative ways wherever they feel good—nipples, neck, ear, nose, booty, and so on. Sex toys can be used alone or with others.

Sex toys are really awesome for a lot of people. They would not have had a projected $29 billion global market in 2020 otherwise.[1] A 2017 study by the business data platform Statista found that 25% of "adult females" in the United States use sex toys several times per week.[2]

Another 2009 study of 3,800 "women" in the United States found that over half of adult "women" report having used a vibrator. Vibrator use was found to be significantly related with positive outcomes when it came to desire, arousal, lubrication, orgasm, and overall function. The study concludes, "Vibrator use among women is common, associated with health-promoting behaviors and positive sexual function, and rarely associated with side effects."[3]

It's often said that vibrators are addictive or that they desensitize your parts. The 2009 study found that only 16.5% of vibrator users reported numbness, that it lasted more than a day for only 0.5% of respondents, and that most reported it as only a very slight numbness.[3] A lot of articles on the internet address the question of whether or not vibrators are addictive. Sex therapists, ob-gyns, and sexperts have all weighed in and the consensus seems to be: if you get used to coming with a vibrator, you might get lazy about doing it other ways.[4,5,6] But that's far from the same thing as addiction.

Sometimes sex toys are also called *sexual aids* because, for some people who rely on sex toys, the term *toys* may make them seem like an indulgence or a luxury. Sex toys can provide what might not otherwise be possible for people with disabilities, for people who have a hard time coming, for people whose partners can't or don't want to use their own parts, and for a whole host of other people for whom sex toys are very, very useful.[7] This kind of difference in terminology and conceptualization—sex toys as sexual aids—can potentially change what insurance companies are willing to cover when it comes to sexual health. Still, *sexual aid* is also not a great blanket term because, for people having queer sex outside of the penis-in-vagina model, *sexual aid* can make it sound like the body parts they're working with are somehow insufficient or imply that sex isn't sex if a real penis isn't involved.[7]

The Five Sex Toy Commandments That Were (Not) Literally Transcribed by Moses on Mount Sinai

1. Thou shalt not stick something in your butt that does not have a wide base that will keep it from getting sucked into and stuck in your butt. The wide base part has to be really strong and wide. You'd be very surprised what can get sucked into an anus. One study that looked at best practices in

getting things out of butts reported objects found in butts including a body-spray can, bottles, dildos, sticks, a water hose, a corncob, and a pointed squash.[8] The vagina has a cervix that closes one end of it so things (bigger than spermies) can't get stuck in there. But the butthole hath not!

2. Thou shalt not stick anything dry in an anus; always lube up!

3. Thou shalt not stick something in a vagina that was just in an anus without washing it first.

4. Thou shalt not use broken toys! As Liz Duck-Chong, trans health promotor, filmmaker, writer, and host of the sex ed and sexual health podcast *Let's Do It*, says: "It is potentially unsafe to use sex toys that are damaged, including glass, wood, or hard plastic toys with chips, cracks, or stress marks. If you are at all unsure or worried about a toy being dangerous, throw it away and buy a new one."

5. Thou shalt not use dirty toys! Be as "dirty" as you want sexually, but don't be literally dirty about your sex toys. Sex toys can be vehicles for bodily fluids, which can transport STIs from person to person.[7,9,10] So use the same safer-sex barriers and precautions you would use with body parts. Also, they can grow bacteria on them if you don't wash them after use. A few studies have found an association between not washing sex toys and BV.[11] So you really shalt keep them clean. Duck-Chong suggests: "When not using them, store cleaned and dried sex toys in an enclosed location protected from dust, dirt, food, or pet debris, and before use, consider giving toys a quick wash in hot water."

Sex Toys Come in Many Different Materials That All Have Their Own Cleaning Requirements, Lube Compatibilities, and Physical Characteristics

Sex-toy hygiene is a social-justice issue. As Duck-Chong put it: "The lack of medical research, understanding, and reporting on sexual behavior outside of heterosexual penis-in-vagina sex has real-world consequences, especially on marginalized populations for whom it's a major hurdle in improving our knowledge about our own sexual health." As we established earlier, toys are an integral part of some people's sexual lives, and they should be studied seriously as such. Not knowing that they can spread STIs or cause BV, or how to clean, use, and store them is a health risk. Unfortunately, there's very little research out there, but here's what is known. This stuff is going to get a little complicated and boring, but it's important, OK?

Nonporous materials like medical-grade silicone, hypoallergenic metals, borosilicate, glass, and acrylonitrile butadiene styrene plastic are generally the most hygienic.[7] Unfortunately, sex toys are a very unregulated industry—nobody's really checking if what the labels say is true—so it can be hard to know if what is marketed as silicone is actually the real thing.[7,12,13] So if you can, it's worth it to buy sex toys from established brands. The majority of sex toys sold are made of porous, cheap jelly rubber (not the same thing as silicone!), which is soft and pliable but possibly toxic because it can contain PVC.[7,14,15] If you do use rubber toys, store them in cool locations to avoid them melting.[7]

Water-based lubes are the safest bet with sex toys and are fine to use with any material or type of condom.[7] Glass, metal, and plastic toys are all smooth, firm, and compatible with all types of lube. Silicone is soft, more like a body part. Silicone toys are not compatible with silicone lube because the chemical interaction can cause the toys to start breaking down.[7] If you use condoms with silicone toys, make sure the lube on the condom is not also silicone-based (most is). For silicone, glass, or metal toys, use a latex condom (as long as you don't have a latex allergy!).[13] But do not use oil-based lube with latex condoms because oil breaks down latex.[7] For porous toy materials like rubber, latex, or jelly, because many of these materials have oil in them, use a polyurethane condom. Oil and latex is just a bad match all around, and combining them can break down both the rubber toy and the latex condom.[7,13] You don't want these materials breaking down in your body while rubbing against your very absorbent mucus membranes!

OK, now in chart form:

Lube Type to Toy Material Compatibility	Rubber, Latex, or Jelly Toy*	Silicone	Glass, Metal, Plastic
Water-Based Lube	✓	✓	✓
Oil-Based Lube*	✗	✓	✓
Silicone-Based Lube⁺	✓	✗	✓

* Do not use with a latex condom
+ It's on most condoms, so watch out

There is almost no research about the best ways to clean sex toys. But there was a 2019 article in the official journal of the American College of Obstetricians and Gynecologists, which gave a set of recommendations for ob-gyns to give their patients about cleaning sex toys. And this is basically what it said:[7]

- You should wash your sex toys with mild fragrance-free soap and warm water to get any discharge/debris off after every use. (Don't submerge anything with batteries or a motor in water.)
- Definitely disinfect before sharing.
- Porous toys are not considered possible to disinfect.
- To disinfect most nonporous toys, you can soak them in a bleach solution for three minutes or in 70% isopropyl alcohol for five minutes. (Bleach solutions' proportions of bleach to water vary depending on how strong your bleach is, but it should come out to 0.5% sodium hypochlorite.)
- Check the packaging of your toy or the manufacturer's website for information about whether or not you can even use alcohol or bleach on the toy's specific material because you can't with everything. (Also, alcohol doesn't always kill HPV.)[16]
- If you sanitize toys using chemical sterilizing agents, wash them again before use.
- Sometimes manufacturers and other websites recommend boiling, but that does not guarantee killing all germs and fungus.

My personal conclusion from all of this is that, wow, sex toys are really not for kids! Realistically, you will have to do some thoughtful, patient research when buying, cleaning, and disinfecting your toys. And still, despite my own weirdness, I recommend you try them. (Real sex toys, not hair clippers.)

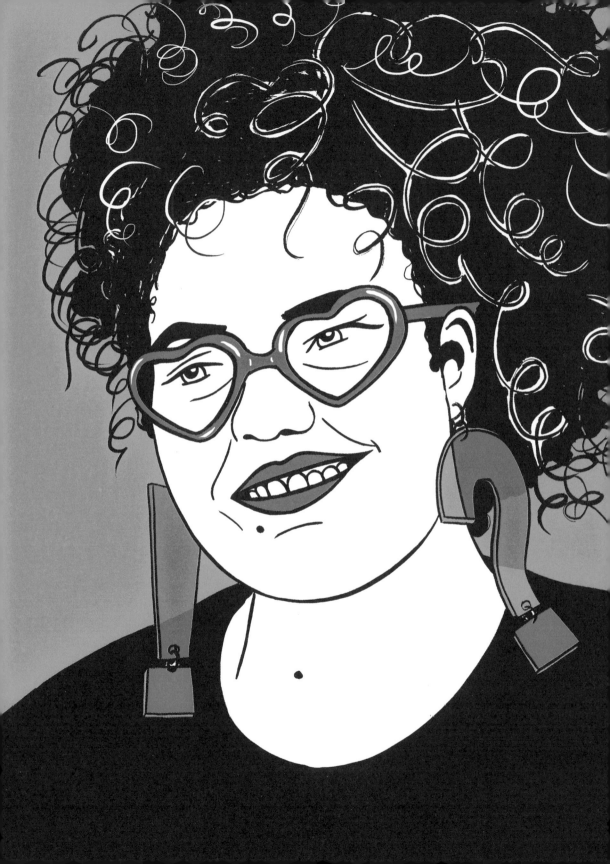

17
Sexuality and Disabilities

Interview with Bianca Laureano, PhD, CSES, MA2

Bianca Laureano, PhD, CSES, MA2, is an American Association of Sexuality Educators, Counselors and Therapists–certified sexuality educator and sexologist. Dr. Laureano works at the intersection of sexuality and disability justice. She is a self-described "disabled, fat, queer, AfraLatina disability justice student and activist." She was the lead educator for the Netflix / Obama family–produced documentary *Crip Camp* about the disability rights movement in the US. She is also the founder and lead educator at the virtual freedom school Ante Up! and the cofoundress of the Women of Color Sexual Health Network.

Dr. Laureano was wearing bright purple lipstick and big, sculptural, gold-frame glasses when we talked over a video call. She has seemingly boundless energy and a gigantic smile. She even warned me right away, "Zoe. I talk a lot." She does. You can tell she is used to talking about sensitive issues. She does it with delicacy and joy. "Positivity" often gets sloppily painted over stories about people with disabilities in a person-overcomes-great-odds narrative that can flatten people's stories. But, really, you can't escape how much Dr. Laureano loves her work. She also seems like she doesn't have an awkward bone in her body. It was a real reminder of the goal state. Or proof that her own doctrine is attainable. Like, she could probably be a cult leader.

She told me intimate stories as if we were BFFs. She made me laugh talking about sex and tear up talking about friends who stepped up to care for her after the death of her mother. It occurred to me about halfway through our conversation that she probably does this with everyone and probably on purpose. What she's doing is leveraging intimacy as a political tool: daring to be *so* human subverts the cultural norms that ask us to leave so much of our emotional selves at home, out of public view. It challenges taboos that make sexuality "inappropriate." By setting the tone, Dr. Laureano gives you space to be your whole human self too. And then she effectively gives you a preview of a better world in the form of a conversation. Here's how (a small fraction of) ours went.

The way you talk about disability is very different from what I've previously heard and seen. How do you talk about the way you talk about disability?

Usually when people talk about sexuality and disability, they're doing it from a medical model of disability, or a social model, but almost never a justice model.

The medical model focuses on diagnosis—finding a cure—and views the doctor as the expert. For example, a sex therapist might give someone a diagnosis and then treat them based on that diagnosis instead of treating them as a person who can speak for themselves and identify what they need.

The social model helps us differentiate between what is disability and what is disabling or debilitating. This model asks if it is the disabled person's body-mind as the problem or if the problem is the way society has created barriers and inaccessible spaces.

In the justice model, disabled people speak for themselves, but take that to another level where we acknowledge that we all have different disabilities and experiences being disabled people, which requires us to engage in cross-disability organizing and cross-disability access. Also, the justice model humanizes disabled people. It says, "We're worthy, we're whole, we're not broken, we don't need a cure."

How do you see people commonly framing sexuality and disability, and how does that need to change?

It's common, unfortunately, that disabled people are assumed to be asexual. That's just wrong. It's an ableist projection of "nobody would want to fuck that person, so they can't be sexual." When people weaponize asexuality, it harms asexual people *and* disabled people. Some disabled people are asexual, but assuming we all are strips us of our body autonomy, of the sexual experience that we want, and of desire.

Also, disabled people experience significant rates of sexual assault, and people don't listen to us or believe us because they think, *Why would someone want to fuck you? I don't believe you were raped.* That's what the #MeToo movement is trying to change, and yet it hasn't been very inclusive of disabled people, even though we've known for decades that rape and violence results in trauma that results in mental health and cognitive disabilities.

People who are institutionalized also experience desexualization. Nursing homes and medical facilities have rules against sexual conduct, which includes consensual sex behind closed doors. A lot of states' consent laws say that people with cognitive disabilities cannot consent to sex. These laws are ableist and rooted in the medical model. They're created by politicians who think that people who are neurodiverse or have developmental disabilities cannot consent. I think that's wrong. What's really happening is that they haven't taken time to get to know neurodiverse people. [Neurodiverse people] do communicate, just not always in the same ways.

If the reproductive justice movement is really about body autonomy, it needs to collaborate with us more. Consider that, for disabled people, abortion is promoted. We're told we shouldn't give birth because we shouldn't pass down our genetic makeup. That's eugenics; it's not something in the past. There are still laws that enable people to forcibly sterilize disabled people, and they're written based on nondisabled people's experiences. If a disabled person becomes pregnant and they have a guardian, that guardian can make a decision for them to terminate the pregnancy without even talking to the pregnant person.

It becomes about the nondisabled person saying, "Well, I have to take care of this [disabled] person and I don't want to take care of a baby too." This happens because the laws, health care, and social security that we have set up to help disabled people are just not comprehensive enough. But, really, we're all dependent on each other in a variety of ways. Sex and disability needs to be framed in a way that acknowledges that all of our bodyminds need support. It's not just disabled people that need care and support and attention. One disability justice principle is *interdependence*, which means we can't do it alone—we need each other to survive.

Can you talk about that term, *bodymind*?
Often when people talk about disability and access, they're talking about bodies and how they move. But that disconnects us from our brains and from people who are neurodiverse, have cognitive disabilities, or [who] identify as mad and who are often very excluded from our movement, especially when it comes to sexuality topics. The reality is that many of us have both [physical and cognitive differences], so the bodymind connection is very important to acknowledge.

Can you also talk about the term *mad*? What does that mean now?
Mad is a term that people who identify as having mental illnesses are reclaiming. It's language that historically led to us being institutionalized, ignored, and traumatized. The story also goes back to the days where women were diagnosed with hysteria for either being too sexually aroused or not sexually aroused enough.

When I read that the old diagnostic criteria for hysteria included both pussies that had too much and too little sensation, I really wondered, how did they measure that? What were their metrics? (See Chapter 7 for more on hysteria.)
Misogyny was their metric. Also ableism. The medical model often has no basis. For example, what does it mean for someone to be "addicted to sex"? That's a contentious conversation in our field. Who decides if a person is too aroused or having too much sex?

It's wild what people get away with in the medical context. We've been medicalized and overmedicated, which pathologizes our experiences and decreases our libidos. Also, people don't always understand how depression itself impacts our libidos, our ability to make social connections, to build intimate relationships. *Bodymind* acknowledges that connection.

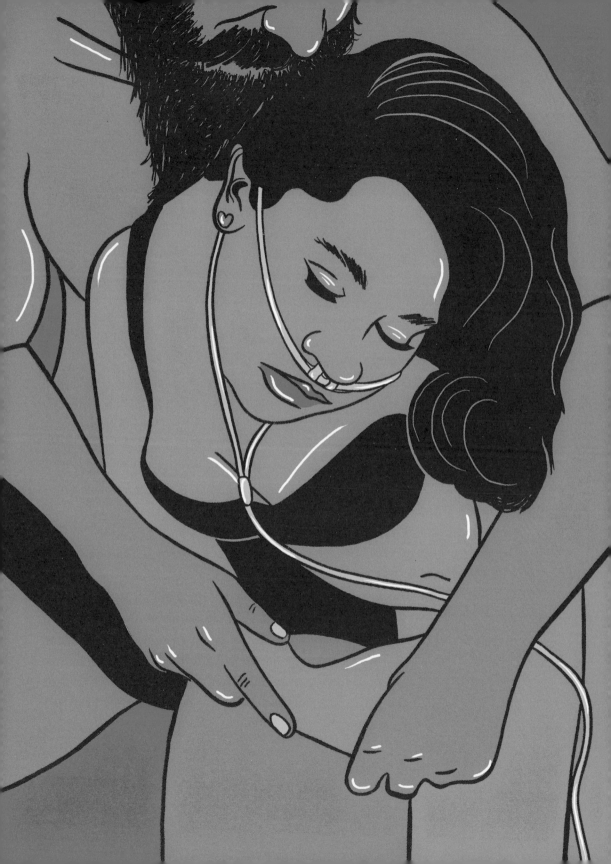

The concept can also help us shift away from sexuality being focused on the genitals. We can have pleasure not connected to our genitals, and nongenital orgasms. Our entire bodymind has the capacity to experience pleasure.

The mind-body connection also explains why accepting your body can be such an important part of achieving pleasure. What do you say to people who are working against body shame and ableism?
It's one day at a time, and some days are better than others. It's a lifelong journey. Body acceptance and self-love are revolutionary acts, especially in a country that doesn't want us to be here. That's why coming into our sexual selves and sexual identities is so important for disabled people. Because it's about saying, "Yes, I'm here; yes, I have sexual expression; and I have the right to engage with that however it looks and feels."

That's really hard, even for me.
Yeah, everyone, disability or not, has something about their body—whether or not they admit it—that they don't like. Many people haven't healed from the trauma of being socialized to think that our bodies are not acceptable. One of the silver linings is that we can all connect in understanding how we've been socialized to hate our bodies based on a white-supremacist ideology [in which] we're supposed to look, sound, move, react, produce, and communicate in a very narrow way. When we understand how that is the root of ableism and how it's deeply connected to anti-Blackness, colonialism, and eugenics [see Chapter 21 for more on the history of eugenics], we begin to understand more fully that ableism is what kills disabled people, not our disabilities.

It helps to think about: Who do you have in your spaces with you? Who are you exposing yourself to? Who do you want to bring in closer, and who do you want to give a little space to because they're not really in service to your care or your healing-focused approach? Who do you want to have a sexual relationship with? Who is worthy of having a sexual relationship with you? Who can show up for you in the ways that you deserve as a person who has been oppressed and whose body is holding, and probably remembering, different types of trauma?

It's also important to acknowledge that some people may not find the healing they're looking for. Some people might not find healing at all. Because that's how ableism and white supremacy work. Even if you're white. Nobody comes out of a white-supremacist culture unscathed.

Assuming that people with a range of disabilities might have a range of mobility and a range of sensation in different parts of their bodies, how can people with disabilities work with their bodies to find sexual pleasure?

Try to be clear about what your body is capable of experiencing. It doesn't have to be all about our genitals. There are heightened sensations in different parts of our bodies, and you need to find those. Sometimes it can look like asking an attendant for a foot rub, or some lotion put on your legs. Then you can experience touch, and you can realize: "Oh, wow, that left big toe, that feels good, something's going on there, and I'm going to remember that, and maybe I'll ask for some of those heated vibrating slippers."

It can be about other things—even smelling new and different scents, if you don't have chemical allergies. Try a bath bomb with glitter in the water. That can be a form of pleasure! Makeup, gender play, dress up—those are all forms too! Even communication is also foreplay!

It can also look like using the internet to watch things. I acknowledge the complexity of porn, and if you're going to pay for it, try to do it ethically and support sex workers. But it's not just porn. I'm thinking about ASMR. Sometimes someone just wants to hear someone eat a bunch of peanuts. That's a form of arousal too.

There's also kink, fetish, and power play, where your genitals aren't even connected. It can be about writing love letters, getting your hair brushed, sending a text message to someone at the time they asked you to contact them. There are so many different ways to engage in power exchange, and it's a common exploration for people. It can be healing for people to be part of consensual planning of a scene, to experience power they don't have every day.

When there's so much ableism and oppression in our lives, this process can feel overwhelming. That's why I tell people to take it one step at a time. Some days you're just gonna be like, "Wow, everything sucks in a bad way." And sometimes you'll be like, "Wow, I got amazing pleasure from feeling the sun on my face and my kneecaps today."

I assume that part of what's hard is having to ask others to make provisions or assist. What do you tell people who want to approach someone about help masturbating?

Being able to ask for what you need is vital and a form of power. It's all about communication and making clear it's a desire that you have.

I also acknowledge that a lot of people don't have privacy. They're not respected. They don't feel like they can ask that of people, which is why sex workers are such an important part of our community. They can show up, and you can say, "I need help masturbating. Can you help move my body in this particular way, at this particular angle? Can you help put this vibrator here? I'll move my hand or make a sound if I need more help." It doesn't have to be about fucking someone. It can be about: "Oh! You need to be on your left side today because you're having pain on the right, so I'll move you over. I'll move your arm. I'll put pillows between your knees." There's a lot of ways to ask for help.

And there's a lot of ways to masturbate. It can be as you eat, it can be the gag reflex, the swallowing gesture. Some people get amazing comfort and pleasure just with warm water running over their body. Some people need help getting into the shower, soaping up, and maybe that's pleasurable. Maybe you can just ask for a detachable showerhead and maybe an assistive device to hold it.

Sometimes it's about asking someone, "Can you lift my hips up onto this pillow and leave me alone for 30 minutes?" You don't need to say what's going on, you can just ask to be positioned in a particular way and do whatever you want to do. Also, we live in a sex-negative world, so sometimes coded language can help us communicate too.

This is why interdependence is such an important part of disability justice. If we're really about pleasure, we really need to go all-in for what pleasure looks like for all of us.

How can props help? What should people look for beyond dildos and vibrators? Also, is the term *sex toys* problematic? I read that some people take issue with it because they actually need them, and the word *toys* doesn't recognize that.

Language is really personal and it also shifts and changes, so it's important to ask people what language they use. I grew up with the term *sex toys* and that's what I feel comfortable with. Also, other language, like *assistive device*, is just not very sexy to me.

Some of the most promoted toys are not accessible because not all of us can move in the same way. That's a common challenge. So it also helps to find sex toys with longer handles.

It's also helpful to know how to use pillows and how to use a lift or a wedge. And suction cups are really great for helping people put something on the floor or a wall or a mirror. Sex furniture can be really helpful too. I have a piece that looks like an ottoman but with a curve in it, and it helps get your body into different positions.

But it's important to think about what we need and what we don't need. Because a lot of sex furniture is very expensive and a lot of the cheaper sex toys use chemicals that are not good for the body. You can use a lot of things that you can find anywhere. I'm sure my kitchen is full of sex toys. [See Chapter 16 to learn more about choosing sex toys made of safe materials and about safely using food as sex toys.] There's sensual play, like prickly and soft things. Get a feather from an arts-and-crafts store. Have someone write on your body with makeup or paint or food.

It's about being creative and using what's available to you in a variety of different ways.

RESOURCES

These resources are recommended by Dr. Laureano:

- The group Sins Invalid is run by queer, trans, and BIPOC folks and has a great disability-justice primer: sinsinvalid.org/disability-justice-primer.

- liberator.com is great for sex furniture, works with disabled influencers, and also makes products in plus sizes.
- A lot of people find the Hitachi Magic Wand vibrator useful because it has a long handle.
- CBD lubes and suppositories are good for people with pain.

Illustration on page 173 based on a photograph from the visual essay about sexuality and disabilities "The Lion Dressed as the Elephant" by Trista Marie McGovern (@tristamariemcg) and Emma Wondra (@emmawondra).

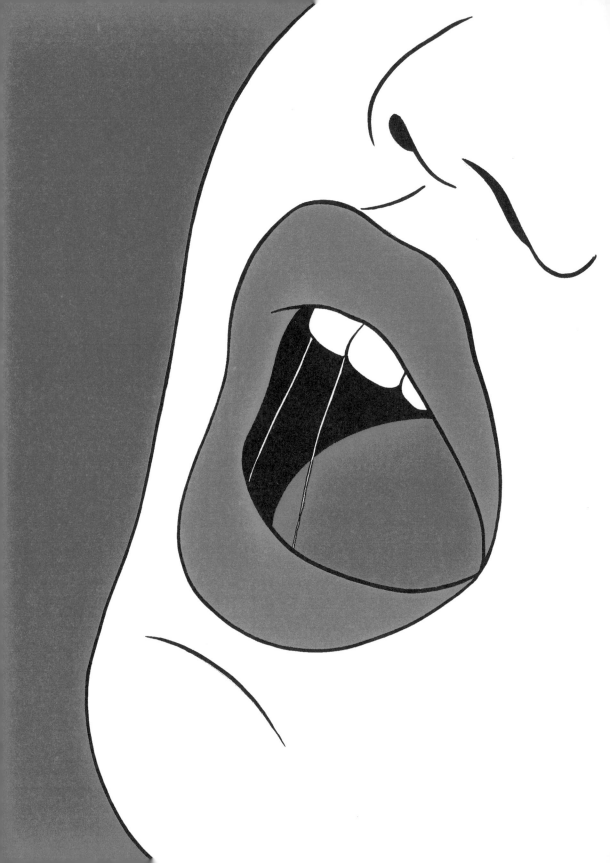

18
Types of Orgasms

THIS IS GOING TO BE A VERY SHORT CHAPTER BECAUSE THIS TOPIC DOES NOT EXIST.

There are a few definitions of *orgasm*. Some focus on the subjective experience—Dr. Emily Nagoski, author of *Come as You Are*, defines it as "the sudden, involuntary release of sexual tension."[1] Some focus on what happens in the body, and those definitions look at the involuntary contractions of the pelvic-floor muscles.[2]

Dr. Nagoski explains that what people perceive as their own orgasms don't always match up with the physical responses, like muscle contractions, that scientists peg as the actual, physical occurrence: "Orgasm—like arousal—isn't about what happens in your genitals, it's about what happens in your brain."[1] That's why the "clitoral versus vaginal orgasm" distinction is beside the point. All efforts to count types of orgasms are. There are either infinite types of orgasms, or one type of orgasm, but nothing in between.

There are an unknown number of parts of the body that people can stimulate to orgasm. A few known ones are the nipples, anus, and mouth.[3] People with spinal cord injuries report having orgasms through stimulation of their lips, ears, neck, and even the hyper-sensitive skin near their injuries.[3,4] People can orgasm in their dreams and during birth.[3] My college roommate once had an orgasm because she was stoned and eating really good Indian food while listening to a really good concert. What do you call that kind of orgasm?

The superiority of the vaginal orgasm was probably Freud's worst idea ever. He wrote that clitoral orgasms are immature, that mature women orgasm through their vaginas, and that, if you can't, something is wrong with you. That is entirely unfounded. Less than a third of people with pussies can reliably orgasm from vaginal penetration.[1]

Freud's brainfart birthed all sorts of bad dynamics: generations of people with pussies felt flawed for being normal. And as Dr. Ellen Støkken Dahl and Dr. Nina Brochmann put it in *The Wonder Down Under*, the idea that people with pussies should be able to orgasm from penetration alone gave cis men "permission to go for it, come, and then happily turn [their] backs as [they] switched off the light. A woman's pleasure was her own responsibility."[5] So can we all collectively throw that idea in the garbage, please?

If you're taking testosterone, your orgasms might change. You may feel more peak intensity and more of a focus on your genitals rather than a whole-body experience.[6] This might be a good or a bad thing for you, or just something neutral and different.

The bottom line is that everybody's orgasms are equally valid and normal and awesome as long as they feel good. Mmmkay?

PS (and this is a PS because Dr. Nagoski is right, this is actually beside the point): A vaginal orgasm IS a clitoral orgasm. It's just a different part of the clitoris getting stimulated. (See Chapter 4 for more on the G-spot and how this works.)

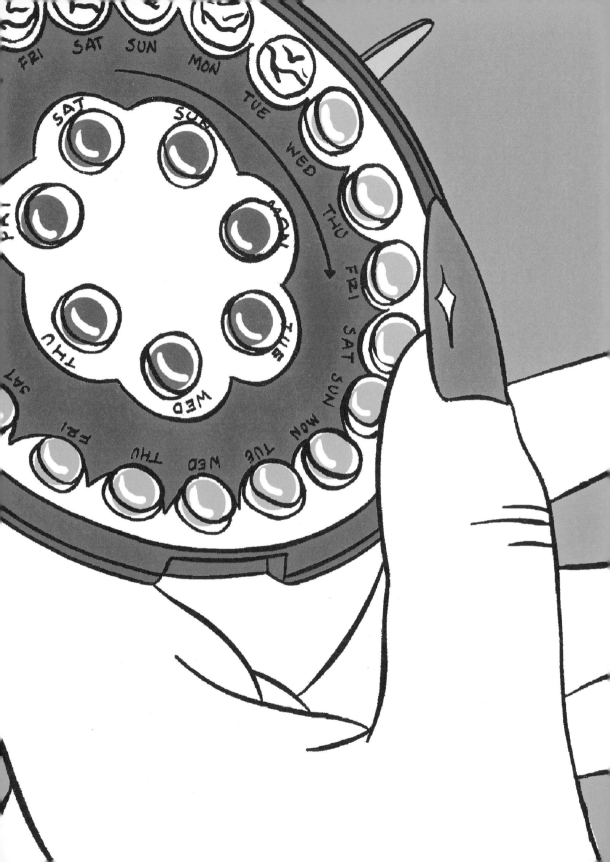

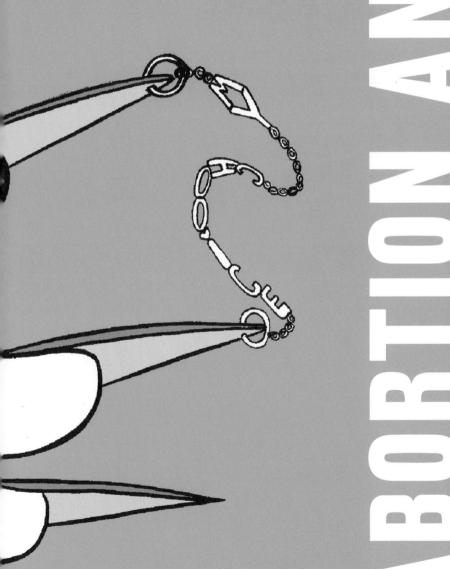

ABORTION AND CONTRACEPTION

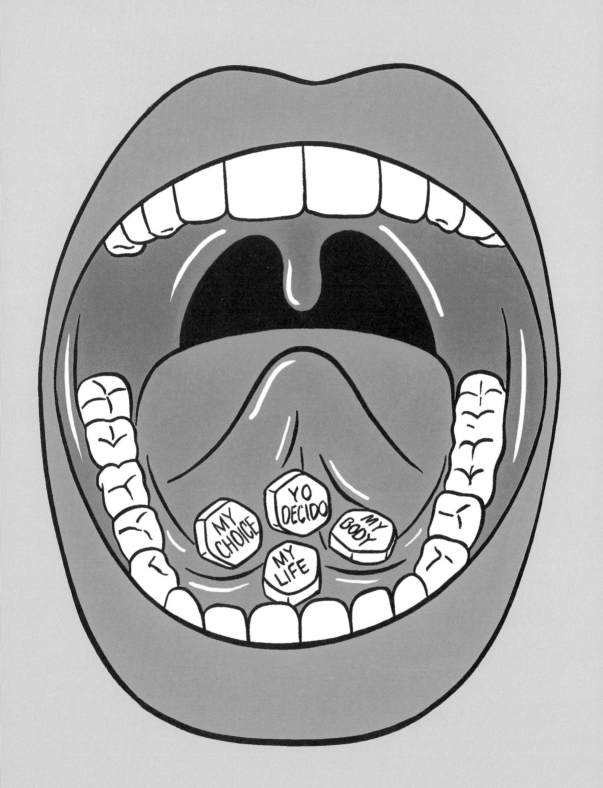

19
Abortion

I'VE NEVER HAD AN ABORTION (WHICH IS VERY—LIKE, *VERY*—SURPRISING TO ME), but about one in four women in the US will have had one by age 45.[1]

Abortion is the intentional termination of a pregnancy. People who get pregnant have been doing it for millennia, all over the world (even when and where it has been illegal). This is presumably because having a baby is an enormous change to someone's life and there are a lot of real good reasons you might not want to or be ready to or be able to have one. Abortion is safer than carrying a pregnancy to term and delivering, and it has no known long-term health effects.[2]

Abortion is controversial because, however tiny the clump of cells is that comes out of a pregnant person's body, that tiny clump of cells might have eventually become a person, so some people call abortion a form of murder. I don't see it that way. But, either way, what abortion accomplishes, other than ending a pregnancy, is that it gives control to the pregnant person over their body and their life. Denying someone the right to abortion does the opposite.

Some people would say, "But abortion takes away the life and agency of the unborn child," and some others would say, "It's not a child," and yet others would say, "Yes, it is," and *this is the argument that never ends, yes it goes on and on my friends / some people started arguing it, not knowing what it was /*

and they'll continue arguing it forever just because it has become a very handy and divisive tool in very high-stakes political battles, used by people with ungodly amounts of money who need a lot of regular people to keep single-issue voting on the question of a pregnant person's right to abortion so that they can keep having ungodly amounts of money.

No, literally. As the *New York Times* editorial board put it in 2018,

> Out of concern for individual freedom, the Republican Party once treated abortion as a private matter. When Ronald Reagan was governor of California, he signed one of the most liberal abortion laws in the land, in 1967. As late as 1972, a Gallup poll found that 68 percent of Republicans thought that the decision to have an abortion should be made solely by a woman and her doctor. But after Roe, a handful of Republican strategists recognized in abortion an explosively emotional issue that could motivate evangelical voters and divide Democrats.[3]

If you ask me, the right to abortion—the right to make decisions over one's own life and body—is a prerequisite for gender equality. But when it comes to your decisions, my opinion doesn't matter, and neither does any other opinion in the world besides (the nine US Supreme Court justices' and) your own.

(See Chapter 29 to read my plea to future us to protect our rights and/or to accompany me down a terror toilet and out the other side to something that is not quite hope.)

What Happens in an Abortion?

Medical abortions, medication abortions, and self-managed abortions are most commonly and safely done before a pregnancy's 10-week mark. Medication abortions can be tried a bit later on in a pregnancy too, although they're not always as effective.[3] Since their approval by the FDA in 2000, medication abortions have become pretty common. In 2017, they accounted for 38% of all abortions in the US.[4]

All of the terms that start off this section can refer to abortions with pills, but *medical abortion* and *medication abortion*, which are the same, mean something different from a *self-managed* abortion. With a medication/medical abortion, a doctor prescribes you some combination of misoprostol and mifepristone, and then you go take them wherever you feel safe and cared for. *Self-managed abortion* just means that a pregnant person is operating outside a medical setting, but more recently, the term has often been used to refer specifically to abortions via misoprostol and mifepristone.

Since misoprostol is less regulated by the FDA than mifepristone, and is still about 85–95% effective in ending a first-trimester pregnancy without mifepristone,[5,6] it's usually the self-managed abortion pill. But the two drugs in combination is also an option when the pregnant person has access to both, and is more than 95% effective in the first nine weeks of a pregnancy (and a few percentage points lower from 9 to 10 weeks).[7]

Mifepristone works by blocking progesterone (the pregnancy hormone). Misoprostol works by inducing contractions to end the pregnancy.

I've heard from friends that these kinds of abortions are pretty painful and feel like shit for most people. Most people will experience bleeding, uterine pain, and cramping. Cramping might last up to three days. NSAIDS like ibuprofen are recommended for that. Eighty-five percent of people report having experienced at least one of the following side effects: nausea, vomiting, weakness, diarrhea, headache, dizziness, fever, and chills.[8]

The good news is that these methods are considered very safe, even when self-managed.[5,9] They are even enthusiastically approved by the World Health Organization for use up to weeks 9–12 of pregnancy, depending on the drug combination.[10]

In-clinic and ***surgical*** **abortions are umbrella terms for *vacuum aspiration* and *dilation* and *evacuation* abortions.** With these options, you go to a clinic or a doctor's office and they physically take the cells out of your uterus using a vacuum aspirator, which is a little sucking tool.

Vacuum aspiration uses only a speculum to access the cervix and then a vacuum to remove the contents of the uterus through a thin tube called a cannula. You may feel a pinch when numbing the cervix, pressure from opening the cervix, and medium to intense cramping throughout.[11] The whole thing takes about five minutes.[3]

Dilation and evacuation is an abortion method for further-along pregnancies—usually in the second trimester. It involves opening (dilating) the cervix more to get bigger pieces of tissue out, using misoprostol or thin rods that expand, called *osmotic dilators*, then using an electric vacuum aspirator. You may feel pressure and cramping during dilation and some tugging during the suction part. You usually get more pain meds and sedation than for a vacuum aspiration.[12]

After about the 24th week of a pregnancy, the common option is called an *induction abortion*. This is where the provider will induce labor, usually with medication. The fetus may be injected, through the belly, to end the pregnancy. Then it will be birthed through the vaginal canal. You may have to do this in a birthing ward of a hospital. Bring someone who makes you feel cared for with you if that's an option. You may have to stay overnight. It is usually not as long or painful as full-on birth, but contractions can last from a few hours to a day.[13]

Induction abortion sounds incredibly emotionally hard—at least to me. That said, however you feel before, during, or after having any form of abortion is valid. Whether it makes you deeply sad, hugely relieved and happy, or you feel . . . nothing, your feelings are acceptable and correct.

How Can I Get an Abortion?

How easy or hard it is to get an abortion depends on where you live. But no matter where you live, there are people out there who dedicate their lives to helping people just like you get an abortion even if you live far away and have no money. They're out there; you just have to find them.

In many US states, abortion is criminalized. There have been at least 21 arrests since 2000 related to ending pregnancies or to helping a loved one do so.[14]

(Wherever you live, definitely do not be scared to seek medical attention after taking abortion pills if you have complications. Especially if you live in a state with restrictive laws, just say you are having a miscarriage and do not say you took the pills—the treatment is the same anyway, and you don't want to put yourself at legal risk. There are no known tests that can detect misoprostol.[15] If you do for any reason need legal help or want to know more about your rights, visit reprolegalhelpline.org.)

In looking for information on the internet about getting an abortion, be careful. There are a lot of sites and apps out there that look very legit and seem like they're trying to help you get an abortion when in fact they're purposely spreading misinformation so you don't get one. These sites are made by the yes-it's-a-child people.[16] Start with the resources below.

RESOURCES

For help procuring various types of abortion services in the US:

- Euki app
- Cara app
- Safe Abortion app from the Hesperian Foundation
- Safe Abortion app from Women on Waves

For more information about medical and self-managed abortions, how to get them, and how to take the pills:

- reproaction.org
- womenhelp.org
- abortionpillinfo.org
- howtouseabortionpill.org
- womenonwaves.org and womenonweb.org
- ifwhenhow.org
- plancpills.org

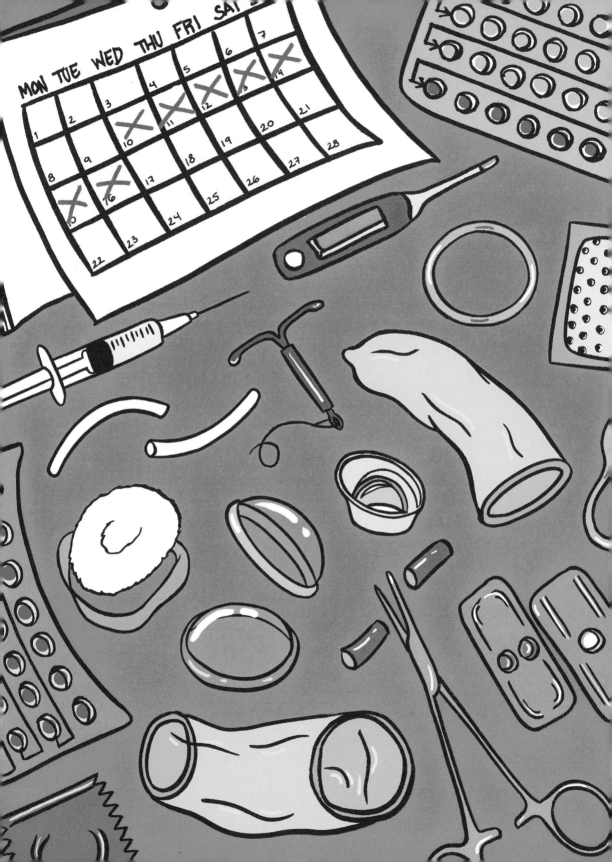

20
Contraception: Options and Phantom Side Effects

IN THIS CHAPTER, I AM GOING TO GIVE YOU A QUICK, VERY BASIC RUNDOWN OF CON-traception methods, and then I am going to talk about that weird and frustrating mystery wherein there is a growing public conversation around people getting depressed and feeling generally awful as a side effect of hormonal birth control, but there actually are a lot of studies on this, and they keep showing that depression is *not* a side effect of hormonal birth control.

Without contraception, a sexually active young adult with a pussy who's having penetrative vaginal sex with a person with a penis, over the course of a year, will have an 85–95% chance of getting pregnant.[1]

Lucky for everyone, unlike so many other topics about pussies, there is a wealth of research on birth control and there are a lot of people and organizations who have made good-quality information about it available. For much of this chapter, I have relied on two amazing resources: Bedsider.org and Scarleteen.com. If you're in the process of choosing a birth control, this chapter should only be a starting point. I highly recommend consulting both.

At bedsider.org/methods/matrix you can compare contraceptive methods side by side in a matrix based on many very intelligently selected factors like "party-ready," "do me now," "mistake proof," "cost," and so on. I'm a huge fan because the tool respects that people have their own reasons for picking their birth control method(s) and that all those reasons are valid. In all my personal experiences around birth control, I felt like I was being pressured and told what to do, so I love seeing this validation of every individual person's knowledge of what is best for them and their agency to do that. I also appreciate that Scarleteen includes recommendations about what kinds of people might benefit from certain types of birth control methods over others, and that it seems to take the possibilities of side effects more seriously than some other internet resources.

Whatever form(s) of contraception you end up choosing, do a lot of research. It's great to use contraception, but it's even better to use it right and to be educated about how it works and what side effects to watch out for.

The cost of each method depends on what kind of insurance you have and how much of access to free and low-cost clinics, like Planned Parenthood, you have. If you have health insurance, first ask your health-insurance provider what your plan covers. If you don't have insurance or if your insurance doesn't cover the type of contraception that you want, look into what kinds of deals or coverage you might qualify for at a Planned Parenthood or a similar clinic.

Contraception for Trans and Nonbinary People[2]

You will still need contraception if you've not had your uterus or both ovaries out and you're doing things that could get you pregnant but you don't want to get pregnant. Neither testosterone nor gonadotropin-releasing hormone (GnRH), which suppresses ovarian function, can be relied on as birth control. If you get pregnant while taking testosterone, your doctors might recommend that you stop taking it because of dangers that it can pose to the fetus. (Psst, trans and nonbinary people who produce sperm: same goes for y'all. Feminizing hormone therapy may change sperm production, but it is still not a reliable form of birth control.)

Most of the methods listed here will not mess up masculinizing hormone therapy, with the exception of combined hormonal contraceptives that contain estrogen, like pills, patches, or the vaginal ring. They *can* mess with the masculinizing effects of testosterone. That does not mean that any hormonal method is off the table. Progestogen-only methods like pills, shots, implants, and IUDs should be just fine and can even provide the extra benefit of allowing you to skip periods if they are not something you want in your life. Emergency contraception is also OK, and testosterone is not thought to interfere with its effects.

Condoms[3]

The first thing I would like to say about condoms is that a few weeks ago out of sheer curiosity, I filled up a condom with water to see how much it could hold. I put it inside of a bucket so that when it popped it wouldn't waste a bunch of water. The condom filled up the entire bucket before popping. The bucket size was 3 gallons.

Anyway. Unlike other methods of contraception, condoms help protect against both pregnancy and STIs. There are external condoms that go on the outside of a penis and internal condoms (sometimes called female condoms) that go inside of a vagina. Both types of condoms can also be used for butt sex but, if you use an internal condom in a butt, take out the internal ring!

Condoms come in lots of sizes and materials, with lots of different types of lube on them. Some have lube that contains spermicide as an extra measure of precaution, but spermicide is bad for your vagina party (see Chapter 32 for more on why). The most common condoms are made of latex and cannot be used with oil-based lube (see Chapter 22 for a list of oil-based lube examples). For people who are allergic to latex, condoms made from a range of alternative materials, from lambskin to polyurethane, are options. Those condoms are not as easy to find, but they're out there!

According to a literature review on the subject, here are some things researchers have found that people do wrong with condoms that make them less effective:[4]

- Not using them for the whole duration of penetration, e.g., "Let me just put it in for a little bit, then I'll put the condom on," a.k.a. the Just the Tip tactic. Lol that is not safer sex.

- Unrolling the condom before putting it on.
- Not leaving a little bit of space at the tip of the condom when putting it on or not squeezing the air out of that little tip part when they do leave that space.
- Putting it on inside out and then taking it off and flipping it right side out before use.
- Using sharp things (including teeth!) to open the package, tearing the condom.
- Lube issues: either not enough lube or using oil-based lube.
- Not holding on to the base of the condom when pulling the penis out after sex.
- Re-using condoms during the same session. (Once there's semen in it, throw it away!)
- Storing them for too long and letting them expire before use.

In this chapter's resources, I've included a cute video link for how to correctly put on a condom. I do NOT recommend simply typing "how to put on a condom" into YouTube: it seems to be an excuse for dudes to put their erect penises on the internet, and consequently, there are one gazillion tutorial videos, and a lot of them are doing it wrong.

Internal Condoms
Used perfectly*: 95% effective
Used typically: 79% effective

External Condoms
Used perfectly: 98% effective
Used typically: 86% effective

Hormonal Methods

Hormonal birth control methods present a small risk of blood clots, which is higher for: smokers; people over 35–40; people who have diabetes; and people who have a history of high blood pressure, cardiovascular disorders, or high cholesterol.[5,6] The other side effects I've listed under these methods are the ones about which there is more consensus. I will address other possible side effects at the end of the chapter.

How Do Hormonal Methods Work?[6]

Combinations of estrogen and progesterone work by stopping your ovaries from releasing eggs. Progesterone occasionally does that, but not consistently. Both combination and progesterone only methods also work to make your cervical mucus thicker so that it's harder for sperm to get into your uterus. Sometimes those hormones also make your uterus a less hospitable place for a fertilized egg to implant itself.

Much of the Development of Hormonal Birth Control Was Horrible and Inhumane[7]

It's important to be aware that, in developing many types of hormonal birth control (like in the development of many medical technologies), drug companies tested them on marginalized people of color, often without consent. As Harriet Washington explains in *Medical Apartheid*:

> The pill, Norplant [an earlier version of the implant], and the Depo-Provera shot were first tested in Mexico, Africa, Brazil, Puerto Rico, and India. Once approved, they were administered to large numbers of girls and women in the US in venues that are disproportionately and, usually, overwhelmingly African American and Hispanic. . . . Many serious effects emerge for the first time during this post-approval stage, when very large numbers of women begin taking a drug. Thus, the immediately post-approval use of contraceptive methods in large numbers of closely monitored poor women of color constituted a final testing arm, so that they were unwittingly participating in a research study.

(See Chapter 21 for more on how racism fueled the development of birth control.)

The Pill[8,9]

You take a pill at the same time every day for three weeks. Then you have a choice. You can take the week of placebo pills (pills that don't contain any medication) that come with most brands and get your period. Or you can skip the placebo week and keep taking the non-placebo pills, in which case you will skip your period. There are many different pills out there that work slightly differently, but they fall into two main categories: combined estrogen and progestin (a synthetic form of progesterone) and progestin-only.

Possible Bad Side Effects: Bleeding between periods, sore boobs, and nausea and vomiting, especially in the first three months, with changes to your sex drive that can last longer.

Possible Good Side Effects: Lighter periods, cleared-up acne, and reduced cramps and PMS.

Used perfectly: 99.7% effective

Used typically: 91–93% effective

The Ring[10]

There are two brands of the ring available in the US: NuvaRing and Annovera. They kind of look like those jelly rave bracelets, except they go inside your vagina and you DO NOT trade them with your friends. You leave them in for three weeks (even while you have sex), then take them out for the fourth week and get your period (probably). The ring releases synthetic estrogen and progestin.

Possible Bad Side Effects: Especially in the first few months, spotting between periods, sore boobies, nausea, and even vomiting. Increased discharge, irritation, infection, and a change in your sex drive that may last longer than three months.

Possible Good Side Effects: Cleared-up acne, shorter and lighter periods, lessening of cramps.

Used perfectly: 99.7% effective

Used typically: 93% effective

The Shot[11,12]

Depo-Provera is a shot of progestin that goes into your arm or butt every three months. The shot is kind of a heavy-duty method. Scarleteen's recommendation about the shot is very sensible:

Because once you get that injection, you not only can't discontinue use for three months, and because side effects of Depo-Provera can continue for many months to even years after use, we usually advise that people try a more easily reversible method of progestin-only contraception first, like the [progestin-only pill]. That way, if you find out you and progestin don't do so well together, you won't have to live with side effects you don't like for so long.

Possible Bad Side Effects: Heavier periods or spotting between periods for 6–12 months, changes in appetite, and weight gain. Less-common side effects include changes in sex drive, hair loss, hair growth on face and body, nervousness, dizziness, headaches, nausea, and sore boobs.

Possible Good Side Effects: Periods can get lighter or go away completely.

Used perfectly: 99.8–>99% effective

Used typically: 94–96% effective

The Implant[13,14]

The implant, called Nexplanon, is a tiny plastic stick that goes into the skin in your upper arm, where it releases progestin. It lasts for up to three years unless you get it removed.

Possible Bad Side Effects: Heavier periods or spotting between periods for 6–12 months. Less common side effects include acne, changes in appetite, changes in sex drive, ovarian cysts, dizziness, hair loss, headaches, nausea, nervousness, sore boobs, and scarring or pain at the site of the implant.

Possible Good Side Effects: Periods can get lighter, lessening of PMS and depression, fewer cramps, improvement in symptoms of endometriosis.

Used perfectly or typically: >99% effective

The Patch[5,15]

The patch is a little square sticker that goes on your body anywhere except your boobs. It releases hormones into your skin. You wear one a week for three weeks in a row with one-week breaks between. The patch is extra not-right for anyone on the list of people who should not use methods that contain estrogen, since it has an extra lot of estrogen. Also, its designers weren't thinking very inclusively: the patch only comes in white-people-color beige and might not work as well for people who weigh over 198 pounds.

Possible Bad Side Effects: Bleeding between periods, nausea, vomiting, and sore boobies, especially for the first three months. Changes in sex drive may last longer.

Possible Good Side Effects: Lighter and more regular periods, cleared-up acne, lessening of cramps and PMS.

Used perfectly: 99–99.7% effective

Used typically: 92–93% effective

Intrauterine Devices (IUDs)[16,17,18]

When my mom's ob-gyn pulled her 10-year-old, flesh-and-goop-covered IUD out of her vagina, he held it up to his ear and said, "Too bad there aren't two! You could make earrings!"

IUDs are little T-shaped or double-fish-hook-shaped doohickeys that get inserted into your uterus. There are hormonal IUDs and nonhormonal IUDs. The hormonal ones are made of plastic, and they release a small amount of progestin. Depending on the brand, they can last from three to seven years. Some people report that these IUDs make their periods lighter and reduce cramps.

The nonhormonal IUDs are made of plastic and a little bit of copper. They can last up to 12 years. They will not interact with masculinizing testosterone therapy but might be less appealing because of possible side effects like spotting between periods and increased bleeding. Some people also report cramps and backaches.

While rare, there can be pretty serious complications with IUDs—like if it slips out, pokes into the wall of the uterus, or becomes infected. Listen to pain in your body. If something hurts, especially after three months, go get it checked out. There have been concerns that the nonhormonal IUDs can spur autoimmune problems, but there's still very little research on this.[19]

(There was a disaster with an IUD produced in the 1970s, called the Dalkon Shield, which was taken off the market after just three years. It harmed hundreds of thousands of people. This gave IUDs a bad rap for many years. But IUDs are *much* safer now.)

Used perfectly or typically: >99% effective

Emergency Contraception[20,21]

These are options for when you get semen in your vagina accidentally (or on purpose but later you *feel* like it was a mistake). Emergency contraception pills are not the same as abortion pills. They cannot terminate a pregnancy; they can only prevent one. To prevent a pregnancy, most forms of emergency contraception must be taken within five days, but the sooner you take it, the better its chances of working.

Plan B and Next Choice are both available in the US without a prescription. If you're nearing the end of the five-day window, you might want to reach for a new option: Ella. You have to get a prescription, and it needs to be taken during the five-day window, but unlike other options, it's just as effective day four as it is day one.

Every time (it's a lot of times, I don't know how many) I've taken a Plan B pill, it has given me extreme diarrhea. That said, I'm a Jew, and almost everything gives me diarrhea, including being stressed out, which I usually am when I'm taking a Plan B pill. Other side effects of emergency contraception can include upset stomach, vomiting, breast tenderness, irregular bleeding, headaches, and dizziness.

When people hear *emergency contraception*, they usually think of pills, but getting a nonhormonal IUD put in within five days of that unwelcome-or-regretted sperm entrance will also lower your chance of getting pregnant by 99.9%.

Within the first 24 hours: 98% effective

After that: 75–89% effective

Methods That Depend on Spermicide

I don't recommend spermicide. Spermicide can irritate your tissues and throw off your vaginal microbiome, which can increase your chances of contracting an STI.[22,23,24,25,26] Spermicide also significantly increases your chances of getting a urinary tract infection (UTI).[27,28,29,30,31]

The Diaphragm and the Cervical Cap[32,33,34]

These are little barrier thingies that you put spermicide on and stick in your vagina, up against your cervix, to stop sperm from getting inside. Cervical caps and diaphragms are both generally made of latex or silicone, but are slightly different shapes. They both kind of look like tiny, weird hats. You'll have to get a health care provider to do a fitting so you can get the right-size device for your cervix. Diaphragms require a prescription, but the cervical cap does not.[35] They're not always easy to get in, and they can get pushed out of place during sex.

Also, they must be washed between uses. Most sites recommend soap and warm water.[36] Another thing to consider is that, if yours is silicone, you might not want to use silicone lube. While this is not something many sites or sources talk about, it is widely known that silicone lube should not be used with silicone sex toys because it will break down the material of the toy. The same logic should presumably extend here. At least one diaphragm company does specifically advise against using silicone lube.[37]

There are a fair amount of studies that found that diaphragm use was associated with UTIs.[38,39,40,41] But 1) they are all pretty old, and current diaphragms on the market may have improved, and 2) these studies may have been observing UTI occurrences based on spermicide use, not the diaphragms themselves (which go hand-in-hand, since diaphragms are supposed to be used with spermicide).

Diaphragm
Used perfectly: 84–94% effective
Used typically: 83–86% effective

The Cervical Cap
Used perfectly: 91% effective
Used typically: 71–86% effective

The Sponge[42]

The sponge is another kind of cervical barrier that uses spermicide. Most sponges have spermicidal foam in them and you have to wet them and squeeze them to activate it. You can have sex as many times as you want while the sponge is in, but it also needs to be left in for another six hours after sexual activity. You can put it in up to 24 hours in advance of having sex (but I would advise against doing that if you don't need to because of the irritating qualities of spermicide).

Used perfectly: 91% effective

Used typically: 86% effective

Fertility Awareness[43,44]

This is a cool method, but it takes considerable dedication and commitment and willingness to admit if it's not right for you. This method is about tracking your menstrual cycle so that you can know when you are fertile. It can be used either to help you get pregnant or not get pregnant. This method is not easy to do with a lot of precision, but the process can help you learn a lot about your body. Counting days between periods to understand how long your cycle is and track its progress is only part of it. People also pay attention to their cervical mucus, their body temperature when they wake up, and the position and texture of their cervix. It takes about six months of charting daily to really get ahold of your cycle and be able to use this method effectively. There are a lot of tracking apps that can help. People with irregular cycles will probably not be able to use this method.

Used perfectly: 95–99.6% effective

Used typically: 76–98% effective

The Pullout Method[45]

The old pullout! It's also called *withdrawal* or *coitus interruptus*. It's when the penis pulls out before it ejaculates and does not ejaculate in the vagina. It's not ideal because you have to trust the person with the penis to pull out in time. When I told my mom this is my preferred method of birth control, she said, "Zoe! Goddamnit. That is the eventually-you-get-pregnant method of birth control!"

Used perfectly: 96% effective

Used typically: 80% effective

Sterilization[46]

If you are, like, so super sure you don't ever want to get pregnant, there is a range of mostly irreversible surgeries that will make pregnancy impossible.

Options include removing the ovaries, removing the uterus, removing the uterine tubes, and interrupting the uterine tubes.

Usually, when the purpose of these procedures is birth control, the most common option is the interruption of the uterine tubes, either by tying them or sealing them closed or cutting them and then tying them off. Sometimes "getting your tubes tied," as it's colloquially called, can be reversed but not always. It should be considered permanent. This surgery, as opposed to removing the ovaries or uterus, will not cause a huge hormonal upheaval in the body.[47,48,49]

OK, So What the Hell Is the Deal with the Phantom Side Effects of Hormonal Birth Control Methods?

At the very pushy urging of the doctors at my college's health center, I started the pill the first week of my freshman year. It made me feel *terrible*. I was emotionally unstable, sad, and disconnected from myself. Once, I cried hysterically in the cafeteria because I waited in line for some chicken but the person before me got the last piece. That moment was a relief actually because it gave me an objective measure of my emotional reactions: something was off. I know with absolute certainty that I don't love chicken that much. But when I went back to the doctors, they twice assured me that it was just freshman year of college—not the pill—making me feel that way. In fact, I specifically remember them saying, "This is the most studied drug on the planet. There are *no* side effects."

I don't know if I started to feel more normal, or if I just got used to feeling terrible. My memories of college are generally bad, so it may be the latter. When I finally went off the pill, I went through another huge emotional upheaval, didn't get my period for about six months, and started growing thick, black hair on the backs of my knees and tops of my toes. I've never gone back on any form of hormonal contraception because *fuck. that.* The whole experience made me feel gaslit by my doctors and scared of intervening with my body.

This is not meant to be a cautionary tale. Many, many, *many* people have a much easier and totally fine time with birth control pills and other forms of hormonal contraception (HC). Indeed, many people *love* HC. And while no other life change has made me feel *that* terrible, it's entirely possible that the emotional instability actually was a symptom of starting college. But also, I'm far from being the only one who's experienced side effects like these. Anecdotal evidence of people feeling terrible on HC is everywhere. There was even a viral *New York Times* video about a person feeling terrible on HC in 2018, called "Birth Control Your Own Adventure" by Sindha Agha (and it's awesome).

Also, the idea that HC could cause depression is totally believable. First of all, sex hormones, like the ones in HC, affect a person's mood in several ways. This is well accepted and has been demonstrated over and over by many studies.[50,51,52] Second, back when HC had way higher doses of hormones than currently available forms do, studies showed that depression was a fairly common side effect (increases in depressive symptoms ranged from 20% to 50%).[50] Third of all, many studies have shown that mood disruption and mental-illness symptoms are still major reasons that people give for why they stop taking birth control.[53,54,55,56,57]

But the research on birth control and depression tells an inconsistent story. There are thousands of studies on the subject, but a few are more highly regarded than the rest because of how they collected and analyzed their data. Four randomized controlled studies (the best, most trustworthy kind of study because it curbs biases in results and uses a control group for comparison, which many studies lack!) looked at whether or not HC causes mood changes, and none of them made a strong case that it does.[58,59,60,61] In fact, one found that HC improved symptoms of depression.[60] And then there are the studies that were not randomized and controlled but that made up for that in scale (a lot of study-sample biases disappear when the group being studied is big enough). One Australian study followed 10,000 people with pussies for three years. Another American study looked at 7,000 people with pussies over the course of 14 years. Still nothing linking HC to mood changes. In fact, both showed a slight decrease in depressive symptoms over time.[62,63]

One huge Danish study that followed 1,061,997 people with pussies from 2001 to 2013 did show that HC use was associated with an increase in the likelihood that someone would start taking antidepressants or get diagnosed with depression at a psychiatric hospital (2.2 and 0.3 per 100 person-years,** respectively, compared with 1.7 and 0.28 per 100 person-years for nonusers), especially among adolescents. Interestingly, it found that the risk of depression increased steadily for the first six months of HC use, then decreased slowly, returning to pre-use levels four years later. Also, rates of depression were higher for users of progestin-only methods than they were for users of combined methods.[52]

A 2019 review of 90 smaller-scale studies on the effects of HC identified a few consistent patterns of HC side effects such as: a decreased ability to read other people's emotions as well as thinking everyone else is feeling worse than they really are; having way more intense emotional reactions (crying about the chicken); getting less pleasure out of things we like; and messing up the way we respond to stress. These feel like validating findings, but the data isn't, like, *super*strong since the studies reviewed are all fairly new and most haven't been replicated. (As the authors remind us, "Results have to be interpreted with caution, as the evidence is observational in most studies, and therefore, we cannot infer causality.")[64]

And still, it's a fucking lot of studies. What this review made me think is that perhaps a lot of studies that look at HC's effects are too focused on *depression* when maybe what we're looking for is just a nebulous combination of smaller, harder-to-pinpoint effects that amount to feeling *weird* and *bad*.

Other recent reviews of studies about hormonal birth control have tried both to explain why so many studies have turned up inconsistent results and to identify any consistencies among studies' results. Their conclusions were[50,51]

1. There aren't enough studies that look at people using HC over a long period of time.
2. Too many studies lumped together people taking different kinds of hormonal birth control and then studied them as a whole rather than looking at the effects of specific methods or doses.
3. Studies define and measure mood changes differently.
4. People's expectations of HC's mood effects might be throwing off the data. If people expect to have mood changes (one study found that 20% of subjects did),[65] and then they don't, they might report their mood as extra good. Also, people with the idea that they might feel shitty on HC might end up feeling shitty just because they expected to feel shitty.
5. A critical mass of studies show that adolescents, people who have a history of depression, and people with previous bad experiences with HC *are* all at a higher risk of developing depression on HC.

Dr. Ellen Støkken Dahl and Dr. Nina Brochmann also reviewed this mystery and some of these studies in *The Wonder Down Under*. They concluded that this whole thing might just come down to coincidence and confirmation bias:

> Depression, mood changes, and irritability are such common phenomena in the population that this is likely to be a trick of chance. If, in addition, you've heard that contraceptive pills can cause mood changes and depression, it's even more likely you'll draw this conclusion, given that [many people report negative effects from placebo treatments if they think those treatments cause negative effects]. Rumors of mood changes spread like wildfire among female friends on Internet forums, and suddenly, you start to see your own experiences in a new light.[66]

They might be right. Their theory is plausible. But based on the data, my personal experience, and the countless conversations I've had with so many people about their similar experiences, I have a feeling that there's more to be discovered. If you're crying about chicken, I don't think you're hysterical. But for more of an explanation, we'll have to wait and see.

_____

RESOURCES

- How to put on a condom: https://youtu.be/Aq42dsjQM14
- bedsider.org
- scarleteen.com/article/sexual_health/birth_control_bingo

*The effectiveness of birth control methods is commonly measured by looking at how many people out of 100 will get pregnant if they are exclusively using that method for one year. So if something is 86% effective, that means 14 people out of 100 will get pregnant within a year of using that something as contraception. But because most birth control must be used in a specific way to be maximally effective, effectiveness gets broken into two groups: used perfectly and used typically. Typical use entails different sorts of common mess ups for each form of contraception, often including just not using it consistently. I didn't go into every way each form of contraception can be used wrong because there are too many wrong ways to list! And like I said, when you pick your method, ya gotta read about how to use it right. (Except I did go into it with condoms because I suspect people don't always know what they're doing but they *think* they know, which is worse than when they know they don't know. You know?)

**Person-years is a measurement that combines the number of people in the study with the number of years they were studied. This measurement is used because the number of people in a study over time can change (like if people drop out). A study that looks at 10 people for 10 years would have 100 person-years of data.

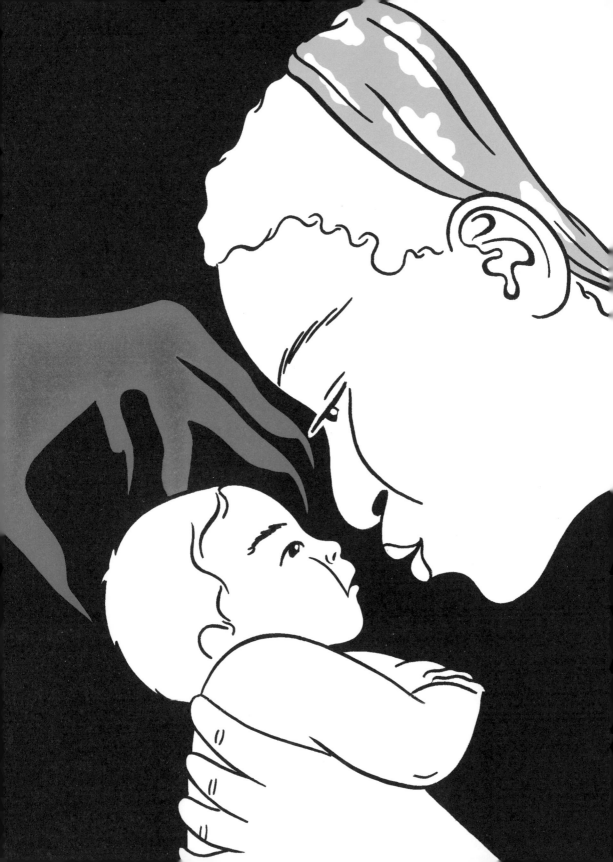

21
The Other Kind of Birth Control

Second-wave feminism gave us a lot of gifts, like access to birth control and abortion and the Equal Pay Act of 1963. We have a lot to thank those ladies for. But damn, their movement was super white and was not paying very much attention to what was going on with people who were not.[1] This is how second-wave feminists came to focus only on abortion—the right not to have babies—at a time when hundreds of thousands of people were being deprived of their right *to* have babies, by being forcibly sterilized—made permanently unable to have babies, often by removing their uteruses.

Our cultural story around birth control usually goes: Birth control is great because it allows people who can get pregnant to decide not to have babies—it increases their agency over their own bodies. Yay for that. But we almost never talk about when birth control takes away the right to have babies—probably because white people who don't have disabilities have not been historically denied that right. And historically, it's usually been white people who do not have disabilities who have gotten to tell our cultural stories.

As Dr. Angela Davis wrote in her 1981 essay, "Racism, Birth Control, and Reproductive Rights": "The abortion rights activists of the early 1970s should have examined the history of their movement. Had they done so, they might have understood why so many of their Black sisters adopted a posture of suspicion toward their cause."[1]

Hundreds of thousands, if not millions, of people have been permanently robbed of their fundamental right to reproduce, and most feminist movements and conversations about "reproductive rights" simply fail to address that. We're going to take Dr. Davis's advice now and look at the violent injustices that continue to happen with "birth control," so that we can be better at fighting for reproductive justice *for all*.

Bullshit Racist Ideas Led to Mass Sterilizations

Forced sterilization as a form of state-sponsored violence in the United States grew out of some racist bullshit that was popular at the turn of the 20th century: eugenics and neo-Malthusianism. Eugenics said that humans should breed ourselves like we breed plants and pets—for "desirable" traits. And you guessed it: non-whiteness, poverty, disability, illness, sexual promiscuity, and having committed crimes were considered undesirable traits. As Harriet Washington puts it in *Medical Apartheid*, "Highly educated persons of good social class were considered eugenically superior," and Black mothers, on the other hand, were considered "sexually indiscriminate[,] bad mothers who were constrained by biology to give birth to defective children."[2] Neo-Malthusianists said, *There's not going to be enough resources to go around if we keep letting poor people have so many babies, so get the poor people on birth control or, even better, sterilized!*[3]

Around the same time, white people started having fewer children. This really freaked out the kind of people we would now call *white nationalists*, which at the time was no mere fringe, extremist group. In 1905, President Teddy Roosevelt proclaimed, "Race purity must be maintained!" and by 1906, he was going around talking shit about the impending "race suicide."[1] Birth control advocates used this logic to promote their cause by framing birth control among the "lower classes" as a means of preserving white supremacy—counteracting the low birth rate among whites by also lowering the birth rates among poorer, nonwhite populations.[1]

One of those advocates was Margaret Sanger, the founder of Planned Parenthood. She raised money for research for the original birth control pills, lobbied politically for their legalization, and coined the term *birth control*.[1] She even helped our IUD-inventing friend from Chapter 4, Ernst Grafenberg, escape Nazi Germany. Sadly, Sanger tended to say Nazi-like things herself. In a 1921 essay called "The Eugenic Value of Birth Control Propaganda," she wrote:

> As an advocate of Birth Control, I wish to take advantage of the present opportunity to point out that the unbalance between the birth rate of the "unfit" and the "fit," admittedly the greatest present menace to civilization, can never be rectified by the inauguration of a cradle competition between these two classes. In this matter, the example of the inferior classes, the fertility of the feeble-minded, the mentally defective, the poverty-stricken classes, should not be held up for emulation to the mentally and physically fit though less fertile parents of the educated and well-to-do classes. On the contrary, the most urgent problem today is how to limit and discourage the over-fertility of the mentally and physically defective.[3]

This human-breeding logic was not only morally disgusting, it was scientifically bullshit. There was no genetic screening at the time, so there was no way to know who carried what traits.[2] Still, eugenicists lobbied for forced sterilization as a public good. Sanger argued for the sterilization of "morons, mental defectives, epileptics, illiterates, paupers, unemployables, criminals, prostitutes and dope fiends."[1] In 1927, the Supreme Court ruled eight-to-one in favor of mandatory sterilization laws. By 1932, eugenicists had successfully gotten 26 states to pass similar laws.[1,4]

In 1939, Sanger, her eugenicist friend Clarence Gamble (a Procter & Gamble heir), and the American Birth Control Federation launched the Negro Project.[5] Gamble's proposal for the project explained that poverty in the American South could be fixed by lowering birth rates among Black people.[5] As Dr. Davis put it: "More and more, it was assumed within birth control circles that poor women, Black and immigrant alike, had a 'moral obligation to restrict the size of their families.' What was demanded as a 'right' for the privileged came to be interpreted as a 'duty' for the poor."[1] By 1941, between 70,000 and 100,000 people were sterilized in the US.[2,5] Throughout the 1940s, Gamble opened over 20 sterilization clinics in the South and Midwest.[5]

Meanwhile, in Puerto Rico

By the mid-1930s, the US government had made Puerto Rico very poor by stealing literally, like, all the land away from the people and turning the island into one giant sugar plantation.[4] And then the government said, *OMG look how POOR all these people are, they should not be able to have any more babies!*[1,5] In 1937, Blanton Winship, the US-appointed, non–Puerto Rican governor of Puerto Rico, passed a eugenics-inspired law legalizing sterilization, to control the "menace of the ever-growing population."[5]

Then during the 1940s, the US industrialized Puerto Rico to meet wartime manufacturing needs with cheap labor. The US government knew that this would cause further unemployment there, so industrialization was, from its start, also accompanied by plans to ship out about a third of the island's population, mostly to New York City, along with a giant national campaign for sterilization.[6,7]

Back in Boston during the 1950s, two scientists named Gregory Pincus and John Rock were trying to develop the first birth control pill with funding from Sanger's friend, the wealthy birth control benefactor Katharine McCormick.[8] But they had two pesky problems: 1) contraception research was illegal in Massachusetts, and 2) as McCormick put it, "Human females are not easy to investigate as are rabbits in cages."[6,8] The testing and prodding involved in their studies was so constant and intrusive, their test subjects were dropping out left and right.[7] So these sick assholes went looking for human test subjects at a nearby mental hospital, lied through their teeth by saying that their proto–birth control might have "calming effects," and started performing experiments on patients under false pretenses.[6,8]

Next, the scientists brought their testing to Puerto Rico because it didn't have legal restrictions on contraception research and it had a network of "family-planning" clinics that had been established for population control in the '30s by the Roosevelt administration. Many of these clinics were later taken over and run as birth control–testing laboratories by Gamble.[5,7] From just 1937 to 1939, Gamble experimented on approximately 5,000 lower-income couples.[7] The trials for Pincus and Rock's pills made many participants sick—22% dropped out because of side effects.[6,7]

While these tests were going on and for many years after the pill was finally on the market, other available methods of birth control were unavailable and sterilization was pushed nationally as the best method of contraception (if not the only).[6,8] While many people may have been misled or pressured into agreeing to the surgery, many more got it because it had simply been culturally normalized and, again, it was the only option for people in dire situations of colonially imposed poverty.[7] By the end of the 1970s, over a third of Puerto Ricans with pussies had been sterilized.[5]

Hold On, It Gets Worse: The 1970s

Back on the mainland, the civil rights movement and the sexual liberation of the 1960s came and went, but tragically ableist, classist, racist sterilizations continued. It wasn't until 1973, when the Southern Poverty Law Center filed a lawsuit on behalf of Mary Alice and Minnie Relf, that the issue of sterilization abuse of marginalized people came to public consciousness in a meaningful way.[1]

Mary Alice, 14, and Minnie, 12, Black sisters, both of whom had intellectual disabilities, were taken by their mother, who was illiterate, to receive birth control shots in a clinic in Alabama. When her daughters were taken away to get the shots she had requested, they were instead surgically sterilized. The case exposed what was still a huge national problem: the presiding district court found that an estimated 100,000–150,000 poor people were sterilized JUST THAT YEAR under federally funded programs.[9]

Nobody knows how many thousands of people were forced into getting sterilized by a widely practiced form of coercion at the time: doctors threatening to take away welfare if people didn't get the procedure.[9]

During this period in the South, sterilizations of Black people without consent and without any medical reason happened so often that they had a nickname: "Mississippi appendectomies." Teaching hospitals in the North also performed unnecessary hysterectomies on poor Black people as practice for their medical residents.[10] One study found that, by 1970, one in five married "Black women" and about the same percentage of "Chicana women" in the US had been sterilized.[1]

The Relf sisters' case was a victory, but it didn't fix the problem entirely. The judge prohibited the use of federal money for involuntary sterilizations and the practice of threatening to take away welfare. The case's publicity also led to the requirement that doctors get informed consent from patients before sterilizing them.[9] Then, in 1973, another big birth control thing happened: *Roe v. Wade.* Yay for legal abortion! But in 1977, abortion opponents scored a win, the Hyde Amendment, which cut federal funding of abortions and ended up causing a lot of states to cut or end funding for abortions.[1]

Sterilizations, however, remained free and federally funded. So with no access to legal abortion, many people turned to sterilization, for which there were abundant sources of funding.[1] Sterilizations actually tripled between 1970 and 1980, partially because hysterectomies were offered as the only option for problems that can definitely be treated without removing the uterus, like fibroids. By 1983, when Black people were only 12% of the country's population, 42% of people sterilized in federally funded programs were Black.[2]

During the same period, there was also a proliferation of well-funded birth control initiatives aimed at Black people even while, as Washington puts it, "health advocates failed to address more pressing African American health issues, such as abysmal nutrition, poor control of infectious disease, high infant mortality, low life expectancy, poor quality health care, scarce mental health care, and even a lack of access to hospitals and physicians." She continues to poignantly explain that this truth "cripples any argument that birth-control clinics were erected with African Americans in mind."[2]

Even after sterilization policies changed, Native Americans were still forcibly sterilized. One government report, which used data from only four cities, found that 3,406 Native Americans had been sterilized without informed consent in just three years, between 1973 and 1976. At the time, that number represented more than 3% of childbearing Native Americans.[11] But according to a study conducted by Native American researcher Dr. Connie Uri of Indian Women United for Social Justice, the real percentage of childbearing Native Americans who had been sterilized without consent by 1976 was closer to 24%.[1] As late as 1977, three Cheyenne people filed a class-action suit against the US Department of Health, Education, and Welfare for having been sterilized after doctors threatened to take away their welfare and lied, saying the surgeries were reversible.[11]

In 1973, Dr. Bernard Rosenfeld, who had been a resident at Los Angeles County General Hospital, coauthored a report about sterilization abuse of Mexican women in the US, mostly migrant workers. He wrote that there was very little informed consent happening and that obstetricians told residents to "strong arm" vulnerable patients into accepting sterilization so that the residents could get surgery experience. In 1978, the Los Angeles Center for Law and Justice filed the class-action lawsuit *Madrigal v. Quilligan* on behalf of 10 sterilized people who reported an array of abuses.[11] Doctors had refused to give them abortions if they did not consent to sterilization.[12] Doctors gave English consent forms to Spanish speakers and told them they were consent forms for cesarean sections. Doctors had people sign consent forms while they were under anesthesia. Those people woke up to find themselves sterilized.[6] Many doctors went ahead without any consent at all.[5,12]

The sterilized people lost the case. But it did, at least, force consent forms to be bilingual and for waiting periods to be instituted between consent and operations.[12] The National Organization for Women (NOW), one of the most important women's rights groups at that time, opposed these waiting periods because they were getting in the way of "the rights of women who wanted to be sterilized immediately."[5] Facepalm. Yes, in the case of abortion, for example, waiting periods have been weaponized to prevent access to the procedure. And today some argue that these same waiting periods for sterilization are outdated and indeed are making it difficult for people who rely on Medicaid for health care to get sterilized during childbirth.[13] But at the time they were introduced, the waiting periods were a helpful measure. I would guess that, at that moment, there were a hell of a lot more people who needed protection from forced sterilization than there were people who absolutely needed immediate sterilizations.

This Shit Is Still Going On

In the 1990s, the effort to stop poor people from having babies began to switch from sterilization to using long-acting reversible contraceptive (LARC) methods like IUDs, implants like Norplant, and injections. Two days after Norplant was approved by the FDA in 1990, the *Philadelphia Inquirer* ran an editorial called "Poverty and Norplant—Can Contraception Reduce the Underclass?" which suggested making better welfare benefits contingent on getting the implant. A huge backlash against the article spurred the paper to run an apology: "Our critics countered that to dangle cash . . . in front of a desperately poor woman is tantamount to coercion. They're right."[14]

And still, between 1991 and 1994, 13 states tried to pass laws that would have paid poor people to get birth control implants, and seven states tried to pass laws that would have made Norplant mandatory for people with pussies who had babies with drug addictions, who had gotten publicly funded abortions, or who wanted to receive welfare. During the mid-1990s, judges in California, Florida, Illinois, Nebraska, and Texas ruled in favor of requiring people with pussies to get birth control implants as part of criminal sentencing, usually as a requirement for reduced sentences.[14]

Both Norplant (which was later taken off the market) and Depo-Provera were pushed on poor, mostly nonwhite communities throughout the 1990s, including huge efforts to get Black teenagers to take them.[4] Norplant, for example, was distributed in school-based health clinics (the first 100 of which were in nonwhite schools), even to middle school students. The drug had never been tested on people so young, and researchers were monitoring how the drug affected the students and reporting back to Norplant's creator, the Population Council. According to its website, the Population Council "conducts research and delivers solutions to improve lives around the world." According to Harriet Washington, it "researches and tests contraceptives on poor women abroad."[2] So, basically, the distribution to school clinics was a giant national experiment using nonwhite middle- and high-school-age kids as guinea pigs.

A 2006 study found that, even then, "low-income women of color were more likely to report being advised to limit their childbearing and were more likely to describe being discouraged from having children than were middle-class [w]hite women."[15] That is racist and gross and is transparently just the moldy remnants of the last century's eugenicist thinking.

In 2016, the National Women's Health Network and SisterSong, an organization that works to "amplify the collective voices of Indigenous women and women of color to achieve reproductive justice," put out a joint statement on the perils of pushing LARCs on poor communities:

Too much LARC zeal can easily turn into coercion, becoming just the most recent in a long line of population control methods targeted to women of color, low-income, and uninsured women, indigenous women, immigrant women, women with disabilities, and people whose sexual expression is not respected. . . . Women report having their opinions ignored and their choices curtailed by clinicians, public health officials, and government programs. . . . We see this coercion play out when a program funds a free IUD but not its removal, when a clinic must meet a quota for LARC use or risk its own funding, and when a doctor tells a woman she's not responsible enough for a method she can control herself. . . . [W]e strongly support the inclusion of LARCs as part of a well-balanced mix of options, but we reject efforts to direct women toward any particular method. Only affordable coverage of all options—and a comprehensive, medically accurate, and culturally competent discussion of them—will . . . meet the health and life needs of every woman.[16]

Providing access to contraception is one thing, but trying to make decisions for people or pushing decisions on them is another. Yes, birth control is a technology that can improve your life if you want it, but so is air-conditioning, and we don't see massive campaigns to get disenfranchised people's houses hooked up with AC, do we? No. Nor do we see campaigns to get disenfranchised people proper nutrition or mental health care. Because the instinct to get people to have fewer kids is just as racist and classist and ableist now as it always has been. If we pushed AC on the oppressed with the fervor that we push birth control, it wouldn't be as offensive, but it would still be wrong and absurd. Offering is OK. Pushing is not. It is preposterous to think we can possibly know what is best for people whose lives are not our lives, whose struggles are not our struggles, whose joys are not our joys.

Oh, and in case you thought the sterilizations were over! In 2013, the Center for Investigative Reporting found that at least 148 people with pussies were sterilized by the California Department of Corrections and Rehabilitation from 2006 to 2010 and that there may have been as many as 100 more cases dating back to the 1990s. Former inmates and prisoner advocates said that the prison medical staff coerced the inmates into agreeing to the surgery, targeting especially those they thought were "likely to return to prison in the future."[17]

And then, in 2020, whistleblower Dawn Wooten, a nurse who worked at the Irwin County Detention Center in Georgia, alleged that a doctor who also worked for the facility was performing hysterectomies on detained migrants without consent. She said, "I've had several inmates tell me that they've been to see the doctor and they've had hysterectomies and they don't know why." When they did understand that the doctor intended to perform hysterectomies, "some of them a lot of times won't even go, they say they'll wait to get back to their country to go to the doctor."[18]

Fighting for People Means Getting Behind Them, Not in Front of Them

The best way to fight for the rights of others is to get behind the people who are already fighting for themselves and to amplify their voices. Not only has white-washed history left out all of the reproductive injustices people with pussies have been put through, but it has also erased the decades of valiant, organized, and systematic work by thousands of activists against those injustices. In trying to stand up for the causes of others, we must remember to take our cues from those affected in trying to understand both what those causes are in the first place and how to help.

The term *reproductive justice* was invented in 1994 by the Women of African Descent for Reproductive Justice, the precursor to SisterSong, a group that formed specifically because they "recognized that the women's rights movement, led by and representing middle class and wealthy white women, could not defend the needs of women of color and other marginalized women and trans people." SisterSong defines *reproductive justice* as "the human right to maintain personal bodily autonomy, have children, not have children, and parent the children we have in safe and sustainable communities."[19] In this case, the cue is to understand reproductive rights as one element in a group of inextricably linked issues, like environmental justice and police violence.

As Loretta J. Ross, survivor of sterilization abuse and one of the founders of SisterSong and creators of the concept of reproductive justice, put it in a speech in 2014:

Reproductive justice was powerful because it brought all of the tenets, all of the little tentacles of the game together in one analysis and said, "You cannot isolate abortion from all the other human rights issues out here, you cannot isolate refusing to let me be a parent from all the other human rights issues." . . . If we're talking about building a movement where everybody's at the table, then every issue must be at the table, and the issue most likely to be kicked off the table is the fundamental relationship between reproductive oppression and white supremacy.[20]

White feminists who do not have disabilities but who do have disproportionate leverage in deciding how the world works: hiiii! We really need to take history into account and expand our efforts and thinking and conversations. Let's move from a *reproductive rights* mostly about abortion and contraception to a broader human rights framework of *reproductive justice.* We must talk about the right to have babies when we talk about the right not to have them. We must talk about racism when we talk about sexism because we cannot smash The Patriarchy without smashing white supremacy. This means holding the lens of history up to all new public health campaigns and legislation, to ask ourselves if what we are really looking at is just the newest form of racist population control. And if it is that, it means saying so, loudly. But it mostly means getting behind organizations that are already doing this work.

To send money to SisterSong, visit https://sistersong.nationbuilder.com/donate.

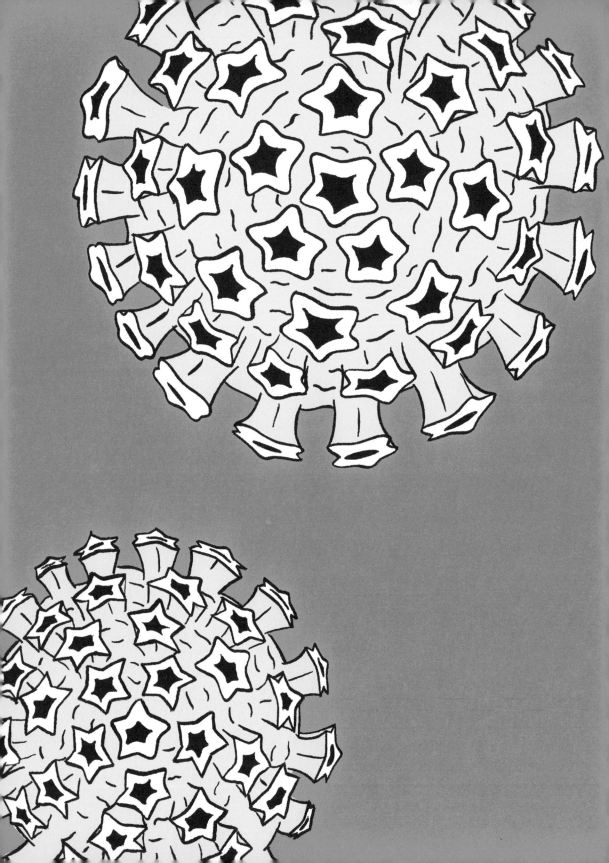

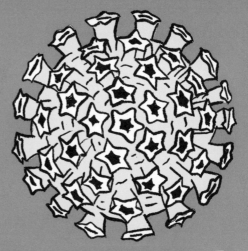

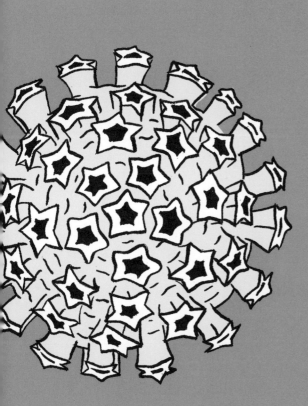

INFECTIONS

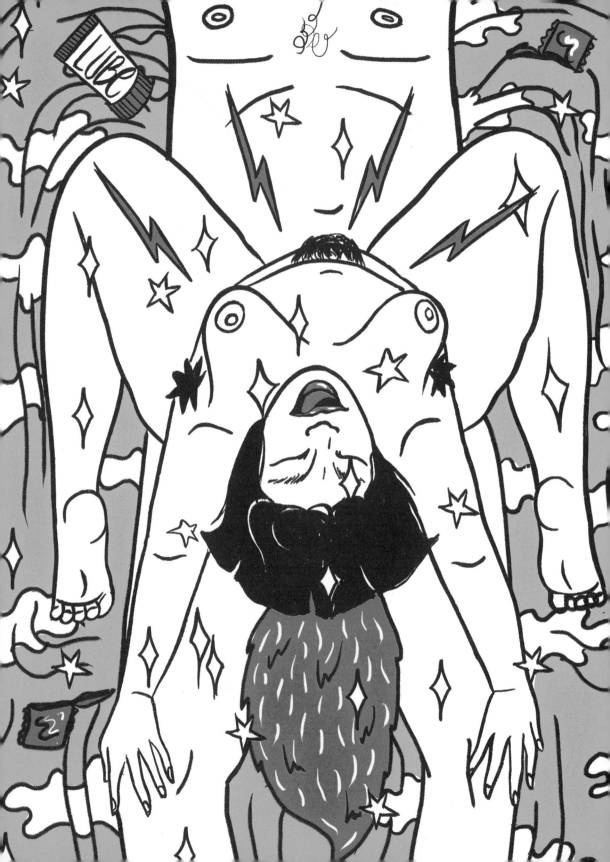

22
Safer/Funner Sex

A NOTE: SINCE I COVER HOW NOT TO GET PREGNANT IN CHAPTER 20, AND HOW TO navigate consent in Chapter 13, this chapter focuses on STI prevention in the context of consensual sexual activitay.

You've probably heard by now that, basically, to reduce your risk of contracting STIs, you need to cover certain body parts with condoms/dams/cots/gloves/barriers to avoid certain parts directly touching and/or exchanging fluids. But this chapter is not going to cover every type of barrier that prevents an infection, nor every type of contact that can transmit or contract an infection. There are many credible sources you can turn to for that information—see the resources listed at the end of this chapter.

I had a very decent sex education, both in school and from my mother. (She once barged in on a hang with my high school friends holding a dental dam that she proceeded to open, stretch over her mouth, and then lick enthusiastically while explaining, "Thbis bis hbow it wborks, okbkayy?!"). And, still, I have a terrible safer-sex track record. Knowing what measures were necessary to prevent myself from contracting STIs did not help me actually take those measures, so I want to talk about strategies and concepts that I think *would* have.

Why Aren't We (I) Making Better Safer-Sex Decisions?

A lot of the times I failed to have safer sex, it was simply because I couldn't get a man to use a condom. Even when I did work up the courage to tell men to put on a condom, I often couldn't put my foot down about it. (And many of those times, I didn't even really want to have sex in the first place but felt the need to go through with it or felt like it was just easier to do it than not to.) I deferred to men and let them do what they wanted because The Patriarchy taught me to. Many studies have shown how traditionally passive, feminine gender roles lead to less condom use and more STI transmission (and also less pleasure).[1,2,3,4,5] It makes a lot of sense. The Patriarchy tells people with pussies: *Be amenable and prioritize the wants and needs of men over yours or else you're an undesirable bitch!* So demanding that a partner use protection can be really, really hard.

But one 2008 study of 430 undergrads in the US showed that learning feminist ideology that deconstructed gender roles helped people with pussies negotiate for condom use (and more pleasure).[6] So maybe when you find yourself in that moment—when you want to ask or insist that someone use protection—it might help to remember why it feels so hard to demand what is your gosh-given right (yet again, The Patriarchy!).

It doesn't matter if it's sex work, a one-night stand, or with a partner you've been having unprotected sex with for years: you *always* have the right to have safer sex. Don't let anyone lead you away from that truth.

It's shocking to think back on how many otherwise "decent" men were entirely willing to push back *very hard* against using condoms when I asked them to. It's a very normalized behavior. But don't let how common it is confuse you: common ≠ normal ≠ OK. Even if the person you're with is "nice" in general, if they push for anything less than the level of protection you're asking for, they're being an asshole. You have the right to request any safer-sex provision in any situation, anytime. (And: "Let me just put it in a little and then I'll put the condom on," a.k.a. the Just the Tip tactic, is not a real compromise, no matter what tone of voice it is uttered in.)

If anyone sneaks off a condom during sex, that is a form of rape—though it may be hard, or impossible, to prosecute in the US. Still, get in touch with the sexual assault hotline listed in this chapter's resources section so you can take steps to get some physical and emotional care.

OK, but what about the many, many times that my failure to use protection was 100% on me? I've always known that condoms should be used for blow jobs, but I have never in my life even tried to put a condom on a penis before sticking it in my mouth. And I've never once used protection with someone with a pussy. To make a nonscientific statement: nobody fucking uses dental dams. And since that's the norm,[7] I kind of just always went along with it. ¯_(ಠ益ಠ)_/¯ (Sorry, Mom.) And you know what? These decisions put me in pretty plentiful company.[8,9]

Once, while conducting interviews about sex and dating culture in the Philippines, I asked a young man if he thought that Catholicism (famously anti–birth control) was the reason people there often opt against condoms. He smiled and said, "I think it's just, 'cause, um . . . it feels better," prompting a bunch of people sitting around us to laugh at how foolish my question had been. It's funny, but it's not a factor to be ignored. In 2013, Bill and Melinda Gates were so convinced that a better-feeling condom would help curb the spread of infections that they offered up $100,000 to anyone who could make a condom that felt good.[10]

So there's that. Protection doesn't feel as good as no protection or, at least, a lot of people have that idea . . . and honestly, while some sex educators may hate me for saying this, I'm one of them. With penis-in-vagina sex, as long as a condom is lubed up enough, it's totally the same for me. But I really never want to put a condom in my mouth to give a blow job. That's just unappealing. And don't even get me started on flavored lube. Also, there's just no way in hell that licking a dental dam is going to be as awesome as getting your face just, like, all up in a pussy. I think it would be a form of gaslighting not to acknowledge that. And yet! All that direct contact is just the way infections get spread.

Because it can seem like protection and pleasure are diametrically opposed, there's a movement in the sex education and public health worlds to start making pleasure a bigger part of the safer-sex conversation.[11,12,13] Studies have shown that when we don't talk about pleasure when we talk about sex, it has a negative impact on people with pussies' ability to negotiate for safer sex.[14,15]

Most sex ed only ever talks about risk and makes sex seem scary. I mean, yes, the risk is always real. That's why it's a new Thing to say *safer* sex instead of *safe* sex. But legitimizing pleasure as a motivation to have sex can help reframe sex from something that we do *for others* to something that we do *for ourselves*, and, therefore, something that should happen in a way that we feel good about. Secondly, legitimizing the desire for pleasure in the first place is important because pussy pleasure is still a taboo that causes shame.

When we talk only about risk, we further the idea that sex is a Bad thing to do, which also causes shame. Fear and shame don't help people make good sexual health decisions. Shame is the key actor that we want to eliminate. We know, for example, that shame and STI stigma lead people not to seek treatment when they find out they have an STI (see Chapter 23). So I think it's very possible that simply feeling ashamed and freaked out is enough to make people freeze in the moment and avoid safer-sex conversations or not stick up for themselves when it comes to protection.

This is sad because not only is safer sex safer, it's *funner*! I know, I know: all of what I've just said seems to contradict that. But protection and pleasure are not actually a trade-off. Because, at the end of the day, don't you have more fun when you're not worrying? I definitely get more pleasure when I'm not stressed about transmitting or contracting an STI because I can be more present in the sensations in my body. I'm not saying I would opt for a condom in my mouth over worrying, I'm saying I would opt for approaching the whole situation proactively and intentionally.

If you're like me and you're like, *No, I'm never going to put a condom in my mouth*, and/or like, *No, licking latex is not the same as getting your face in a pussy*, then safer sex comes down to being informed, assessing risk consciously, and deciding which dicks to stick in your mouth and which pussies to stick your mouth on. Let's talk about what goes into those decisions.

The Risk Spectrum

Risk exists on a spectrum. Some things are riskier than others, in terms of STI transmission: penis-in-vagina-without-a-condom sex is riskier than, say, making out with someone; sticking your face in the pussy of someone who has had sex with lots of people since last getting tested is riskier than sticking your face in the pussy of someone who just got tested and has told you their status.

Sex educator Melina Gaze explained to me that people's comfort with risk also exists on a spectrum. You might be a very risk-averse person who does not want to take any chances with STIs, or you might feel like the benefit you get from not using protection is worth the risk of contracting an infection. Where you are on that risk spectrum is different from person to person, and it can also be different for any given person from moment to moment.

Rather than making decisions in the moment, or being horrified by your decisions after you make them (lol, my life), be proactive about these considerations and know where you stand. It's helpful to actively think about both where you have historically stood on that spectrum and where you'd ideally like to stand on it in the future. Getting out ahead of yourself can help you make decisions you feel better about in the moment.

There are factors that can lead you away from where you'd like to stand on the risk spectrum. For example, alcohol, which—LOL, WOW—um, *really* changes the amount of risk I'm willing to take.

I'm not going to tell you to not get drunk. But maybe try to develop some kind of negotiation mechanism with yourself? Try to have a mindful moment before making sexual contact, and be like, *OK, so this is my drunk self, but I am going to decide to make safer-sex decisions as if I were not drunk!* I never did this with safer sex, but I did manage to stop pretending I was rich and taking cabs home from bars when I was living in New York City and actually broke as shit. So I believe in the technique.

Other factors can come into play too. What if you really like someone and really want them to like you back? Or what if the chemistry is randomly fire and things are super hot in the moment? Or what if you are depressed? Or what if you are ecstatically happy? Take a moment and check in with yourself and remember where you've decided you want to stand on the risk spectrum. Also check in with yourself about whether there is some factor that consistently leads you away from your ideal spot on the risk spectrum. Figure out if it's something you can address.

Everyone has a right to take risks, but no one has a right to intentionally impose risk on others. Everyone also has the right to have sex that is exactly as safe as they want it to be. So it's a cool idea to talk about where you are on the risk spectrum with your partners and to mutually decide what level of risk you want to take together. If a partner wants to take less risk than you, then you should adopt their bar for what you decide to do together.

Talking About STIs Before Sex Can Be Seriously Awkward but You Should Do It Anyway

My asshole ex, The Waxer from Chapter 1, didn't disclose to me before we had unprotected sex that he knew he had herpes, even though I asked if he had any STIs. I was furious when he finally told me because he had made the decision for me. There had been no informed consent, and therefore, what he did—intentionally give me false information to make me more likely to have unprotected sex with him—is a form of coercion.

Here's where it gets more complicated. When I met my now husband, I had never had an outbreak, but I had also not been tested for herpes. I did not tell him before we had unprotected sex that I had been exposed to herpes. He didn't ask, but I should have told him anyway.

If you have an infection or if you think you've been exposed to an infection and haven't been tested or gotten your results yet, you should tell people if you're going to be doing activities that could give them that infection. Like I said, a person has the right to decide for themselves if they want to take a risk. This idea is part of informed consent (see Chapter 13 for more on what that is and why it's important).

I know disclosing can feel horrible and put you in a very vulnerable position. But don't let awkwardness make you avoid the disclosure conversation altogether because besides the fact that you should tell them for *them*, informed consent through mutual disclosure is in *your* interest too; you don't want to get an additional infection. (If you think it will be more than emotional vulnerability, i.e., that the person might physically harm you, do what you need to do for your personal safety, even if that means not disclosing.)

This stuff is difficult and not always clear-cut. But here's a rule of thumb that might help you make good decisions: Be generous. If you're not sure if you should tell a partner something or not, tell them. (Again, your physical safety comes first though!)

Asking, "Are you clean?" is a shitty way of trying to have a disclosure conversation. First of all, the term *clean* perpetuates stigma—are you dirty if you have an STI? Also, it's a yes-or-no question and one that is, in the vast majority of cases, almost impossible for anyone to truly know the answer to. You need more information than a yes or no to make an assessment about what kind of risk engaging sexually with someone represents. Also, people are more likely to lie to you if they think you will judge them.

Bringing it up in a way that doesn't shame anyone for having an STI can help both: 1) up your chances that the other person will be honest, and 2) not contribute to overall STI stigma in the world. You can go first. Offer your most recent STI testing history, level of risk taken since that round of testing, and any STIs you know you have or think you have been exposed to since testing. Then ask the other person to disclose the same. They have the right not to, and may not, in which case you'll have to factor the lack of information into your risk assessment. If you want to ease in before getting down to the very personal details, you could ask someone how they feel about safer sex and testing in general.

If someone tells you they have an STI, the least awkward and most respectful way to respond is probably to just thank them for telling you. You can ask if they are receiving treatment for it and try to assess what will or won't put you at risk of contracting it. You can take your time to decide and respond. If you decide you don't want to have sexual contact with that person, consider that the rejection will likely feel shitty for them no matter how nice you are, so try to be sweet about it!

If you're planning to meet someone off an app, you might take advantage of the less awkwardness of communicating over the internet to have the disclosure conversation before you meet up. Sure, it might spoil the illusion that you're "not really there to see if you want to have sex with each other," but that particular awkwardness might be less than the awkwardness of having a disclosure conversation in person or especially after you've already started hooking up. Even if you're not sure you want sex, having had that chat can't hurt. Having a disclosure conversation does not have to mean you're definitely going to have sex.

I was a pretty giant slut for about 15 years and literally zero people ever initiated an STI-disclosure conversation with me. So I'm going to make the very scientific conclusion that you are probably going to have to start these conversations yourself if you want them to happen. (See Chapter 13 for more on consent and awkwardness.) I won't tell you it's cute or fun or something that can be made sexy. It's just really important.

Disclosing HIV in the Context of Sex—Not the Same

HIV is a different case. It carries a lot of stigma, but there are medications (antiretroviral therapies) that, when taken correctly, make a person with HIV's viral loads completely undetectable, which means that the virus is completely untransmittable. According to the National Institutes of Health, there is an "overwhelming body of clinical evidence" to back up this fact.[16] Because the stigma is so much stronger than with other STIs, disclosing an HIV-positive status can have much more serious ramifications. There is a growing movement against the idea that people with undetectable HIV should have to disclose their status. We don't make people disclose that they have diabetes—because the other person isn't going to get diabetes from sexual contact. This is why it is especially fucked up that people who have HIV that's untransmittable can, in some states, be criminally prosecuted for not disclosing their status.[17]

My friend Jesus Herrera is HIV positive, and he doesn't feel the need to disclose for the sake of the other person's health, since he knows he can't transmit the virus, but does so anyway for a different reason: "Based on the other person's reaction, I know how educated they are on the subject. It's a filter I use to see who is supportive, who is ashamed, who I would be willing to spend more time with. That said, I have a high level of self-esteem and a privileged life. People who don't but are still undetectable and are just trying to live normal lives—I think should have every right to not say anything."

One Quick Safer-Sex Technique-Thing

USE. LUBE. USE SO MUCH LUBE. SQUIRT THAT SHIT EVERYWHERE. USE IT AS TOOTHPASTE (JK). But seriously, not enough people talk about lube in the context of safer sex. Lube not only makes everything feel way better, it makes it safer because it reduces friction and possible micro-tears in tissue and breakage in barriers, which means fewer entry points for any possible STIs. (Spit is not as good as lube at doing lube's job! Also, it can spread infections.)[18]

Some people use oils, like coconut oil or CBD-infused oils, which have gotten popular recently, marketed as lubes. Oil is NOT compatible with latex, so using oil-based lubes with most condoms/dental dams/gloves is not safe. Here are some things to NOT USE with latex condoms:

- Cold cream/hand cream/body lotion
- Olive/peanut/corn/sunflower/canola/coconut/baby oil
- Butter/margarine
- Cocoa butter
- Massage oil
- Petroleum jelly (e.g., Vaseline)
- Any vaginal medications you may be using that contain mineral oil[19]

A few more weird lube-safety things you might not think of:

- Check to see if you are allergic to anything in a lube before you use it.
- Don't use a lube with lidocaine or benzocaine, which are numbing agents, if you're not using that lube because of a chronic-pain problem. If something causes pain during sex, being able to feel it is safer than being numbed.[18]
- Don't use lube with spermicide. That shit is not good for your vagina party. (See Chapter 32 about why.)
- Using lubes with sex toys is a little complicated. See the table in Chapter 16 for more on what lubes can be used with which materials.

Let's Normalize Masturbating Next to Each Other

All of this chapter has been about activities that can spread infections . . . but what about activities that can't spread infections?

There are so many things to do with people that can give you a lot of pleasure and are unlikely to transmit infections. One of those things is to masturbate next to someone. The first time Melina mentioned this to me as a safer-sex practice, my head exploded. I can think of so many times when, had I simply been like, "Hey, want to masturbate next to each other?" both the other person and I would have had a way better time.

How many times have I wanted to have a fun experience with someone and get off but not quite felt comfortable sharing fluids with them, and then proceeded to have paranoid and not-that-enjoyable sex with them anyway? How many times was I horny enough to want to come but not exactly horny enough to really want to have sex with the person I ended up having sex with, even if

I enjoyed their company and did feel safe sharing fluids with them? How many times did I find myself with a partner with whom I had terrible chemistry and we both exhausted ourselves trying to get each other off, to no avail? How many times had I just been kind of fucking tired but also, yes, still horny enough to want to come but, like, quickly? Damn! I could have been masturbating!

Really, though it may still be uncommon, I think that, if presented with the option, a lot of people might be stoked. Kind of like how when you cancel on people, they're often secretly elated.

Even if you make out with someone while you're both masturbating, it's still less of a risk than penetrative sex. You can scale risk up and down with the amount of contact. Like, you could masturbate each other too and avoid sharing fluids by washing hands or even wearing gloves between touching yourself and your partner. There's also sexting and phone sex, which, without doing the research, I feel confident saying have a 0% risk of transmission, unless you stick your phone up someone's vagina or butt, in which case . . . I'm not sure that qualifies as "phone sex" anymore.

RESOURCES

For information on barrier methods and what kinds of contact transmit STIs:

- scarleteen.com/article/bodies/safe_sound_sexy_a_safer_sex_howto
- pussypedia.net/articles/safer-sex-barrier-methods
- ourbodiesourselves.org/book-excerpts/health-article/top-ten-safer-sex-tips/
- ashasexualhealth.org/safer-sex-toolbox/
- cdc.gov/hiv/basics/hiv-transmission/increase-hiv-risk.html

Safe Sex for Trans Bodies—an amazingly detailed primer from the Human Rights Watch Campaign Foundation and Whitman Walker Health:

- assets2.hrc.org/files/assets/resources/Trans_Safer_Sex_Guide_FINAL.pdf

A guide to safer sexting for teens that's good for everyone:

- plannedparenthood.org/learn/teens/bullying-safety-privacy/all-about
  -sexting

If you have been sexually assaulted or want to talk to someone about sexual assault:

- Rape, Abuse and Incest National Hotline
    1.800.656.HOPE (4673) | www.rainn.org
- National Domestic Violence Hotline
    1.800.799.SAFE (7233) or 1.800.787.3224 | www.thehotline.org

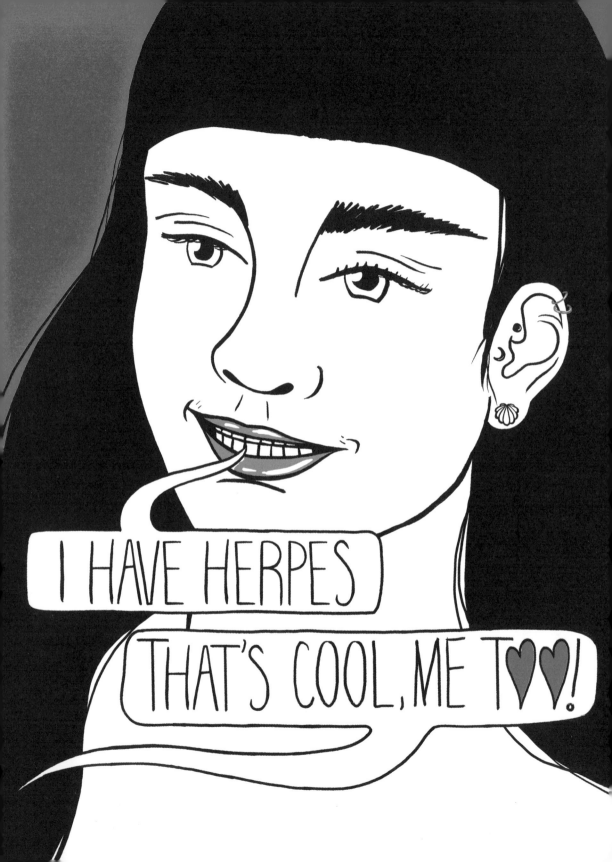

23
STI Stigma and Shame

STI STIGMA IS OUTDATED AND LITERALLY BAD FOR EVERYONE'S HEALTH. I PRO-pose we cancel it. It is caused by taboos that we collectively enforce. We believe them, so they are real. That is why STIs are embarrassing. The cool part is that if we don't believe them, they become not real. If people unsubscribe to the taboo around STIs, they will become less embarrassing, cause less shame, and be less bad for our health.

A Fake History of STI Stigma That We Don't Need

A long list of major publications have run almost-identical articles, all titled something like *How Big Pharma Helped Create Herpes Stigma to Sell Drugs* and all based on the same very few bits of evidence. (I would call out these major publications, but they happen to be the same publications that I hope will run articles promoting this book.) I will tell you about those very few bits of evidence shortly, but first I want to get on a soapbox real quick.

People, we do not need STI stigma to have been invented by Big Pharma to decide it doesn't serve us anymore and tell it to have a nice life. In fact, we have an even better reason to do so. We know how common STIs are. We don't stigmatize people for contracting the common cold, yet we stigmatize people for contracting very common STIs. Because we don't shame people for getting any single other kind of infection, what the shame around STIs really comes down to is shaming people for having sex, which . . . we're all past that, right? It's very silly. OK, moving on.

The story about herpes stigma being invented by Big Pharma would truly suit my political motivations—to stick it to The Man—were the story not so flimsy and overblown. Here are the facts: There was a company called Burroughs Wellcome that developed Zovirax (now known as aciclovir), a drug for herpes, in the 1980s. Their then head of research and development wrote years later that, at the time, the company's marketing department didn't believe there was a market for the drug.[1] So, in 1986, the company began an aggressive marketing campaign, running full-page ads in national magazines from *People* to *Playboy*. The ads did not mention the drug. They just told readers that herpes can be treated. A spokesperson from Burroughs told a newspaper at the time, "The intent is to encourage people with herpes to visit their physician . . . because [herpes] had a reputation for being an untreatable, incurable disease."[2]

And . . . that's the whole thing. I think this story is very far from amounting to "Big Pharma invented herpes stigma." I think the story got so much traction because it's exciting to think we've discovered The Man doing some shady shit. But, as readers, we have to be careful to maintain healthy skepticism with stories that our hearts want to root for. Just because something challenges widely accepted truths about culture or big institutions does not mean it is well reported or true.

Here's just one reason to believe herpes stigma was alive and well before Burroughs Wellcome: in 1986, the *Sun Sentinel* published an article commenting on the Zovirax ad campaign. The first sentence reads, "In the early 1980s, fear of herpes approached hysteria."[2] I would definitely classify *nearly hysterical fear of something that is fairly benign* as evidence of existing stigma. Here's another: four years before the ad campaign, in 1982, *Time* magazine ran a cover story about herpes, called "The New Scarlet Letter." Here's another: all three of my living grandparents say there's been stigma around "venereal disease" for as long as they can remember. It's likely that STI stigma in Western cultures is at least as old as sex stigma (which is, like, at least as old as the Old Testament), since humans have known since ancient times that STIs were caused by sex.[3] So while Big Pharma may do a whole lot of evil shit, blaming it for STI stigma is a red herring. We need to look inward to move onward.

STI Stigma Is Bad for Everyone's Health

Of course nobody wants to have an infection that causes painful sores on your genitals. It's not like I expect people to celebrate STIs. But social stigma makes the physical sores a mere fraction of an STI's symptoms. The anxiety and shame people experience around STIs makes having them way, way worse than it needs to be.

One study with a modest sample size reported that 62% of people with genital herpes reported "severe psychological distress." Severe psychological distress can make any physical symptoms you're having get way worse and weaken your immune system, which can make it harder for your body to fight any STI you might have contracted.[4]

There's also a mountain of evidence that stigma and shame cause people both to not get tested for STIs and then, once they have tested positive for an STI, to not seek care or to delay seeking care.[5,6,7,8,9,10,11] We would presumably rather forgo treatment that would make us feel better and protect our bodies and keep us from possibly infecting others than deal with the embarrassment and social consequences of having an STI. When we make that decision, we effectively choose to avoid judgment that is unfair in the first place over protecting our own health and one another's. This is so facepalm and so sad.

Let's Undo STI Stigma

I know that knowing, understanding, and being able to talk about *why* something is bad doesn't necessarily make that thing easy to #unsubscribe from. For example, just because 16-, 20-, or 25-year-old me could have articulated perfectly well that sex negativity is puritanical bullshit, and just because based on that political belief I gave myself license to have a lot of sex doesn't mean I didn't also feel shame around the sex I had or the number of sexual partners I had. I still have an ugly little patriarchal black-hatted Puritan that sits on my shoulder occasionally and calls me a slut. And without any data to back me up, I'll go out on a limb here and say: I don't think I'm the only one.

My point is that undoing STI stigma is going to be hard, even if we can explain to ourselves why we should undo the stigma. The easy part is how we treat others: we can stop making jokes about STIs and we can refrain from making fun of or gossiping about anyone else's STI. The harder part is how we treat ourselves. I'm not going to tell anyone with an STI, "Just stop being embarrassed!" I know it's not that simple. I've had some supremely awkward moments disclosing HPV, and the stigma that HPV has is nowhere close to the stigma of other STIs like herpes and HIV. But having someone react badly to any disclosure can sting and stick with you.

Still, we should try to #unsubscribe from the stigma around STIs, both for others and for ourselves. We should always keep in mind the goal of letting go of the shame.

One thing that helps me kill the shame monsters is to remember how irrational and unfair this stigma and imposed shame is, and to summon my indignance: hell no, The Patriarchy will not make me feel bad. I have shit to do!

Another thing that has helped me move past STI shame is to talk casually about my HPV with friends, and especially meeting others who talk publicly, openly, and directly about their STIs. Chatting with my friends about my HPV has helped me move past the shame not just because in this way I've learned that most of my friends have HPV too but also because saying it out loud helps normalize it. I find that the more I say it, the less weird it feels.

But the most powerful thing that has helped me overcome shame is meeting other people who have genuinely gotten over theirs. Once you get over your shame, you have the superpower of helping to heal others of theirs.

That's why talking publicly about your STIs is a subversive public service, an act of resistance, and something we can all do to smash The Patriarchy. I learned that from Caitlin Donohue, journalist and author of *She Represents: 44 Women Who Are Changing Politics and the World*, who wrote in a 2014 article for *Rookie*, "Today, if someone were to call me names for being STI positive, I would never apologize but, instead, bid them adieu like any other asshole in my life. It's a pretty good deal when I think about it: Yeah, I caught herpes, but I got rid of jerks . . . and got to join my very first secret society! Although I'm very glad the secret's out now."[12]

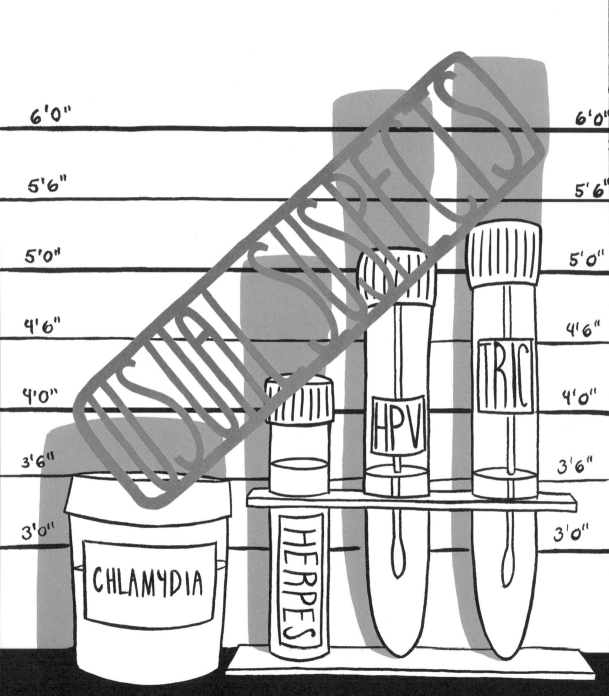

24
The Usual Suspects

I'm not sure we should call STIs *sexually transmitted infections*. STIs are just infections that you most commonly get from sexytime. We could just call them *infections*. What other kinds of infections do we name after how they are transmitted? Have you ever heard of *Dirty ATM Button Followed by Eye Rubbing Infections (DABFBERI)?* No. It seems shamey and kinda rude to be like, *You have this infection and YOU GOT IT FROM SEX*. Unnecessary, amiright? Anyway, there's an array of infections out there that you can get from sex. We're just going to review a few of the usual suspects.

A Note to People with Pussies Who Have Sex with Other People with Pussies (PWPWHSWOPWP)

Yes, there is research that showed that rates of some STIs were lower among PWPWHSWOPWP.[1] But it is old! And now there are a lot more PWPWHSWO-PWP, and many of those PWPWHSWOPWP don't exclusively HSWOPWP.[2] That may mean more pussies on the sex market but it also might mean more STIs in the PWPWHSWOPWP germosphere because all kinds of folks are in the mix. The Lord giveth, and the Lord taketh away, y'all! I've not seen a single public health institution recommend fewer safer-sex practices or less testing for

PWPWHSWOPWP. So however few penises you come into contact with, it's still good to be STI-knowledgeable and alert.

Chlamydia

Since 1994, chlamydia has been the most common STI reported to the Centers for Disease Control and Prevention (CDC).[3] Chlamydia is a bacterial infection that is treatable with antibiotics. In 2016, 1.5 million people in the US tested positive for chlamydia.[4] And between 2014 and 2018, cases in the US went up by 15%.[5]

Chlamydial infections in pussies most often do not have symptoms.[3,4] When they do, they will be different depending on where the bacteria are living. You can get pain in your urethra, anus, or cervix. You can get itchy. It can hurt to pee. You might also have a change or increase in discharge.[4] It's a good idea to get tested for chlamydia if you have any of the symptoms mentioned above, and often even when you don't. Because, left untreated, it can cause pelvic inflammatory disease (PID), which can be very painful and lead to fertility problems.[3,4]

Human Papillomavirus (HPV)

Human papillomavirus (HPV) is a mega-common viral infection with over 100 different strains, about 40 of which infect genitals.[6] At least half of sexually active people will get HPV at least once.[7] One survey cited by the CDC found that, during 2013 and 2014, 42.5% of US adults had it.[8]

Here is a nonscientific opinion: We are all WAY too freaked out about HPV. Public health campaigns have drilled it into our minds that HPV is running rampant and can cause cancer. I know way too many people who have freaked the fuck out about getting it. But here's the truth: It is not a particularly dangerous infection. It is often entirely without symptoms.[6] Yes, some strains can cause cancer, but it usually takes more than 10 years of no treatment for cell changes from HPV to become cancerous.[9] A whopping 90% of HPV infections will clear up on their own within one or two years.[6,10] Ya just need to let your doctor keep an eye on it. That's all!

That said, yes, some strains can cause warts. They are contagious, but not harmful beyond the anxiety and shame they can provoke.[6,11] Also, only a small fraction of HPV infections cause warts. One 2013 review of international studies found that, overall, between 1 and 4% of people with pussies had warts caused by HPV.[11]

There are vaccines available for HPV. Vaccines are helpful, safe, and save lives. The HPV vaccine does not have dangerous side effects, despite what you might hear on the playground.[7] That said, many insurance companies won't cover it past age 26 because the CDC doesn't think it's particularly helpful for people any older, anyway.[12] It's pretty expensive without insurance. Here's the good news: If you are getting Pap smears every one to three years, you probably don't need to worry about whether or not you have HPV. (See more on why in Chapter 25.) Besides the vaccine, there's really no other way to protect against getting HPV. Condoms help but are not a sure bet.[7]

If your Pap smear shows irregularities, still no cause for alarm. If you've been diligent about your smears, the first instance of something irregular is almost certainly nothing to freak out about. Your doctor will probably want to do a colposcopy, which I've had and is truly not scary. Basically they just get a really good look at your vagina and cervix with a light and some pussy-binocular thingies—it takes all of, like, 15 minutes.[13] Then, if they see anything they want to look at more closely, they may take a little sample of it so they can get it analyzed. If they do that, and they don't love what they see, guess what, you STILL don't need to get freaked out. They will likely want to do either cryotherapy (using cold) or LEEP (using a little electric wire) to get rid of the funky cells. Both treatments are over 85% effective, and neither requires a hospital stay. Also, neither should be more than mildly painful. Some people even say they don't hurt at all.[14,15] After treatment, it will be important to go get checked out to make sure the funky cells are gone.

There has been some research that has shown decreased sexual pleasure and satisfaction after LEEP procedures. The last review of studies on the topic hypothesized that these effects were caused not by LEEP but instead by the psychological stress of having been diagnosed with and treated for a stigmatized infection: "Treatment of vulvar and cervical dysplasia can contribute to a sense of loss of control over one's body and anxiety concerning personal and genital health, can influence body image and self-esteem, and can raise questions of trust and loyalty in sexual partnerships. All of these factors can be detrimental for a woman's emotional, sexual and overall well-being."[16]

I have mixed feelings about their explanation. It might be totally true. Their scientific reasoning for arriving at it by scrutinizing the design of each study that showed negative effects checks out. As I explain in Chapter 23, STI stigma does cause lots of psychological stress that can exacerbate physical symptoms. And we know that kind of stress is bad for sexual pleasure. But this explanation is also ringing the hysteria alarm bell in my brain—even if it's not blaming people with pussies. I just worry it lets Science off the hook for investing in more research about the physiology of the issue, into making sure LEEP is safe. Especially because there's lots of anecdotal evidence out there—people telling their own stories who say they experienced a physical change in their bodies after the procedure. The literature review concludes that more research is needed. It is, indeed.

Herpes

As Patty McInnis wrote for the "Herpes" article on Pussypedia.net, "Staying ignorant about herpes is kinda like if you wanna slice of pizza, but aren't sure if you have enough cash and you're too scared to check, so you just don't. And you don't get any pizza, even though you actually had enough money for a whole pie."

Herpes has an outsize stigma in relation to how harmful it is to your body, which is: not very.[17]

There's two kinds of herpes: HSV-1 and HSV-2. It used to be said that HSV-1 was "oral herpes" and HSV-2 was "genital herpes," but researchers have found that HSV-1 can live on both your mouth and your crotch.[17] HSV-2 lives only on the crotch.[18] Both are transmitted by skin-to-skin contact, which can happen even when the person spreading HSV-1 or HSV-2 has no symptoms. Once you have herpes, its symptoms come and go in bouts called *outbreaks*, when little sores that look like blisters or pimples appear.[17] The outbreak may be burny or itchy. The first outbreak is usually the worst. In some cases, you may get a fever, headache, or swollen glands. Subsequent outbreaks are usually less intense and uncomfortable.[17,19] There are antiviral drugs that you can take to help with symptoms, to reduce the number of outbreaks you got, and to reduce your likelihood of spreading the infection to others. These drugs don't cure herpes, but they do help.[19] With or without drugs, over time you will probably get fewer and fewer outbreaks.[17]

If you get herpes, you're in extremely good company. About half of the US population has HSV-1 and almost one in eight people have HSV-2.[20]

Trichomoniasis

Trichomonas vaginalis is the bacteria behind the world's most common non-viral, bacterial STI. It is a sneaky, tiny beast. The national prevalence of it among people with pussies is only 3%, but that figure is 14% for people around ages 13–19 and 27% for the country's "urban, inner-city population" (which is a rude, fancy phrase people use to avoid saying "poor people who are not white"). Among people with pussies who get trichomoniasis, 85% of them have no symptoms at first, but a third of them will have symptoms within six months of infection. Symptoms might include weird-colored or weird-smelling discharge, pain from peeing, and abdominal pain.[21] Trichomoniasis itself isn't that dangerous, but researchers have found that it can greatly increase someone's likelihood of getting and transmitting HIV.[21,22] Luckily, trichomoniasis is treatable with antibiotics.[23]

A Note About Gonorrhea, HIV, Syphilis, and Hepatitis B and C

Yes, you could get these STIs, but they are not the "usual suspects" because they are very uncommon among people with pussies. We're not going to review their symptoms and treatments here because I spent most of my life with an intense fear of all these STIs, which never actually translated to awesome safer sex or testing practices. We know that, in general, fear and shame do not lead to better self-care when it comes to STIs (see Chapter 23). Also, this is one of the few topics for which there is plenty of good information on the internet (check out Scarleteen, the CDC, and the Mayo Clinic).

So I'm going to go over how uncommon these STIs are, and then I'm going to tell you to have safer sex and get tested more often. OK? OK.

- **Gonorrhea:** In 2018, about 0.144% of people with pussies in the US got gonorrhea.[24]
- **HIV:** During 2018, only 0.0048% of people with pussies in the US got infected with HIV.[25]

- **Syphilis:** In 2017, only 0.0023% of people with pussies in the US got infected with syphilis, though this rate rose 21.1% during 2016/17 and might still be going up.[26]
- **Hepatitis:** Between 2015 and 2018, 3.4% of people with pussies had ever had hepatitis B.[27] Hepatitis C rates are going up because of the increased needle sharing that came with the opioid crisis, but, still, in 2017, only 0.009% of US people with pussies got it.[28]

One thing to keep in mind about these numbers is that most are based on reported cases, which means a lot of people's infections don't get counted. Also, if you are sharing needles or are having sex with people with penises who have sex with other people with penises, you are likely at a higher risk for the infections mentioned above.

And now to the PSA I promised: Don't dwell on being freaked out about STIs. There are a lot of them out there. Even more than the ones on this list. Some are almost impossible to avoid, some you are incredibly unlikely to encounter. Yes, you might get one. And while that will almost certainly not be a fun part of your life, it is highly unlikely that any STI will kill you or even take away your chance of having a long, fun, happy sex life.

Fear and anxiety are just drains on the energy and attention you need to be a more awesome caretaker of yourself. Focus on learning about, engaging in, and then asking partners to engage in safer-sex practices (more on this in Chapter 22). Focus on getting yourself to get tested with a frequency that corresponds to your personal level of risk—as well as you can assess that (more on this in Chapter 25). Focus on self-respect and how to put that into action. And wash your hands after using ATMs!

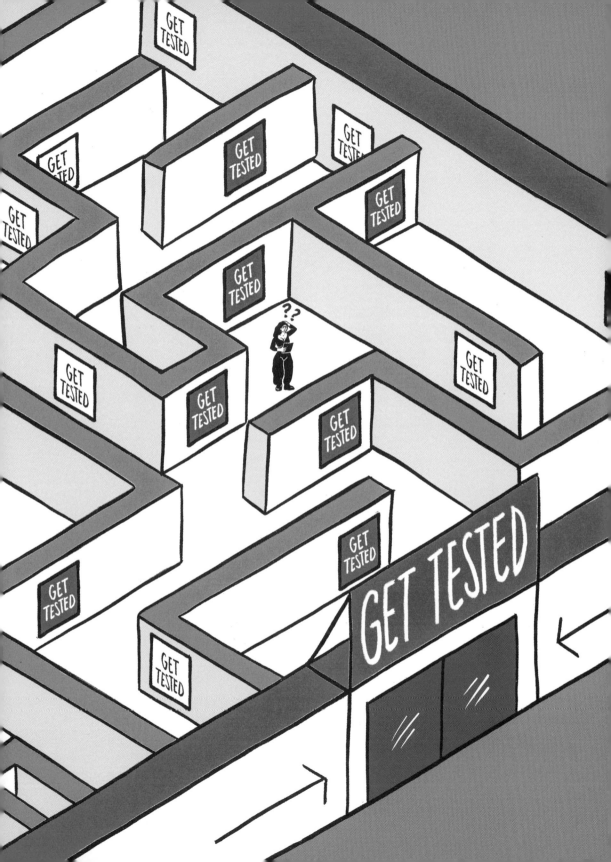

25
What to Get Tested For and When

THE MESSAGING OF *GET TESTED OR YOU'RE FAILING AT ADULTING* HAS BECOME a kind of abusive voice in my head, and I want to tell you that if you're suffering from guilt because you don't know how exactly to obey that voice, you are not alone. Get tested how often and for what?!

Disclosure and testing are heavily, insistently recommended by public health professionals, but there's also a lack of norms and protocols around both practices.

There are materials online for health care providers to help them recommend what patients should be tested for, but precious little information for actual human people trying to figure out for themselves what the hell to get tested for and how often. And then there are a lot of recommendations out there that are just not realistic. *Our Bodies, Ourselves*, for example, recommends getting screened before each new partner. I'm a huge fan of their book and project . . . but I need, like . . . 17 more ellipses here . . . to express how impractical this recommendation is.[1] It's a common recommendation, actually, but it fails to acknowledge how rarely sex is a preplanned activity. *Girl Sex 101* recommends getting tested about two weeks after each new partner or every six to eight months if you're otherwise healthy,[2] which also kind of breaks my brain.

And, still, most sources don't specify what to get tested for.

The First Few Times I Tried to Get Tested for STIs Went Like This

Zoe: Hi, I'm a grown-ass, responsible-ass bitch, and I would like to get tested for STIs.

Clinic person/doctor: OK, for what?

Zoe: I don't know. Everything?

Clinic: Everything? Like, including what?

Zoe: Um . . . [*Lists all the STIs she's ever heard of.*]

Clinic: OK, that's going to be seven tests and one million dollars.

Zoe: OK . . . I guess just herpes and HPV?

Clinic: Do you have herpes symptoms?

Zoe: No.

Clinic: OK, you probably don't need that test, then.

Zoe: Oh, OK. I guess just HPV, then?

Clinic: We don't really test for that; because of your age we just assume you have it.

Zoe: Well, what do you usually test people for?

Clinic: Depends. You have to confess to every bad thing you've ever done, and then we'll tell you what to get tested for.

Zoe: OK . . . [*Ends up paying a lot of money to get tested for chlamydia and gonorrhea, which she was already 99.999% sure she didn't have. Leaves feeling like a poorly behaved child and still really wondering if she has HPV or herpes.*]

We hear so much about how common herpes and HPV are and about how easy they are to unknowingly spread. We hear about how HPV can give you cancer. But when we show up to get tested, doctors tell us, *Meh, you don't really need to get tested for that.* What the actual fuck?

What's going on is that the things that give me (and maybe you) anxiety are not the same things that motivate the public health institutions that make testing recommendations.

Herpes

The reasons it's not recommended to get tested for herpes if you don't have symptoms are

1. Both false positives and false negatives are possible.[3,4]
2. Testing positive for herpes doesn't generally deter people from having unprotected sex and spreading it anyway.[3]
3. The stigma and shame from a positive result can be worse than the infection itself.[3]

The CDC's official screenings recommendation page says: "Testing should be considered . . . especially for women with multiple sex partners.*"[5] BUT it specifies that "portions of this table marked with an asterisk are considerations and should not be interpreted as formal recommendations."

So, basically, the official advice is: *You probably don't need to get tested for herpes but you might want to.* Are you starting to feel less bad that you were confused on this issue?! Even official public health sources are extremely convoluted in their recommendations.

If you want to get tested to soothe your anxiety, go ahead. But because tests for herpes aren't that reliable, results might give you a false sense of security.

HPV

At least half of all sexually active people will get some form of HPV at some point,[6] but in 9 out of 10 cases, the infection will go away on its own within two years.[7] HPV usually does not cause any symptoms, but some strains cause warts and others can cause cancer.[8]

The American Cancer Society, the US Preventive Services Task Force, and the American College of Obstetricians and Gynecologists recommend people ages 21 to 29 have a Pap smear every three years to test for cervical cancer cells and precancerous cells.[8,9,10] It is NOT recommended to get tested for HPV unless funky cells are detected in your Pap smear.[8] The idea is: they don't care about knowing for sure whether you have HPV or not; since you probably do, testing for it is a waste of resources; they just want to make sure that, if you do have HPV, it's not causing chaos on your cervix.

If you're 30–65 years old, it's recommended to either get a Pap smear every three years, or just an HPV test every five years, or a Pap smear combined with an HPV test every five years for average-risk* people.[8,9,10] All the aforementioned institutions agree these are equally effective strategies. If you are at higher risk,* take that into consideration and go for testing more often. How *much* more often depends on . . . a lot of subjective measuring. I say do it however often hits that sweet spot between your wallet and your time constraints and your anxiety levels. If you're under 21, over 65, or if you've had a hysterectomy with complete removal of the cervix (that was not because of cancer or high-risk precancer growth), it's not recommended to get tested at all.[9,10]

The fact that HPV can cause cancer is thrown around a lot in public health campaigns meant to scare us. In my experience, the scare campaigns worked. Way too well. I put off having a pelvic exam for an entire extra year after I knew I had HPV because I was so terrified that, when I did go in, they would tell me I had cancer. Every time I started thinking about making an appointment, I would end up thinking about how I was going to say goodbye to all my loved ones and about what I would do with my last few months of life.

Then I learned that it usually takes more than 10 years for cell changes from HPV to become cancer.[8]

So you really don't need to be as anxious as I was about it. Contrary to my personal belief, public health institutions are actually a more helpful authority to believe than the vicious little gnome that skips in circles around my brain all day singing jingles about how everything's going to kill me. If you really want the test at any point, ask for it when you make your Pap smear appointment. Otherwise, stick to the recommendations above.

HIV

The language used in most materials for health-care professionals about when to screen for HIV is "at least once, then repeat according to level of risk." "At least once" is a bizarre recommendation because, like, WHEN is that one minimum time during the course of a lifetime?! The CDC recommends testing everyone who comes in for STI testing for HIV unless they opt out.[5] This is a public health strategy for reducing the number of people who carry HIV without knowing it (and not a measure of how common HIV is). The Mayo Clinic says if you're higher risk,* get tested once a year.[4] That sounds good to me.

STIs That You Would Think Have Super-Intense Symptoms, Which You Would Probably Know If You Had, but That Are Recommended to Get Tested for Even If You Don't Have Symptoms, Which Is Kind of Confusing

Chlamydia is the most common STI in the US and often does not have symptoms. And it will really fuck you up if left untreated. Gonorrhea is not very common, but it also sometimes doesn't have symptoms, and will also fuck you up if left untreated.[4] That's why these two are the ones you'll probably get tested for most. In an ideal world, yes, you'd test for at least chlamydia between partners. It's definitely a good idea to get tested for it after unprotected sex. Minimally, it's a good idea to get tested annually for both, especially if you have HIV, are under 25, or are higher risk.* You probably don't have to worry about syphilis unless you are a very high-risk* person, but the CDC does recommend testing for it if you are HIV positive or pregnant.[5]

The Confessional Interview

When health care professionals ask you all those questions about *how much sex do you have and in which holes and with who and how many times and do you take drugs and have you ever killed anyone?!?!*, they're trying to assess your risk in order to advise you about what to get tested for. Unfortunately, they also often throw in a lot of judgment and ignorance, especially for queer, trans, and gender-nonconforming people. Doctors are people who spent enormous chunks of their lives studying in medical schools that almost never teach sex positivity. If you find yourself in front of a judgmental person who is asking you to divulge your sex life in detail, try (so much easier said than done, I know) not to let this make you feel bad about yourself. Take a deep breath, remember that you love you, say, "OK, BOOMER," very, very quietly, and then speak up, and be as honest as possible. Their moral assessment of you is way less important than their informed medical assessment!

For trans and gender-nonconforming people who may have had to deal with an array of health-care-related awfulness beyond mere judgment and subpar care, you might want to seek a health care provider that's trans- and gender-noncomforming-friendly. (See the resources section at the end of this chapter.)

*Calculating Your Own Level of Risk

Risk is a subjective assessment made by health care professionals based on a combination of factors that are determined by public health institutions. These risk factors include your age, number of sexual partners, the types of sex you're having (i.e., oral, anal, vaginal), consistency of condom use, your history of STIs, whether or not you are a sex worker, and any drug use—especially needle sharing. If you're 25 or younger and sexually active, you're automatically high risk.[11] Race is also a factor. One result of racism is health inequality. This has meant that Black people and, to a lesser extent, Latinxs may have a higher risk of contracting STIs.[1,12]

I wish I could give you an equation for calculating your own risk, given these factors. There isn't one. Try to assess yourself realistically without judging yourself. *High risk* is a statistical term, not a moral condemnation. Yes, a doctor might be able to make that assessment more objectively than you, but you have to bring your own fine ass in to get tested for a doctor to even have a chance to assess you anyway.

PS to people with pussies who have sex with other people with pussies (PW-PWHSWOPWP): I've not seen a single screening recommendation that says y'all are at less of a risk of contracting STIs. That idea is dated. We are all in the same cute li'l STI boat.

Occasions When You Should Super Definitely Get Tested—Maybe for Everything, or Maybe for What a Doctor Thinks Is Necessary

- If you have any weird symptoms like pain, discharge that's different from normal, a different/new smell.
- If a recent partner starts to have any weird symptoms.
- If a partner you had unprotected sexytime with tells you after that they have an STI.
- If you suspect for any other reason that you've been exposed to an STI.
- If you're pregnant, get tested for HIV and hepatitis B early in the pregnancy. If you're higher risk,* throw in a chlamydia and gonorrhea test too.

- If you find out you have HIV, get tested for everything else too, and then get tested again at least once a year or more, depending on your level of risk.
- When you've just gotten out of a long-term monogamous relationship and you're ready to start seeing other people. I know that sounds weird, but it's better to get checked than to assume you're clean since your partner may have cheated on you. ☹

Also, know that some STIs don't even show up on tests for a while after you get them. This is called the *window period*. Getting a test during that period is a waste of money and time. Infections' dormant periods range from as little as one day for gonorrhea to up to 20 years for syphilis. Because of this, if you think you may have been exposed to an STI, you might want to wait to get tested. If anything happens that you think might have been particularly high risk, testing three weeks after will be long enough to know whether you've caught gonorrhea or chlamydia.[13] If you know a specific STI you might have been exposed to, look up its window period and wait that long. If you've been sexually assaulted, go to a doctor as soon as possible, but they may also have you come back for testing after a few weeks.

It works somewhat differently with HIV since it has a longer window: 10 days to three months depending on what kind of test you can get. The 10-day ones are expensive and not widely available. The three-month ones are the most common.[14] Regardless, if you think you've been exposed to HIV, go to a health care provider immediately, like in a matter of hours or just as fast as you can, so you can get this amazing medicine called postexposure prophylaxis (PEP) to help you not get infected.[13]

$$$$

If you don't have amazing health insurance—which you most likely don't if you live in the United States—testing can be really, really expensive, especially if you want to get tested for everything! Most of the big insurance companies do have some STI testing coverage. If you have insurance, find out what your plan covers. And when you're at a doctor's office, ask what kind of bill you're going to get hit with *before* you go through with tests, so you don't get surprised with an extra mortgage on your way out. There are clinics that have testing for free or cheap, but they're not always that easy to find. Planned Parenthood is a great place to start looking. You can also search the CDC's Get Tested portal, listed in the following resources. Most big cities in the US have at least one place that offers testing absolutely free. Google: "free STI testing + [your city or nearest big city]."

RESOURCES

- plannedparenthood.org/health-center for finding a Planned Parenthood near you
- tools.plannedparenthood.org/std/intro for figuring out if you should get tested
- gettested.cdc.gov for finding free STI testing near you
- radremedy.org search for local health care services that are trans and gender-noncomforming friendly

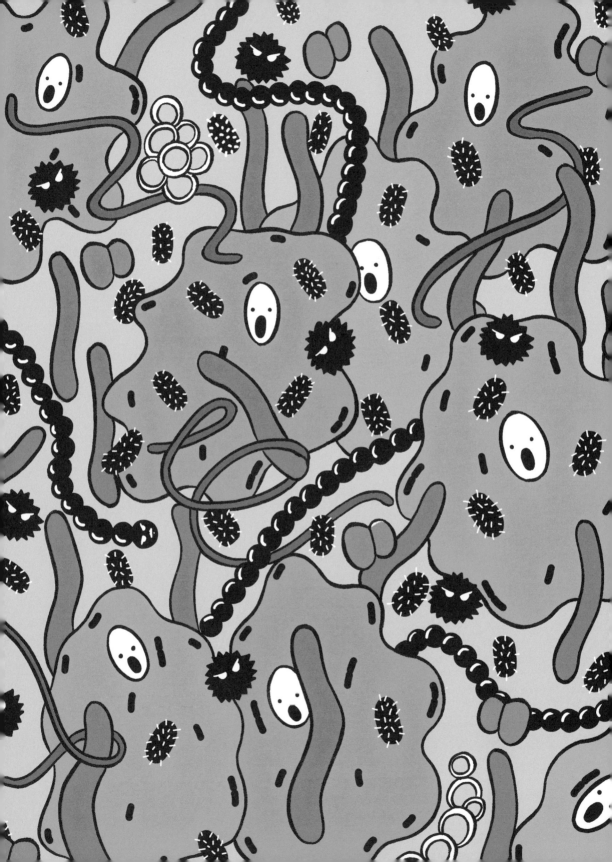

26
Your Vagina Party: The Microbiome, BV, and Yeast

THERE'S A BACTERIA PARTY GOING ON INSIDE YOUR VAGINA RIGHT NOW. BY WHICH I mean, there are a bunch of bacteria living in your vagina. That is normal and healthy and it is called the *vaginal microbiome*, but I like to call it the *vagina party*.

There are cool kids that keep the party fun: bacteria mostly from the *Lactobacillus* family with some really cool names like *L. crispatus*, *L. gasseri*, *L. iners*, and *L. jensenii*.[1] And then there are the bad-kid bacteria that can cause infections and kill your party's vibe, like *Gardnerella*, *Atopobium*, *Mobiluncus*, *Prevotella*, *Streptococcus*, *Ureaplasma*, and *Megasphaera*.[1] Sometimes a type of yeast, *Candida*, which is a fungus, also shows up to the party and puts a damper on things.[2]

Lactobacillus has a way of keeping most of the bad kids out of your vagina party most of the time; it makes lactic acid to keep the vagina at a pH level that the bad bacteria don't like.[3] It also creates a kind of protein called *bacteriocin* that slows the growth of the bad bacteria.[4] I imagine it like this: In my vagina party, I play reggaeton and dance a lot and the few boring, bad *Gardnerella* kids at the party are too cool to dance and don't invite the rest of their bad-kid friends to the party because, to them, the party sucks. They hate reggaeton and the joy of dancing makes them feel vulnerable. That's my vagina party at its optimal state.

But sometimes, for a variety of reasons, a bunch of bad kids will crash the party anyway. And they basically bring cocaine and then, all of a sudden, the whole party is just the bathroom line and people manically talking about themselves and you can't even pee anymore. (I hate cocaine.) And also those kids play techno, which really kills my vibe both in real life and in my metaphorical vagina party. If this extended metaphor is starting to confuse you, the whole point is just that it's not good when too much bad bacteria or yeast colonizes your vagina.

If too many bad bacteria crash your vagina party, then you get bacterial vaginosis (BV).[5] If too many yeast crash, then you get candidiasis—more commonly called a *yeast infection*.[6] (If you are in a Spanish-speaking country when you get a yeast infection and need to ask for yeast infection medicine at a pharmacy, you will have to tell the kind pharmacist that you have *hongos vaginales*, or "vaginal mushrooms.") When any vaginal infection gets bad enough to cause symptoms, the umbrella term is *vaginitis*, which means "your vagina party is not very fun right now."[7]

What Happens and What to Do When Your Vagina Party Is Not Very Fun

When there is too much yeast or bad-kid bacteria at your vagina party, your vagina might get stinky, itchy (try not to scratch! I know, I know, but that can make it worse),[8] or red, or have weirdly colored or textured discharge. It might hurt to put anything in there.[6,9] Parties that have too much fungus (yeast infections) and parties that have too much bad bacteria (BV) result in very similar symptoms, so it can be hard to tell which group of bad kids has colonized your party without getting a test.

Knowing who's at your party matters because treatments differ. At least one small-ish study shows that people are not very good at diagnosing what kind of infection they have.[10] Many times, a mild BV or yeast infection will clear up on its own.[11,12] There's no definitive marker of when you need to intervene, but waiting can be a risky game. I'd say, if your vagina is stanky, if your discharge is weird, or if your symptoms are uncomfortable or not going away, it's best to go see a doctor.

Do not be embarrassed. According to one large-scale study cited by the CDC, at any given time, about 29% of vaginas of people ages 14–49 have BV.[13] And at any given time, about 20% of vaginas have too much yeast living in them.[2] As many as 70–75% of people with pussies will get a yeast infection at some point in their lives.[10]

Being too embarrassed to seek treatment is not the plan. Trust me. My vagina party once got so bad that I could smell it through my pants for like a week. And you *know* that if you can smell it, other people can too. This was an entirely preventable situation. I could not bring myself to walk into a Buenos Aires pharmacy and utter the words *hongos vaginales*, so I waited for the bad kids to just get tired and leave my vagina party. They did not. They just kept inviting more of their bad friends. They basically turned my vagina party into a coke-fueled techno rave. It was so itchy that when I walked into a friend's kitchen and saw a bottle brush hanging out next to the sink, I fantasized about stealing it and . . . yeah. I didn't (and nobody ever should). Eventually I went to a doctor, got some meds, and within a few days, my vagina party was fun again. The point is: just go to the doctor if at all possible.

If you can't go to the doctor because, like the vast majority of US residents, you are hanging on by a thread financially, have terrible health insurance or none at all, and the mere thought of a doctor bill gives you a panic attack, which itself feels worse than your itchy vagina . . . you can try over-the-counter yeast infection creams like Monistat to see if your symptoms go away. They're fairly safe to use even if you don't actually have a yeast infection.[14] If your symptoms don't go away, then, *really*, go to a doctor so they can test you and prescribe you the right medicine. A BV infection left untreated can increase your risk of contracting STIs and even lead to pelvic inflammatory disease, which can affect fertility, which is also much more expensive to treat than a shitty vagina party.[13]

Why the Bad Kids Sometimes Crash Your Vagina Party

Levels of yeast and bacteria fluctuate for many reasons, including hormones. Hormone levels shift with puberty, the menstrual cycle, pregnancy, and menopause. When there's more estrogen in the body, the vagina's skin stores more glycogen. Researchers think that lactobacilli eat glycogen and use it to produce lactic acid.[3] So it makes sense that changes in levels of estrogen can, therefore, cause changes in your vagina party.

Hormones and the vagina party also change during and after pregnancy. The microbiome is important during pregnancy because, if it gets messed up, there's an increased risk of preterm birth. Science is still not entirely clear on why. Also, scientists think that the parent's vaginal microbiome is something that helps get the baby's gut microbiome up and running. During pregnancy, the pregnant person's vagina party becomes less diverse, and more full of *Lactobacillus*. With the party attendees staying more consistent, it also becomes more stable. This might be because there is more estrogen in the body during pregnancy, which, as I mentioned earlier, makes more glycogen in the vaginal wall skin, which makes more *Lactobacillus*. There's an increased risk of yeast infection during pregnancy, which researchers think may be because yeast, similarly to *Lactobacillus*, eat glycogen. After pregnancy, estrogen levels fall, *Lactobacillus* levels fall, and bad bacteria that can cause BV increase.[15]

If you take testosterone, that will change your vagina party and lead to less *Lactobacillus*, which can lead to increased risk of BV.[16] The good news is that this imbalance can be treated with estrogen that gets administered right to the vagina in a way that will not mess up the effects of gender-affirming hormone therapy.[17]

Now here's something weird and confusing: Whether the rate of vaginitis increases or decreases after menopause remains unclear. Many sources say that the risk of both BV and yeast infection increases with menopause.[7,18,19,20] But a few others say the opposite.[21] One study found that rates of BV fall even though the population of *Lactobacillus* in the vagina also falls.[22] The study called this "the paradox of the postmenopausal condition."[22] Two studies found that postmenopausal people who had estrogen hormone replacement therapy (HRT) for menopause symptoms had significantly more yeast infections than those who didn't, even though HRT restores *Lactobacillus* growth.[22,23,24] This also may be because glycogen feeds yeast as well as *Lactobacillus*.[24] The only thing we can know for sure is that Science still has a long way to go in explaining how the microbiome works.

Another thing that can cause yeast infections is taking antibiotics. Again, nobody knows exactly why. If antibiotics kill lactobacilli, presumably that reduction in good bacteria would cause BV, but it doesn't.[14] Yet still, taking antibiotics causes yeast infections about 28–33% of the time.[10]

Sex is another factor. Because sex can introduce new things—saliva, fingers, toys, penises, semen—into the vagina, it can also introduce new attendees to your vagina party. There is evidence that BV can be transmitted from pussy to pussy during sex.[25] And there is also evidence that more sex and/or more sexual partners can lead to BV.[26,27,28]

With yeast infections, it's harder to say. Many studies have found that yeast is not sexually transmitted.[8,26,27,28,29] I only found one study that showed a strong association between intercourse and yeast infections,[30] which was not nearly as many as I expected to find. That said, there is some evidence that oral sex and masturbating with (anyone's) saliva is more strongly associated with yeast infections than intercourse is.[8,30] In fact, multiple studies found that neither number of sexual partners nor how much sex someone had was associated with yeast infections.[8,26,27,31] It seems like common sense that sex would lead to yeast infections, but the research says it doesn't.

Cue Carrie Bradshaw voice

I couldn't help but wonder: If it turns out that having lots of sex is actually not very associated with yeast infections, is the idea that sex could cause yeast infections just another old, sexist narrative about people with pussies who have sex being dirty?

Racism Ruins Vagina Parties

Another thing that can throw off your vagina party is racism. Studies have shown that Black and Hispanic vaginas tend to have a higher pH and less *Lactobacillus* than those of whites and Asians.[32,33,34,35] Black people with pussies are twice as likely to be diagnosed with BV, which, aside from bad pregnancy outcomes, is also associated with increased risk of contracting STIs.[1,34,35] These differences are not surprising. It is well established that racism and poverty wreak havoc on health outcomes in a ton of other bodily systems.[36,37]

And yet, the studies that look at microbiome health differences among racial groups do not go ahead and say, *That's because of racism*. In fact, many researchers ignore racism as a probable factor altogether (except one who, at least, conceded, "It is likely that numerous confounding factors associated with socioeconomic status influence the development of BV"),[34] preferring to look to genetic differences to explain the health gap. Like this study:

> This . . . suggests that although most Asian and white women are "healthy," a significant proportion of asymptomatic Hispanic and black women are "un-healthy"—a notion that seems implausible. . . . The reasons for these differences among ethnic groups are unknown, but it is tempting to speculate that the species composition of vaginal communities could be governed by genetically determined differences between hosts.[32]

It's interesting that they chose the word *tempting*. There's such a long, ugly history of Medicine exaggerating genetic differences, especially in Black people (another example of how our cultural narratives about things influence the way we do Science about them), that it's always worth it to stop and examine when we come across this happening. Too often, as Harriet Washington explains in *Medical Apartheid*, citing race-based genetic differences is a way of letting ourselves off the hook (indeed, it *is* always tempting to let oneself off the hook) for the causes of racism-based bad health outcomes. As Washington puts it: "Locating black violence in the genetic complement of black boys nourishes excuses to abandon social therapeutic approaches. What good is better education, better nutrition, and a more nurturing home and school environment to a born monster?"[37]

To their credit, the researchers quoted previously were trying to explain, by doing Science, why such a large proportion of people with "unhealthy" conditions in their vaginal microbiomes might not have symptoms of BV. So let's assume that they're right for a second and that vagina parties naturally differ by race. We're still looking at racism playing out in medicine. Joan Combellick, PhD, MPH, MSN, CNM—a researcher who has studied the microbiome, whom I interview in Chapter 27—told me, "There's tons of factors that can influence your microbiome. We mostly only study white people. So who's to say what BV really is if there are no symptoms?" She told me about one Black patient who complained that the BV treatment she received had taken away her signature scent. "We all define our bodies so differently." So if the researchers are right about racial and genetic factors causing variations in vaginal microbiomes, that means the problem is not nonwhite pussies' variance, the problem is that we have been using white pussies to define what's medically "normal" and "healthy" and what's not for people of all races.

Researchers can't come out and say, *This is because of racism!* because Science doesn't work like that. You need a lot of direct evidence to claim causality. But here's the cool thing about me not being a scientist: I can go ahead and say it. It seems abundantly likely that higher rates of BV among nonwhite pussies has something to do with one or more of the following factors caused by racism and/or poverty: tons of stress, lack of access to nutritious food, lack of access to medical care, being forced to live in a polluted environment. With current research, we can't know for sure. But I'd bet my fucking dog on it.

Keeping Your Vagina Party Awesome

Mostly, the best way to keep your vagina party awesome is just to let it do its thing. Your vagina knows how to keep itself clean. Definitely don't put soap in there. It can mess with your pH level, which is kind of like the measure of how good the music is at your vagina party.[38] My mom didn't tell me not to soap the crack of my vulva until I was like 25 years old and had been suffering from chronic yeast overgrowth my whole life. (I forgive you, Mama.) Since the day I stopped soaping the crack, my vagina party has been infinitely awesomer. (See Chapter 32 for a list of things besides soap that your vagina definitely does not need, which includes anything with perfume in it, douches, deodorants, steams, and egg-shaped rocks.)

Another thing you can do to keep the party going is not stick dirty things in your vagina. Cardi B was right when she said, "You gotta tell bae, 'Your shit smell like mustard.'" I know that in the heat of the moment it can be very uncomfortable to tell someone, "Your shit is stinky, please go wash it." But is it more uncomfortable than a week of itchy vagina? If you suspect something is dirty—because it stanks, it was just in your anus, it has fuzz on it, or any other reason—you should stop the action and wash it, whatever it is, before sticking it in your vagina. (And if they're hands, just wash them. Hands tend to be dirty.)

Some people take probiotic supplements, a commercially available form of good bacteria, for vaginal health. A very limited amount of evidence suggests probiotics can improve the health of already healthy vaginas and help prevent infections.[39,40,41] While research has shown that probiotics have promise for treating and preventing recurrences of BV, the available studies are not very substantial, nor consistent in the bacterial strains they studied.[41,42] Probiotics do not seem to help prevent yeast infections that arise from taking antibiotics.[10]

Any study on probiotics for vaginal health uses specific strains of bacteria, in very specific amounts. So even if a study shows promising results, those results would be very hard to re-create for yourself by buying probiotics. It's hard to know what you're really buying with dietary supplements in general because of the way they're (not very) regulated by the FDA. In 2017, when the FDA inspected 656 facilities that produce dietary supplements, they found regulatory violations in more than half the facilities.[42] Studies have found that commercial probiotic products often misidentify what bacteria they contain.[43,44] Good probiotics are expensive AF, but if you have money to throw around and are set on trying to use them for your vaginal health, go for the ones that say they contain *Lactobacillus rhamnosus* GR-1.[41]

Some people, in lieu of probiotics, put yogurt in their vaginas to treat yeast infections. Once, a friend had a yeast infection, and her girlfriend was helping her put yogurt into her vagina when she started laughing and subsequently squirted it all over her girlfriend's face. Anyway, yogurt in the vagina as a yeast-infection treatment does not work because the lactobacilli in yogurt are different strains than the most common ones in your vagina party.[40] That said, it is possible (though not advisable) to use the *Lactobacillus* in your vagina to make yogurt. In 2015, Cecilia Westbrook, a ridiculously cool MD/PhD student at the University of Wisconsin–Madison, made yogurt out of bacteria from her own vagina, which she said was "tangy."[45]

A note on yeast infections and cotton versus non-cotton underwear: I've found a vast array of responses to this debate. Some say that panties made of synthetic materials, like polyester, don't breathe and thus create a warm, moist environment that is great for growing yeast.[46] Others say that people who wear non-cotton underwear do not show increased risk of yeast infections.[10,28] So I say wear whatever underwear you like and can afford.

??????????????!

As you may have noticed by now, there are many question marks when it comes to the vaginal microbiome. In the gut, the microbiome has a role in digestion, the immune system, and the production of vitamins. According to a *Scientific American* article from February 2020, "Scientists believe microbes play equally important roles in the vagina but have not yet been able to elucidate their functions." Why? You guessed it! Because vaginas are not studied enough, because . . . The Patriarchy. "Research on [vaginal microbiomes] is lagging behind that done on the microbiomes of other parts of the body."[47]

There's light on the horizon, though. In 2020 (otherwise a very bad year), researchers at the University of Maryland School of Medicine announced a new tool with a very cool name, VIRGO (Human Vaginal Non-redundant Gene Catalog), which will be able to map the DNA of the organisms in the vagina party with a fine-ass resolution never before achieved.[47] Better late than never.

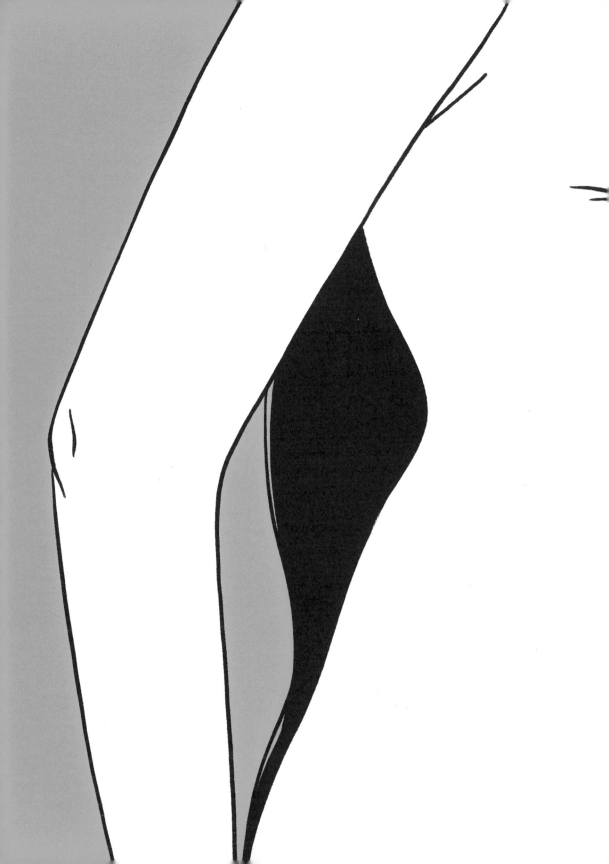

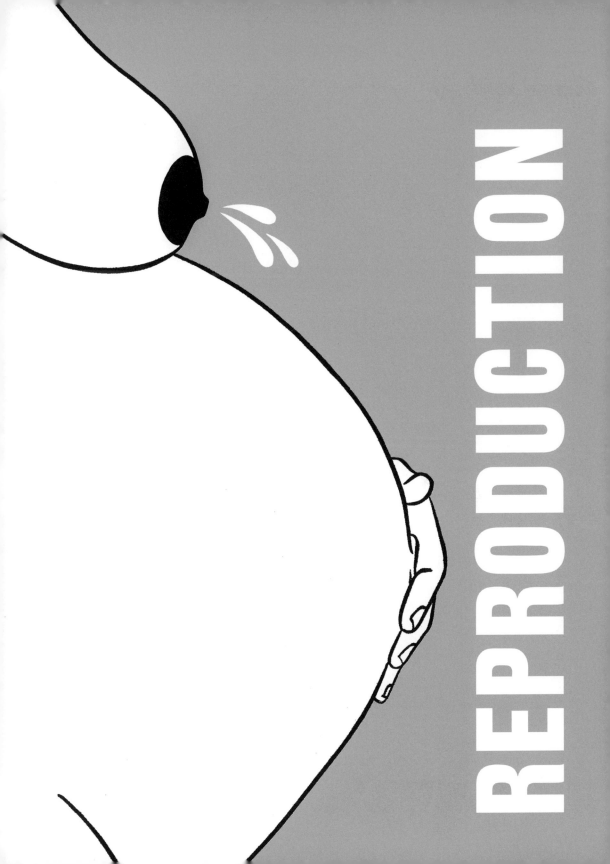

REPRODUCTION

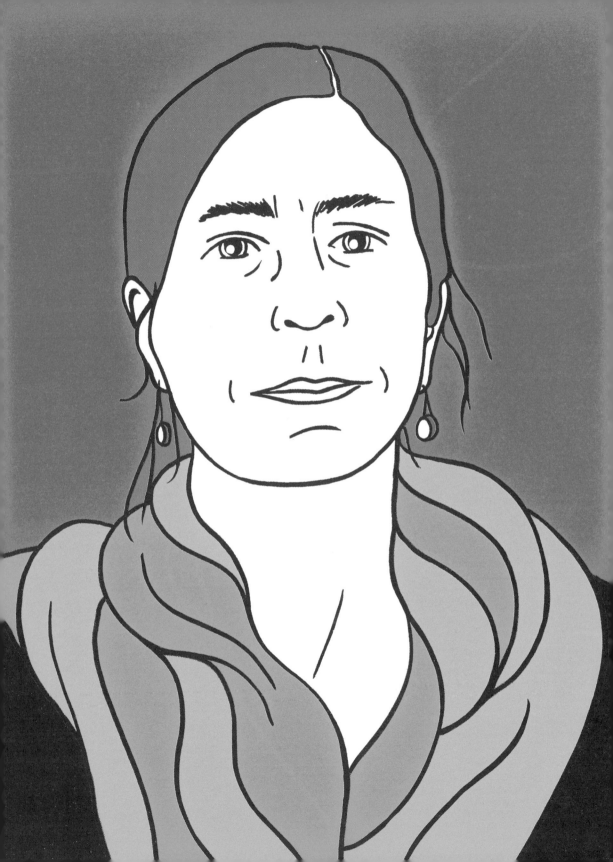

27
Birth

Interview with Joan Combellick, PhD, MPH, MSN, CNM

Birth—when a baby comes out of a pregnant person's uterus and into the world—is both incredibly normal and completely fucking magical. Like, Jesus, have you ever seen a birth?! I never have IRL, but every birth video makes me cry like a baby. (If you never have, throw on the music video for "Vos Sabés" by Los Fabulosos Cadillacs.) In the US, the physiological process of birth is one of the few topics most sex ed does cover. And yet, the full reality of it—the logistical, the emotional, the historical—we keep stashed away somewhere in our cultural attic, maybe in the same hidden box as death.

A lot is wrong with the way birth happens in the US. Profit-driven medical practices cause doctors to intervene too much, even when it's not medically necessary. Hospitals do everything they can not for the health of people giving birth and their babies but rather to get the most possible people in and out and to avoid lawsuits.[1,2] For example, to speed things along, too often, doctors give drugs that cause stronger contractions. They also perform episiotomies—cutting from the bottom of the vagina down toward the anus, which can be very painful to recover from—more often than necessary. And they perform more C-sections than might be necessary. (Of course, there are also some amazing ob-gyns who work in hospitals. I know and love a few of them.) The US also has extremely high rates of both newborn death and maternal mortality, especially for Black and Indigenous people, compared to rates in similar countries.[3,4] These problems have caused people to seek alternatives. Between 2004 and 2017, the number of people in the US who opted for home births (usually with a midwife) over hospital births increased by 77%.[5]

Birth is a ginormous topic about which many entire books have been written, and trying to fit it into one short chapter is kind of like . . . trying to squeeze a baby through a cervix hole (it's called an *os*!). So I called in an expert on getting babies through cervix holes (plural is *ora*!). Joan Combellick, PhD, MPH, MSN, CNM, is a professor, nurse, and midwife who teaches at the Yale School of Nursing and has studied everything from the relationship between trauma, chronic stress, and birth outcomes to the effects of birth interventions on babies' microbiomes to how people make decisions about giving birth during COVID.

I didn't tell her before we spoke that for months I'd been thinking obsessively, even dreaming vividly, about giving birth as I—in my very anxious, Jewish, maximally catastrophizing way—prepare to try to get pregnant. Still, talking to her was exciting and reassuring. At first I was intimidated. She has 12 letters after her name! And good posture! As she sat down in front of a big landscape oil painting that matched her outfit, I awkwardly began our interview by telling her that I'd wanted to talk to a midwife because I wanted someone not just with facts but with strong opinions. Then I immediately realized that may have been offensive. To my great relief, she laughed a little and validated my hunch. "Yes, I think we have the reputation of having a lot of opinions, and there is some truth to it," she said. But hers are the best kind—those informed by three decades of research and practice.

What is a midwife? Why should people seek one out? How can people find one?

A midwife is an expert in the normal physiologic event of birth. In the US, we mostly work in hospitals in collaboration with doctors, who are the experts in complications. Around 20% of women experience some level of complication, but the vast majority of women can have a "normal," undisturbed physiologic birth, especially if they do not receive intervention that is not medically necessary. In the practices I've worked in, we see people throughout their pregnancy, during birth, and postpartum as well. Some practices will require that you also meet with a doctor at least once. But otherwise, an ob-gyn or maternal fetal medicine specialist will [only] get called in if there's a complication. Midwives also see people who aren't pregnant, for preventive care like cancer and STI screening, contraception, menopausal care, or for problems like painful sex or pelvic pain.

In the United States, we do harm with too much intervention applied too soon rather than the too-little-too-late problem that many women living in lower-resource countries have. So to the extent that we can within our current health care system, we midwives try to protect against over-intervention, to support the normal physiologic event of birth.

To find one, google midwives in your area. They should have a mechanism where you can meet before you decide to transfer your care to them. Ask them questions. Express your fears. State your assumptions about the care you will receive. For example, people usually ask about what kinds of pain medication they will have access to and how much access they will have to their midwife: Are they on call all the time? What do others who have worked with her have to say about her? Check out who she is. What training does she have? There are different levels of certifications for midwives. I encourage people to get someone who is trained and licensed.

What do you wish more people knew about birth?

That birth is a normal physiologic event and how to deeply embody that. I've worked with people who grew up in the US and many people who did not, and I think that women who grew up here often really intellectualize the experience. They read everything. They make a plan. That's great. They do need to think through their issues and learn and understand the whole process. But we are short on recognizing that we are mammals. Connect with that! Set aside your screenplay of how this should go, and understand that there are no guarantees. You can't say how it's going to go. Nor can your midwife. Just have this deep fundamental trust that your body is built to do this. Many women in labor get to a point where they say, "I can't do this!" And I always feel like, *Finally! Fantastic!* Because you need to get to that point to do it. You need to stop trying to control it with your brain and let your body take over. It's going to feel impossible for a while, but it's going to happen and you'll be great! I would like for women in the US to try to be their animal selves a little bit more.

Also, remember that we midwives and health care providers are in service to you, the people getting care. You're not in service to us. Make sure that you have the opportunity to say what you need and want and have that responded to.

What do you think about the current trend toward giving birth at home?

Just a little over 1% of women deliver at home. Home births are growing in popularity. During COVID, even Governor Cuomo was talking about it. I'm doing a study right now on women's experience[s] of birth during coronavirus, and it's fascinating to hear about the decision-making around place of birth because it brings up so much of why women are not well-served by the maternity-care system in the US. We are three to six times higher than our peer nations in maternal deaths. It's very common that those countries have much more robust options for home births. Home births and birth centers [in peer countries] are connected to hospitals. They make the transfer easy. The UK published their national health guidelines that say that, for women who have had a vaginal birth previously and are low-risk, they can be as safe at home as they are in the hospital, and [under the care of a midwife] are more likely to have a vaginal birth and less likely to have an episiotomy or blood transfusion. [These countries] are supporting those options. In the US, we have very limited options.

What would you say to people like me, who like the idea of a home birth but are freaked out that something bad will happen?

I would say, delve down deeply into your fears. Working through and understanding those fears and talking to whoever you're seeing for your care about them is a very important process. We have a culture of fear in the US and mistrust in our bodies during pregnancy and birth. We focus on, *OMG, what if this thing happens? It's probably gonna happen.* We don't have within us a lifelong experience of having seen other women give birth. We have birth very closeted. We don't know what that power looks and feels like and why it might be a great thing even if it's the hardest thing you ever do.

What happens in the case of a complication during a home birth?

One reason you might go to the hospital is to get some medicine if your labor is not progressing. If the baby's fetal heart tones don't sound good, you might go to be in an environment where you'd have access to a C-section. But there are things like bleeding after you have the baby—if it's severe enough you'd transfer, but midwives have things that can help with that. [A midwife] should have a relationship with a hospital. In EU countries, hospitals have connections to the home birth process. Here, midwives might be struggling with that. You don't want to end up being dumped into an emergency room. You want to understand what the transfer would be like, and make sure the home-birth midwife can go in with you. The midwife will make a transfer plan for you. That's an established part of that practice. Also, you should know beforehand if your midwife brings oxygen with her and if she is certified in neonatal resuscitation.

Why do so many people seem to feel like they need to do birth the "right way"? Why do you think there's pressure to have an ideal outcome?

Growing up with the identity of being female, we feel we're failing all the time. We don't say, "Look at me! I did this thing!" Shaming and blaming happen all the time with women who get C-sections. There's no failure there. If anything, it's harder. Midwives can be guilty of prioritizing one kind of birth experience, and we need to be able to say, "Hey, do you want an epidural?" But it can even come from your best friend—that "too bad you had a C-section." Forget that! These women labor first and then they have surgery. They are superhuman! But we don't send those messages at all. We should promote claiming the great thing you did, not diminish it.

Also, people need to be able to tell their stories. Sometimes when I go to parties and say I'm a midwife, there are 70-year-old women (and men too) who are still processing their birth stories. We need to give people the space to process. We need to say, "Wow, that was great!" We need to say, "Cool, you did that, that was fantastic." In midwifery culture historically, we did home visits to check in and allow people time to process their whole birth experience, to be able to say things like, "I failed." And for us to be able to say things like, "No, you didn't fail, but tell me all about why you feel that way."

The word *process* makes me think of trauma. Is birth traumatic?

I don't want to overlook that birth is traumatic for some people. But the trauma doesn't necessarily arise from experiencing complications. Research shows that it's more about the way people are treated. Trauma happens more often not when people need interventions but when they're not told: "Here's the situation, here's what we may have to do, this is what we need to do now, and you still have a choice about how this happens."

Just like end-of-life care, beginning-of-life care is a normal human process. We've seen system changes in the US with end-of-life care and recognition that people have a right to decide how their end-of-life experience happens, to bring that experience home and out of institutions and away from over-medicalization, to support their experience with pain relief, and to be in the midst of their families. They've actually made more strides than beginning-of-life care. We need to start giving people options so that they feel they are in charge of their care, wherever they choose to give birth.

That makes sense. My grandma told me about how she was given an episiotomy without warning or consent and even drugged despite her specific request not to be. It seemed like what really upset her more than the pain of recovering was having been disregarded by the doctors. What's your opinion on episiotomies?

They're almost never needed. When they are, a woman needs to be told, "Here's what I'm seeing, I need to speed up this last part of your labor, the baby's not coming, I'm thinking about doing an episiotomy. Is that OK with you?" There *is* time to have that conversation. I think it's bullshit when people say, "There's no time to talk." Including the woman in that decision that involves her body allows her to be an active participant in her care.

Having said that, whether you have an episiotomy or there's lacerations from delivery, it's important to know that those can be completely and thoroughly repaired and to let women know that stitches are going to go away on their own. We need to give anticipatory guidance—things like: frozen witch hazel pads can feel really good on the stitches, it's going to be swollen for a while, it's going to burn when you pee, use this squeeze bottle so you dilute the pee

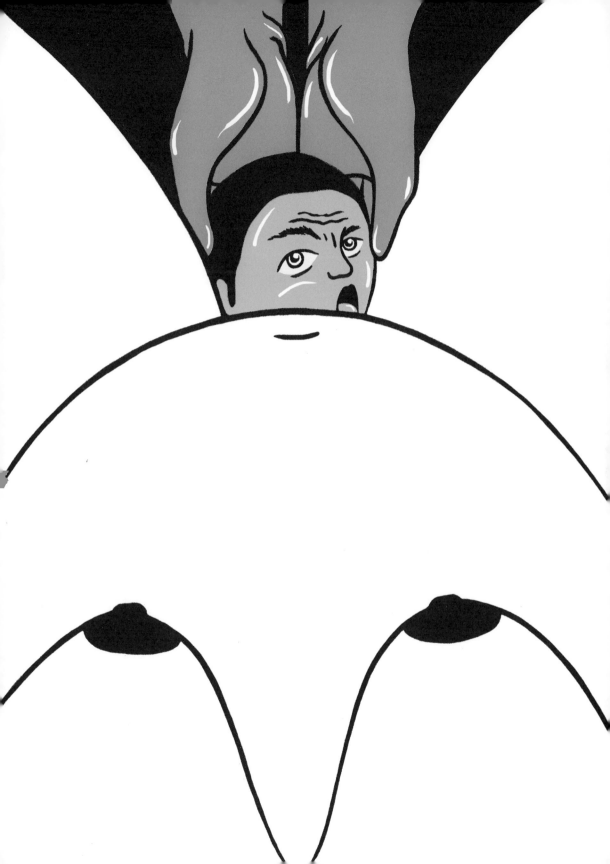

for a few days. Some people have penetrative sex again pretty soon and some people don't, and all of that is totally fine and normal, including a feeling that you don't want to have sex for many months or a year. We need to give more reassurance at the granular level to explain that vaginal tissue is incredibly vascular and will heal very quickly, well before [episiotomy] stitches dissolve or fall out. We need to say, "This is what I'm doing, here's why I'm doing it, this is why your body is so ready to heal from this."

Are there any current birth trends that you would say are particularly awesome or bad?

As long as the mom and baby are safe, I don't have a problem. Eat your placenta if you want. Deliver in whatever position you want. I do have doubts about free birthing [a movement for birthing without any trained attendant]. I think it comes from a place of fear of intervention. But I love this picture I have from the 12th or 13th century, from Angkor Wat, that shows someone giving birth with a support person behind them. We have helped each other to give birth forever. Giving birth without anyone experienced, that's just too harsh and dangerous in my view. I don't recommend it. There are very simple interventions that can prevent severe harm or death. Don't do it alone without access to those things.

What makes your work political?

Birth is a huge, powerful experience. Maybe people-slash-men, in some instinctive way, are afraid of that power. Our world has been controlled politically, medically, historically by men in boardrooms, doctors in their call rooms. And particularly in the US, our maternity-care history is fraught with dominance and control and non-person-centered decision making.

Midwives have been marginalized, and that hasn't helped our birth outcomes in this country. I think that's what leads us [midwives] to sometimes be loudmouthed, opinionated people. Most countries with better maternal mortality statistics have a higher midwife-to-doctor ratio. They have many more midwives than they have doctors. And in the US, we have many more doctors than midwives.

**Why is the maternal mortality rate so high in the US,
and why is there such a huge racial disparity in it? What
needs to be done about it?**

The increasing rate [of] the last five years is stabilizing, but it's still outrageous. I don't want to truncate the whole issue because it is very multifactorial, but there is a lot of evidence that midwifery care is associated with better outcomes for both mother and baby.

Midwifery care tends to be less accessible in BIPOC communities. Black women in the US are three to four times more likely to die in pregnancy-related events than white women. Indigenous women are only slightly less likely [than Black women]. In New York City, Black women are 12 times more likely to die in childbirth-related events than their white counterparts. A lot of this conversation becomes, *What's wrong with Black women's bodies? Why are their health statistics so bad?* I believe that a lifetime of chronic stress and trauma can lead to an increased risk of complications. But having said that, none of these complications are new. We know how to manage high blood pressure and diabetes. There's room for addressing complications better. There's research that shows that, in New York City, it's not necessarily a problem of Black women and their bodies; both Black and white women do worse in primarily Black-serving hospitals. It's about the care that we give.

We need to ask ourselves about the quality of our care at every level. Are we coordinating care well? Are we communicating? Are we educating women on what danger signs are so that they seek care when they need it? Are we believing women when they show up and tell us what they think is wrong? Chronic stress and trauma are significant and can manifest as problems, but I reject that women with complications should internalize that as feelings of "there's something wrong with my body." It's so common to hear health care providers say, "Well, we can't have better outcomes because we take care of high-risk people." What we really need is to be better at what we do, be more person-centered, and believe what women tell us about their bodies.

Our health care system incentivizes a higher number of visits. I used to work at a community health center and had to see one patient every 15 minutes. So I would kill myself trying to still give individualized care. We incentivize quantity and profit over quality, and that has a lot of ripple effects. Also, we don't have universal access to health care, and that's huge.

Do you know if there is any work being done around assisting trans men in the birth process?

I would really like to hear more from trans men who have given birth about what they need and want. The first trans patient that I had, about 10 years ago, showed up with a CD on which he had compiled everything that was known about giving good care [to trans patients]. And it was terrible that he had to do that for his care provider, but I was so grateful. I hope trans men get beyond having to do that, but at the same time, I would really like to hear their voices about what they need and want. I'm sure there are so many ways we fall short.

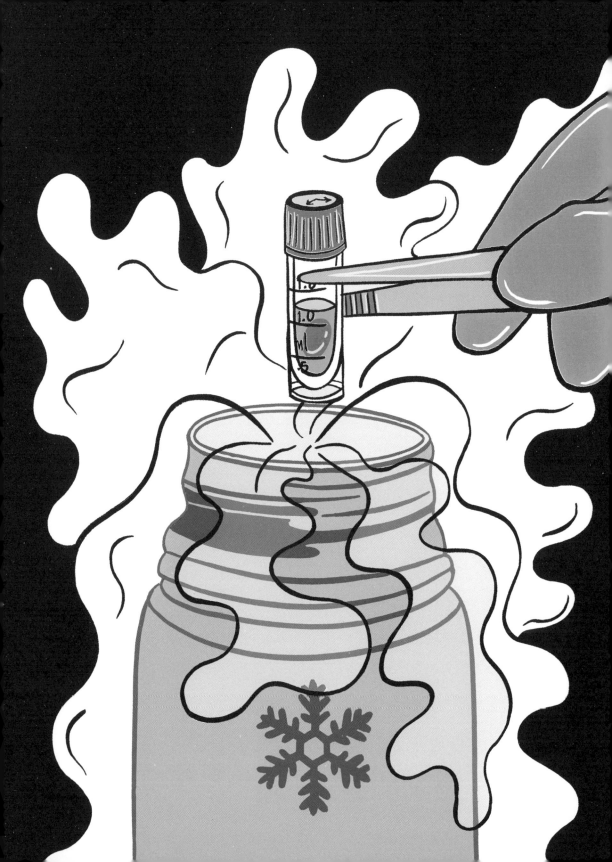

28
How Babies Are Really Made: Reproduction Inc.

THAT STORY ABOUT A MAMA AND A DADDY THAT WERE IN LOOOVE SO THEY PENIS-in-vagina'd 'til Daddy's sperm went racing to pierce Mama's egg is sooo 1999. And it's not entirely accurate. First of all, the fastest-sperm-gets-into-the-egg story is off. And it's one of my favorite examples of how gender narratives infiltrate science and change the way we see biological realities. Second of all, there are so many more ways that babies get made now. People with pussies are having babies older, and many people are making babies outside of cis-heterosexual relationships. So lots of technology comes into play.

The Sperm and the Egg Story: A Story About Stories and Science

Here's the story we usually hear:

The sperm shoot into the vagina, then they all race to the egg, and the fastest sperm wins and gets inside the egg.

Now read that sentence back to yourself in the voice of a four-year-old boy.

Do you notice how it sounds like something a four-year-old boy would say? The problem with this story is that it is told in a way that reflects gender narratives more than it reflects reality. The reason it sounds like a small child's narration is that gender narratives are simplified stories. Stories like: Boys race because they are naturally competitive! The fastest is the best! The boy penetrates the girl! These stories are the glasses we use to see, even in Science, so it makes sense that when scientists saw sperm swimming toward an egg, they said, "Look! They're racing! And the fastest sperm penetrates the egg and wins!"

But that was not what was happening. In reality, it's a much more collaborative process. Sperm don't, for example, go racing up the vagina, through the cervix, and straight to the egg. They get lost, hang out, and get trapped in different places along the way.[1,2] They are often stored for up to 5–10 days before being released to continue on their slow journey to the egg in which undulations in the uterine tubes also help them reach the egg.[1,2,3] And it's not that the "best"/fastest sperm "wins." It's true that the sperm with defects are way less likely to be the winner, but among the healthy sperm, it's actually more up to luck.[1]

A Useful Thing to Know to Help You Get or Not Get Pregnant

To dispel a common myth, the day of ovulation is not the best day for conception. You're more likely to get pregnant in the five days leading up to ovulation. This is because the spermies live for three to five days in your cervical mucus and the egg can live for 12–24 hours after ovulation starts. So, hypothetically, the most fertile two days of a menstrual cycle are the two days before ovulation.[4,5,6]

When the Right Timing Isn't Enough: Reproduction Inc.

For a lot of people, it's going to be a lot harder to get a baby than just squirting the sperm in on the right day of the month. Some people are in a relationship with a person who has the same parts as they do, so they'll either need to acquire sperm or an egg. Some people's parts don't do what they're supposed to do. Many people with pussies are waiting longer now to have babies, so their bodies might need some help to conceive. This has led to the development of an enormous and growing industry called *assisted reproductive technology* (ART).

According to a 2020 report by the market research firm Reports and Data, ART was a $24.21 billion market in 2019 and will grow to be a $50.71 billion market by 2027.[7] Use of ART in the US has doubled in the last 10 years.[8] The number of people who have frozen their eggs in the US went from 475 in 2009 to 6,207 in 2015 and is still on the rise.[9,10]

These are some of the technologies and processes that make up ART:

- In Vitro Fertilization (IVF): When an egg is taken out of the body and fertilized with sperm in a laboratory. The fertilized egg is then returned to that person or another person's womb to grow.[11]
- Surrogacy: When somebody gestates someone else's baby in their womb, made with their own egg but with the sperm of someone from another couple, usually for money.[12]
- Gestational Carriers (often also called *surrogacy*): When somebody gestates someone else's baby in their womb, made with both sperm and an egg from other people, usually for money.
- Egg Donation: When someone donates or sells their eggs to another couple trying to conceive.[13]
- Egg Freezing: When someone freezes some of their eggs to be injected via IVF for pregnancy at a later date.[13]

All these processes can be extremely expensive. IVF cycles cost about $10,000–$15,000 per cycle, and many people need a few cycles to succeed. Additional associated costs of medications can be between $1,500 and $3,000 per cycle.[14] Egg freezing costs about $6,000–$20,000 per cycle and then about $600 a year for storage.[15] Surrogacy costs around $60,000–$150,000 in the US.[16] Whether or not insurance covers ART depends on the state. Most states do not require that insurance companies cover ART.[17] So, needless to say, ART is not available to just anyone.

And even for the price, not all these processes have high rates of success. Success rates for both egg freezing and IVF vary considerably based on many factors about the person trying to conceive and their body. If we want to get an idea of average success rates, we can do a little math. Based on the CDC's *2017 Fertility Clinic Success Rates Report*, during 2017, people in the US underwent at least 196,850 cycles of IVF with the intent to conceive immediately (as opposed to eggs that were taken out and frozen). Those cycles produced 68,908 live births (of one or more babies at a time). So, on average, 35% of IVF cycles resulted in births.[8] It's hard to say how many births result from IVF with frozen eggs. Estimates of the chances of giving birth range from 29.7% for people who froze 10 eggs after age 36 to 61% for people who froze 10 eggs before age 35.[18,19]

So Is ART Good or Bad?

(Dare you to ask someone that at the next art event you go to.)

There has been a huge amount of feminist theorizing over these technologies with a wide range of takes about whether ART ultimately helps or hurts.

The pros are obvious: Even with its costs and limited success rates, ART makes people really happy because it gives them babies. It has made some people I really care about really happy. It allows people with pussies to have babies when they are ready, and that gives us more control over our lives. ART also allows both people who are not in couples and couples who are not in cis-hetero relationships to have babies. And that is all awesome. By all measures, when people really want a baby and can't have one, it's extremely sad, and being able to get one is extremely awesome and something we should all be in favor of helping happen for as many people as possible.

At the same time, ART (much like its homonym, art) has a lot of ways of reproducing inequality especially when it involves—as it often does—richer people seeking services from people that are much poorer than they are. Surrogates, for example, are usually people with low levels of education who are working in low-paying jobs.[20] It is even common for people to travel to poorer countries to reduce the cost of surrogacy, which opens up a host of potentially exploitative factors. As Surrogacy360, a project that promotes ethical surrogacy arrangements, explains:

> International commercial surrogacy arrangements almost always take place between intended parents in wealthier countries and surrogates with fewer economic resources, often in nations with few or no regulations. Because of the power imbalances and the challenges related to crossing national borders, and also because surrogacy contracts have historically given more decision-making

power to intended parents, surrogates' health and rights are often not protected or guaranteed.[12]

Egg "donation" in the US has some Big Exploitative Energy too. To start, it's mostly not donations. As Tamar Lewin pointed out in the *New York Times* in 2015:

> Reflecting a distaste in the United States for the idea of selling body parts, the women providing the eggs are referred to as donors, and at least theoretically are paid not for their eggs, but for the inconvenience, discomfort and health risks involved in the process of harvesting. That process requires weeks of hormone injections to stimulate the ovaries, and endurance of ultrasounds and surgery.[21]

In 2016, two former egg donors successfully sued the American Society for Reproductive Medicine (ASRM) and the Society for Assisted Reproductive Technology (SART)—two groups that establish industry norms in ART—for setting caps on payment for egg "donors."[22] The groups argued that the caps they set were meant to curb exploitation by limiting the appeal of the exchange.[21] But it's hard to ignore that by paying "donors" less, middlemen were able to pocket more money from the people buying the eggs.

Some have argued that ART as an industry has become a way to pathologize infertility and to construct that pathology as an individual and "female" problem despite plenty of male infertility that exists in the world.[23,24] This obscures structural forces like environmental pollution, unsafe working environments, and medical practices that can all worsen infertility.[25] Focusing on individual bodies takes the responsibility away from those responsible for infertility in the first place.[24,25,26] Another concern is that ART might make it hard for people experiencing the painful reality of infertility to have closure on the matter, especially when they are going through repeated pregnancies and miscarriages.[27] Some have argued that framing ART as an individual choice fails to consider that infertility and childlessness are still patriarchal taboos that could potentially push people into ART for the sake of avoiding stigmatized childlessness.[24,25]

We Don't Know If a Lot of ART Practices Are Safe

One cool thing is that it seems like freezing eggs does not lead to an increase in anything coming out weird. The babies seem to be born normal and healthy at the same rate as babies that were not made from frozen eggs.[28,29]

But IVF, egg freezing, and egg donation involve people taking drugs that first suppress and then stimulate their ovaries to release eggs, which are collected either to later be donated, used in IVF, or frozen. And there has not been nearly enough research into the long-term health implications of taking those drugs for us to know if and how it will affect people's bodies.[30,31] There's also no way to know how much effort fertility businesses make to fully explain how much we *don't* know to people considering undergoing these treatments, which begs the question of whether or not there's enough informed consent happening.

And Still

I can't bring myself to judge anyone who's doing what they can to have a baby. If when the time comes for me to get pregnant, I can't, I'm pretty sure I would do fucking anything to conceive, including buying eggs from someone poorer than I am if I had to. ART makes families happen for people who want families. And that counts for a lot. Samara Zuckerbrod, who wrote the "Egg Donation" article for Pussypedia.net, wrote her dedication to the person who gave the eggs that made her. It reads:

> My father is an older, single gay man, which made it difficult for him to pursue more common means of making a family, such as adoption. So, he turned to egg donation and surrogacy, and eight months later, my twin sister and I were born. Speaking as an egg donor baby, I am very thankful for my egg donor, though I don't personally know her, for helping my father create the family he wanted. If, whether as a donor or recipient, you choose to pursue egg donation, please be aware of the potential risks, but also the great rewards![32]

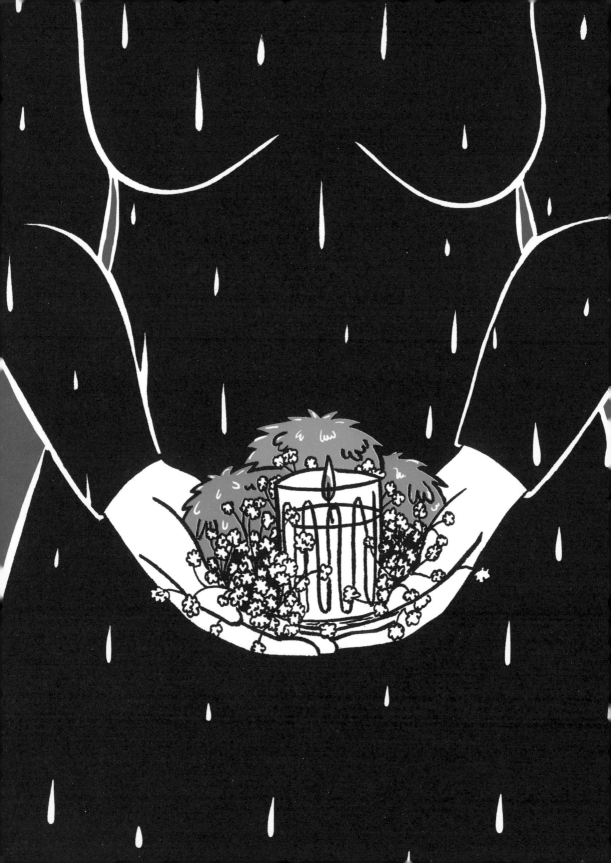

29
Miscarriage

A MISCARRIAGE IS WHEN A PREGNANCY SUDDENLY ENDS AND THE EMBRYO OR FETUS dies before 13–20 weeks.[1,2] After that, it's called a *stillbirth*.[1] Miscarriages most often happen in the first 13 weeks of pregnancy.[3]

Sometimes people know they've had a miscarriage because there is a lot of bleeding and/or cramping and/or abdominal or lower back pain. (These symptoms don't always mean a miscarriage has happened, but you should call your health care provider and get checked out ASAP if you experience them!)[3] Sometimes there are no symptoms, and people don't know it happened until they go in for a checkup.[4]

Miscarriages Are Way More Common Than People Think, and We Should Start Talking About It More So That People Can Stop Feeling So Alone and Ashamed About It

Miscarriages happen a lot but don't get talked about very often. That makes them seem like they don't happen a lot. But they do. It's impossible to know how often miscarriages really happen, since they can happen before people even know they're pregnant.[1] Among known-about pregnancies, they happen 10–20% of the time.[1,3] That's up to one in five pregnancies! And the risk of miscarriage goes up with age. For people under 30 it's about 12%. For people between 35 and 39, it's about 25%.[4]

As Dr. Ellen Støkken Dahl and Dr. Nina Brochmann put it in *The Wonder Down Under*, "Miscarriage is as common as successful pregnancy." Counting the first few days after an egg has been fertilized—even before a pregnancy test can detect a pregnancy—it is assumed that only half of those fertilized eggs turn into pregnancies.[5] The authors suggest that, considering this fact, even though pregnancy tests are now able to detect super early pregnancies, it may not be a good idea to test so early if you're trying to get pregnant: "It may not be wise . . . because most miscarriages happen in the first few weeks after fertilization, before your next period is due. . . . If you wait two extra weeks, until week six of the pregnancy, the risk of miscarriage has fallen to 10 to 15 percent."[4]

When I learned how common miscarriage is, I was shocked. And I suspect most other people would be too. One 2013 study of "men and women across the United States aged 18–69 years" found that "of those who had a miscarriage . . . 47% felt guilty, 41% [felt] that they had done something wrong, 41% felt alone, and 28% felt ashamed."[6] I bet people wouldn't feel so bad if they only knew how truly common it is.

As Dr. Dahl and Dr. Brochmann say, "Many women are left feeling isolated, with an unjustified sense of shame and guilt, at a time when they're most in need of support and consideration from the people around them. Let's start talking to each other!"[5]

What If I Have a Miscarriage?

If you have a miscarriage, there is no right way to feel about it. It might be very hard for you, or it might not, and both are legitimate. As Ash Harlan, a certified nurse-midwife (CNM) and my childhood bestie's bestie, who I once went on a very nice hike with, wrote for the "Miscarriage" article on Pussypedia.net:

> It is important to know that there are many different ways someone may process a miscarriage. Cultural values, religion, family, and life experiences can affect the way someone reacts to miscarriage. Mourning is normal. Holding a ceremony

and naming the baby is normal. Feeling a sense of relief is normal. Wanting to move on and try for the next pregnancy soon is normal. Wanting to wait, or not try for another pregnancy is normal. . . . [W]hether or not the pregnancy was desired or if an abortion was planned does not determine what the "right" reaction is. The range of emotion is vast, and no response [is] wrong.[7]

The word itself—*miscarriage*—kind of sounds like it's the carrier's fault. Like they mis-carried. That's not true. There are a lot of things that can cause a miscarriage. About half happen because something has gone awry with the development of the fetus, and that just happens because the creation of a human is a super complex process and a lot can go wrong. A gazillion strands of DNA separate and recombine during fetal development, and sometimes they just don't match up right.[2] And that is no pregnant person's fault.

Sometimes miscarriages can also happen as a result of chronic illnesses like diabetes or thyroid disease.[1] That is still definitely not any pregnant person's fault, which is worth saying because some people blame other people for having diseases, which is baloney, and also because I don't want any person who lost a pregnancy because of a chronic illness to feel like it is their fault. Because it's not.

The Criminalization of Miscarriage

Smoking and alcohol also increase the chances of a miscarriage,[1] but that does not make someone who engaged in those behaviors and then had a miscarriage a murderer. This may seem obvious, but it may become *cringes with rage* an important legal battle soon. As the Supreme Court shifts conservative, it is likely that a long-fought battle will be settled: whether or not a fetus has the full rights of a person. If the Supreme Court decides that it does, we are not only likely to see *Roe v. Wade* overturned but also criminal cases brought against people who have miscarriages. And we know that poor people and BIPOC who have miscarriages will likely be targeted the most. They already are.

Anti-abortionists and fetal-personhood proponents have long victimized Black people to further their cause. The *New York Times* Editorial Board wrote in a 2018 series on "Women's Rights":

The crack epidemic of the late 1980s and early 1990s [popularized] the idea of fetal rights. Many Americans became seized with the fear—fanned by racism and, as it turned out, false—that crack-addicted black mothers in inner cities were giving birth to a generation of damaged and possibly vicious children. This false fear supplied considerable force to the idea that the interests of a fetus could come in conflict with those of the woman carrying it—and that the woman may have forfeited any claim on society's protection.[8]

Anti-abortionists villainized Black mothers to get people on board with the idea that fetuses needed protection. Now, decades later, to establish fetal "personhood," anti-abortionists have been bringing criminal cases against poor and BIPOC people who have had miscarriages all over the country, using them as sacrificial lambs and sometimes even sending them to jail—even when they have other, living children to take care of—to create legal precedents that will eventually make a fetus a legal person and help overturn *Roe v. Wade*.[8,9,10,11,12]

Harriet A. Washington explains in her book *Medical Apartheid*: "The myth of the crack baby also helped to fuel criminal prosecutions against pregnant drug users, three-quarters of which have been filed against women of color."[13]

National Advocates for Pregnant Women, a nonprofit that "works to secure the human and civil rights, health and welfare of all people, focusing particularly on pregnant and parenting women, and those who are most likely to be targeted for state control and punishment—low income women, women of color, and drug-using women," says that in cases like these, about 7 out of 10 "women" charged cannot afford a lawyer.[8,14]

Please Accompany Me Down My Mental Terror-Toilet and Then Out the Other Side to Something That's Not Quite Hope

I wrote this chapter during the very days that the US Senate was scurrying to confirm anti-abortionist Amy Coney Barrett to the Supreme Court. My fear about these issues was and continues to be visceral. I fear that the Supreme Court will establish fetal personhood and overturn *Roe v. Wade*. I fear that making abortion illegal will be just the beginning of a longer process of stripping people with pussies of our bodily sovereignty. It benefits The Patriarchy to control our bodies because taking away our bodily autonomy makes it possible to strip us of all of our other forms of power. And The Patriarchy, God, it never ever stops working.

I sat writing this at my living room table, in bright Mexico City sunshine, conjuring up dark, *Handmaid's Tale*–like dystopias and wondering if I will be brave enough to resist and at what cost while watching iridescent green hummingbirds drink nectar from orange aloe vera flowers right outside my window. And to ward off the terror I felt in my stomach and the anxiety I felt in my chest, I tried to formulate my call to action to you and to myself.

The first part we already know—we must follow these issues in the news, we must call and email our government representatives, and we really must vote.

Just as importantly, though, let's always notice the hummingbirds. Please let's tether ourselves to beauty and not flush ourselves down dystopian toilets like I was that day. Working yourself up and down like that just wrings the energy out of you. It also does nothing to prepare us for the creative and brave actions that we will have to take to protect our rights and one another—the actions I can't imagine right now because I'm too busy worrying and writing this book.

I remember one unworried day I spent with my grandpa on a cold, gray beach when I was a teenager. He lay on his side directly in the sand, propped up on his elbow watching the sky. He told me how hummingbirds have an incredible ability to slow themselves down, to lower their body temperature and heart rate and breathing to conserve energy. That's how their tiny buzzing bodies endure long, seemingly impossible journeys.

We should really always notice the hummingbirds.

To donate to National Advocates for Pregnant Women, go to https://www .nationaladvocatesforpregnantwomen.org/.

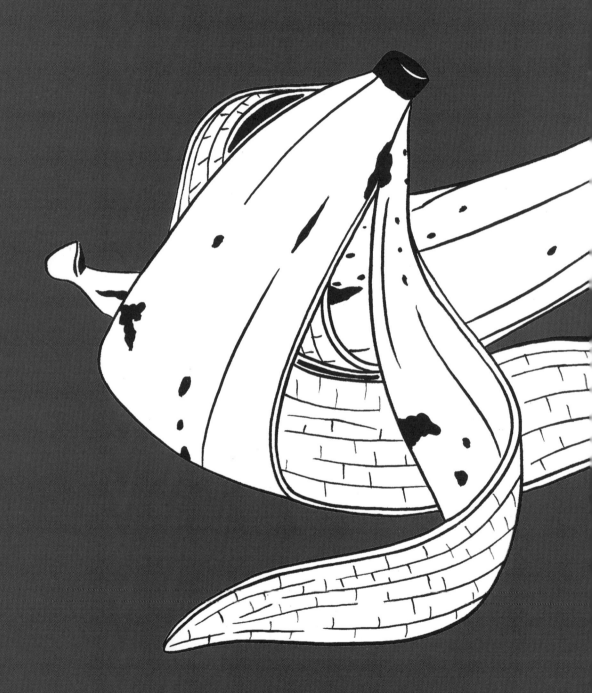

SHIT THE PATRIARCHY TRIES TO SELL YOU

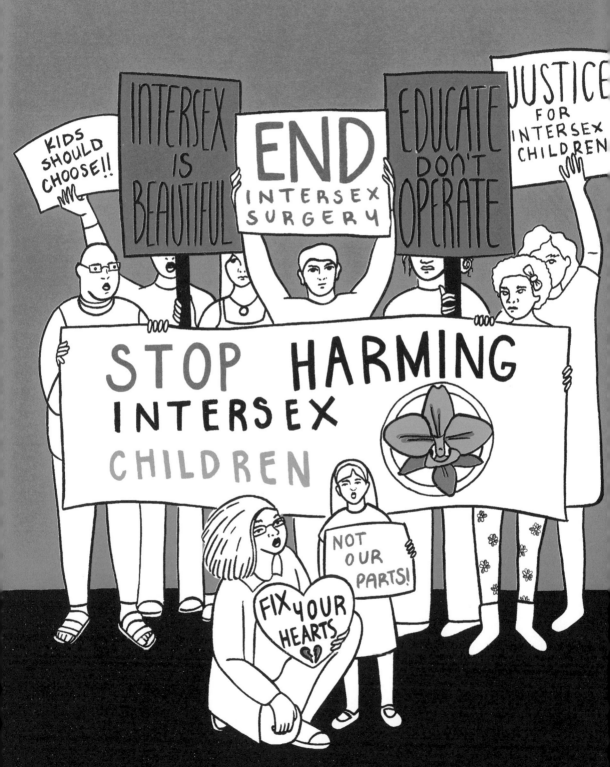

30
Intersex Surgery and the International Movement Against It

Interview with Laura Inter

Intersex bodies have sex characteristics that do not fit into what is usually considered "male" or "female." That does not mean those bodies necessarily pose a health risk or a problem. Still, doctors perform extreme surgeries that often have long-lasting physical and psychological effects on intersex babies and children before they can give meaningful consent in the name of making their bodies more "normal," of fixing the "problem" that their bodies don't fit into predetermined categories. Actually, our cultural obsession with categories is the problem—not intersex bodies, which are often perfectly healthy and functional.[1]

Because of the work of the Intersex Justice Project and the allies that have joined them, two major US hospitals—Boston Children's Hospital and Chicago's Lurie Children's Hospital—have committed to stop performing intersex surgeries on babies. Two out of all the rest of the hospitals in the country (/world) is not enough, but it is an exciting start. The international grassroots movement for intersex rights has gained a lot of traction in raising awareness around the issue. Human Rights Watch,[1] the World Health Organization,[2] three former US surgeons general,[3] and the United Nations Human Rights Office of the High Commissioner[4] have all made statements against nonconsensual intersex surgery.

I first learned about the movement to end intersex surgeries in 2014 from Pidgeon Pagonis, an intersex activist from my hometown, Chicago, and co-founder of the Intersex Justice Project. I asked them out on a date (slid into the DMs) because they're hot. I didn't know much at the time about their work, and I'm pretty sure I made some really ignorant comments on that (first and last) date. I'm still learning from Pidgeon, though, and continue to have a big crush on them, but now more because of their incredible, tireless activism to protect the rights of intersex people.

When I wanted an article about intersex bodies for Pussypedia.net, Pidgeon put me in touch with Laura Inter, founder of Brújula Intersexual (Intersex Compass), a Mexican collective that works with activists all over Latin America and in Spain toward two main goals: to change medical practices on and social representations of intersex bodies and to facilitate a supportive community for intersex people and their families.

Brújula Intersexual maintains an online database of intersex information and reports of abuse of intersex bodies. The group also produces and distributes educational content in Spanish, collaborates with human rights organizations in generating reports, advises state- and federal-government bodies on public policy, and conducts workshops. The site's tagline is: "Intersex people do not need to change their bodies; society needs to change its mind."

Laura Inter keeps a low profile. There are no pictures of her on the internet, all her work is published under a pseudonym, and she almost never talks about herself, which, in the age of social media, is not just rare but radical. When I asked her why, she gave me the most low-key gangster answer imaginable:

> I've never seen the sense or use in posting my photos or what I'm doing on social media. It's dangerous to be a public figure in the world of activism because it can lead to pride and self-importance, which would hinder my work and my life in general. I like to lead a simple and quiet life. Plus, being an activist or doing any human rights–based work in Mexico is dangerous. Many environmental and LGBT activists have been assassinated. So I'm trying to avoid risk.

Also, being anonymous is a form of protest against the overexposure of intersex bodies. From the time we're babies until we're able to say, "Enough!" we have dozens of doctors and medical students surrounding us, observing and touching our most "intimate" parts—even taking pictures. We are also overexposed in the media where our bodies are a spectacle. The goal of "visibility" does not mean someone in front of a camera, but rather to make visible the violations of our human rights.

Here's what the work Laura risks her life to do is all about (in translation from the original Spanish).

What does *intersex* mean?

Since 2006, the official term for intersex variations is *disorders of sex development*, but we consider that term [to be] pathologizing. Intersex is a variation in body shape and composition. It is not a pathology. It's common for intersex variations to be seen as "deformities," but, actually, these variations are well within the natural process of genital development. Intersex is often thought of as a "third sex," or as something related to a nonbinary gender identity, which is also incorrect.

Someone can be born with typical female genitals but also with internal testicles. Or people can be born with genitals that look like they're between typical male and female, for example: a clitoris that's bigger than "normal," a penis that is smaller than "normal," the lack of a vaginal opening, or a common duct where the urethra and vagina open. People can be born with a genetic composition called *mosaic*, which means that some cells have XX chromosomes while others have XY or their chromosomes can be XXY or X0. There is no single intersex anatomy. Some people don't find out that they have intersex variations until puberty when an expected change doesn't play out exactly as expected for a man or a woman.

What kinds of surgeries are performed on intersex bodies to "normalize" them?

In almost the whole world, the medical protocol for people with intersex variations includes medically unnecessary "normalizing" genital surgeries on babies who are unable to provide consent or to understand what these interventions represent or what their consequences are. The medical establishment defends these practices by claiming that they help people avoid problems in social relationships. But actually, these interventions just exacerbate the discrimination and violence that intersex people face as a result of stigma.

When a baby is born with genital differences, or what doctors call "ambiguous genitalia," it will most frequently be assigned female because, according to doctors, it's "easier to build" a vagina surgically than [it is to "build"] a penis. So usually they'll do one of two surgeries.

The first is a reduction in the size of the clitoris, a clitoroplasty, which can even mean removing the clitoris completely. This is usually performed before the baby is a year old, justified on the grounds that it "helps the parents bond with their babies." The second is a vaginoplasty, which is usually performed after a child is 10 years old, although we know of cases where they've been performed much earlier. This is for when there is no vaginal canal or when doctors consider the vaginal canal to be too short or narrow to be penetrated by a penis. To build or lengthen it, surgeons use tissue from other parts of the body, like leg skin, the tissue inside of the cheek, or intestinal tissue.

Using intestinal tissue has a lot of risks, including digestive problems, infections, bad odor, constant flow from the intestinal graft, perforation of the intestines, intestinal adhesions in the place where the intestinal tissue was taken, and even serious chronic problems such as tissue necrosis, which can be fatal. In the case of taking tissue from the leg or back to form the vaginal canal, we have seen cases of infections and hair growth inside of the vagina created by surgery. In the case of taking tissue from the inside of the cheek, there's risk of scarring in the mouth, which can become annoying or painful and implies a risk of infection.

After vaginoplasty, whether or not other tissue was used to lengthen the canal, doctors commonly recommend the use of vaginal dilators, which are metal or plastic tubes of various thicknesses and sizes to keep the vagina open and "functional." Either someone has to put them in themselves, doctors do it in the hospital with or sometimes without anesthesia, or parents have to do it.

If the baby is assigned "male," medical protocol includes multiple surgeries and hormonal treatments that aim for the child to have a penis that is the size—at the doctor's discretion—"necessary to penetrate a vagina." They also try to make sure the penis urinates from its tip rather than from its base, so the person can pee standing up. If the boy does not have descended testicles, the procedure may include testicular grafts of various materials.

These are complex procedures that require multiple surgeries—most of which are performed to repair problems left behind by previous surgeries. We know of a case of a 16-year-old boy who had genital differences at birth but no health problems. He underwent his first surgery when he was a year old, and to date, he has undergone 14 surgeries and requires more due to complications. He still urinates sitting down.

Needless to say, for people forced into these "treatments," there can be serious physical and psychological harm, including partial or total loss of genital sensation, urinary incontinence, pain, recurrent infections, scars, bleeding, adhesions in the surgical area, lifelong dependence on hormone replacement therapy, depression, anxiety, post-traumatic stress disorder, and trauma comparable to that of victims of sexual abuse, among others.

What are the main problems people with intersex bodies face?

After these surgeries are performed, it's common for doctors and hospitals to refuse to release our medical records. They deny us our right to the truth.

Globally, there are very few trained psychologists and specialists who can offer dignified, informed, and efficient care to intersex people. It's all too common that we go to the doctor for problems unrelated to our intersex characteristics, and the doctor ends up fixating there anyway and asking inappropriate questions. By doing this, they neglect or delay attention to the health issue that the person was seeking care for in the first place.

And finally, when intersex people are mentioned in the media or in legislation, it's rare that intersex people or organizations are actually consulted, which means that our actual needs and the specificities of violence that we experience go unaddressed. Sometimes laws and recommendations are explicitly contrary to our cause. It also contributes to the spread of myths, misconceptions, misinformation, and stigmatization.

What is the alternative to performing these surgeries? How should doctors treat intersex bodies?

The coherent solution would be to educate people, so there's less discrimination, rather than modifying healthy bodies without consent. We should start talking about intersex bodies in schools. Doctors, the media, governments, and society in general need to start listening to the voices of intersex people.

Ideally, we would be giving kids with intersex bodies the opportunity to grow up with an intact body and without the physical and psychological trauma of "normalizing" surgeries and treatments that violate their human rights. It is just not appropriate to intervene on the healthy body of a minor, without their consent, for "aesthetic" reasons. We should wait for intersex girls and boys to make decisions about their own bodies when they are fully aware of the possible consequences those decisions may have on their life and health.

Also, intersex people who have already suffered these procedures should be entitled to their medical records and to compensation for damages.

How did the global movement against surgical intersex surgery form, and what is that movement like right now?

In the 1950s, surgical "treatments" for intersex variations began to be medical protocol in US hospitals. In time, these protocols were adopted in hospitals in practically every country in the world. The intersex movement emerged in the US with the Intersex Society of North America (ISNA) in the early 1990s, when intersex people who were born in the 1950s and who suffered from these protocols were old enough to discover what had happened to them and to speak out against these human rights violations.

That pattern repeated in other countries, and now there are groups and organizations of intersex people all over the world demanding their right to their bodily autonomy and integrity. Brújula Intersexual was the first organization led by intersex people in Mexico. It was founded on October 27, 2013, and from its foundation, a Spanish-speaking intersex community began to take shape that did not exist before. Now there are many more projects and organizations in various Latin American countries and in Spain.

How can people support the intersex justice movement?

Inform yourself, with intersex-led organizations, about who intersex people are and the problems that we face. Follow intersex organizations on social networks, share their publications, attend their events, or—if you are able—financially support them. You can also simply ask them what their needs are and how you can help. Help other people understand that there is a huge amount of diversity in people's bodies and that everyone is valuable. You never know who might be listening.

What do you want other intersex people to know?

You are not alone. You can find people with similar life experiences, support, information, and a beautiful community. It's always possible to heal.

RESOURCES

For people with intersex variations and their families:

- brujulaintersexual.org
- vivirintersex.org
- intersexyandrogino.wordpress.com
- intrsx.org/index.php
- intersexjusticeproject.org
- interactadvocates.org

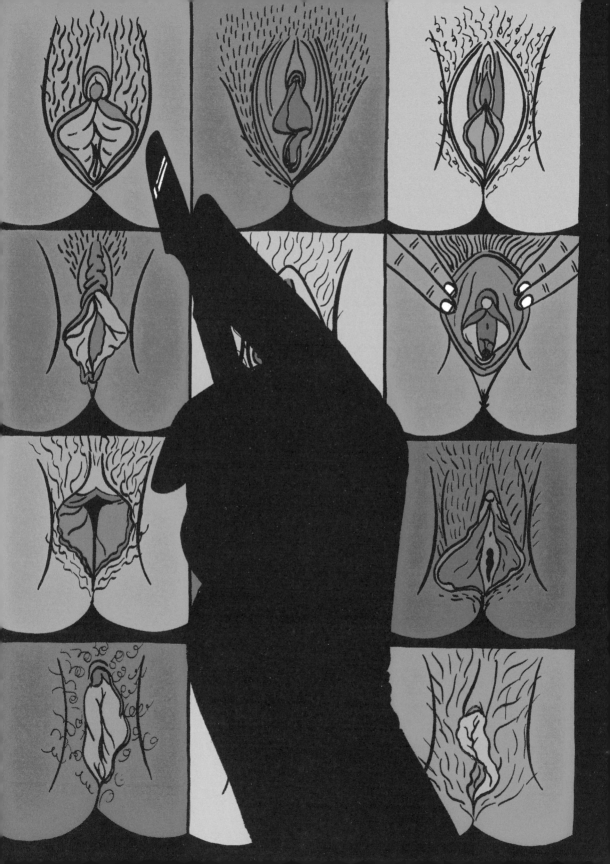

31
Pussy Plastic Surgery

SOMETIMES PUSSY PLASTIC SURGERY IS CALLED *FEMALE GENITAL COSMETIC SURGERY* (FGCS), which assumes all pussies are "female." Sometimes it's called *vaginal rejuvenation*, which makes me want to barf because it evokes the idea that pussies need rejuvenation, reinforces the narratives that people can "wear out" their pussies by having sex or "ruin" them by having children. They can't. Also, it's calling the whole pussy the *vagina*, which—for the millionth time—is wrong. FGCS can include changing the size, shape, or texture of the mons, inner or outer labia, clitoral hood, G-spot, vagina, or any other pussy part.

Some people get these surgeries to remedy physical discomfort, during sex or just during life, that results from the shapes/sizes of their pussy parts—like if your labia are big enough that they chafe on your pants.[1] Some people do it as a follow-up to gender-affirmation surgery, usually to make more defined labia.[2] Some do it to reverse a previous, nonconsensual genital mutilation. Sometimes, it treats prolapse or incontinence.[1] That's all good and well. But very often, these surgeries serve aesthetic purposes, or aesthetically driven emotional purposes, which I would *not* say is all good and well. That's what we're going to focus on here.

FGCS has gotten way more common recently. Labiaplasties, for example, increased more than 50% between 2014 and 2018 in the US.[3] In Australia, labiaplasties performed in the public health system alone tripled between 2001 and 2010.[4] In the UK, labiaplasties performed by the National Health Service doubled between 2002 and 2007.[5] In 2017, the International Society of Aesthetic Plastic Surgery reported that labiaplasty had increased 45% globally from 2014 to 2015, making it the world's fastest-growing plastic surgery.[6]

Why, God?

One study that looked at posts in online communities about FGCS found that "emotional discomfort regarding self-appearance and social and sexual relationships was found to be the most frequent and most prominent motivation for considering labial reduction surgery."[7] But why are people so distraught about their labia and convinced that others will be too?

Almost every pussy in mainstream porn is small, taut, neat, tucked in, hairless, pink, and symmetrical. They are internal, contained, and diminutive because they are manifestations of The Patriarchy's desire for our bodies to be passive and powerless. Many porn pussies have been digitally altered to be literally infantilized.[8] And yet, porn pussies are not just considered the new ideal. Tragically, many people probably think they represent what is common. (It's easy to look around and see that most people don't have model bodies, but many people with pussies rarely ever see other people's vulvas.)

One small-scale UK study of people who sought out labiaplasty found that most interview subjects reported thinking that their labia were abnormal.[9] But another small-scale UK study found that the labia of the vast majority of people who elect for labiaplasty were a "normal" size presurgery. This study acknowledges that "definitions of normal are problematic" since there's a lack of data about normal labia sizes and there is no universally accepted clinical limit for what normal-size labia are.[10] But really, a measurement used to define "normal"-size labia might just be a red herring. The idea that "normal" is important comes from The Patriarchy. The real goal is to overthrow the authoritarian regime of "normalcy" in favor of whatever-the-fuck-your-labia-look-like-is-perfect anarchy.

It's not just The Patriarchy and porn that abstractly, passively sell us this idea of the porn pussy as "normal." It is also actual human beings who sit in front of computers and actively think about how to make people feel badly enough about their pussies to spend thousands of dollars on unnecessary and painful and potentially risky surgeries.

One review of studies that documented and analyzed FGCS-provider websites and marketing tactics found that websites and advertisements consistently use misleading medical terminology like *labial hypertrophy*, which means "labia that are too big," that has no actual established standard attached to it and no established risk factors to your health and is basically Not a Thing. Many FGCS providers use before-and-after photographs to make it as clear as possible: if your inner labia hang below your outer labia, you have a disease.[11] They insist that the porn pussy is not just culturally favorable but medically, objectively, scientifically "normal." Imagine telling cis men they had a disease if their dicks weren't the size of a porn star's.

These websites go on to use abusive language to describe super-common characteristics, like calling pubic fat "unsightly," and inner labia that hang past the outer labia "oversize," "awkward," and "unappealing." Then they talk about how "aesthetically unpleasing" genitals cause shame and embarrassment, "feeling freakish," and "devastating effects" on someone's life. And, of course, they say that surgery is the solution.[11]

In case you're not mad yet, a bunch of the sites get into this awful bull-diarrhea wherein they tell people with pussies to "do it for men." Like, basically, *If your pussy feels loose or your labia are hangy-downy, men won't like it.* As the authors of the review keenly noted, this kind of marketing reinforces the idea that people with pussies should passively exist for men's pleasure.[11] It tells people with pussies to cut off sensitive, pleasure-generating tissue to make themselves more sexually pleasing to men.

It's easy to imagine that someone who may not previously have had shame about their pussy would feel shame after visiting these websites. Their implied logic is that the body parts cause shame because those parts are inherently Bad. But it's The Patriarchy's impossible norms that cause shame, not labia. And it's the assholes writing and making money off of this shit who are Bad. They are selling shame to make money. That should be way more shameful than having literally any size labia ever.

FGCS Is Not Considered Safe

Now, guess if most marketing materials realistically describe the risks associated with these procedures.

Good guess: no the fuck they don't.[11]

And they really should because there is not enough data for these surgeries to be considered "safe." In a 2020 statement on FGCS, the American College of Obstetricians and Gynecologists wrote that these procedures "pose substantial risk and their safety and effectiveness have not been established." The statement goes on to say that people "should be informed about the lack of high-quality data that support the effectiveness of genital cosmetic surgical procedures and counseled about their potential complications, including pain, bleeding, infection, . . . altered sensation, . . . and need for reoperation."[1]

According to the Royal Australian College of General Practitioners, other potential risks and complications include "scarring, resulting in lumpy irregular margins of tissue or [inversion] of inner lining of labia, . . . removal of too much tissue, resulting in pain with and without intercourse—for example, clitoral hood reductions where too much clitoral tissue remains exposed and rubs on to undergarments and causes pain and discomfort; tearing of scar tissue during childbirth following previous FGCS procedures; psychological distress; [and] reduced lubrication."[8]

Some FGCS procedures (often the ones marketed as "vaginal rejuvenation") are done with lasers as well as some procedures that are meant to help with vulva or vagina pain caused by vulvodynia, GPPPD, or menopause symptoms. But none of these procedures are recommendable.

As far as the safety of these laser treatments goes, the FDA released this statement in 2018:

> To date, we have not cleared or approved for marketing any energy-based devices to treat these symptoms or conditions, or any symptoms related to menopause, urinary incontinence, or sexual function. The treatment of these symptoms or conditions by applying energy-based therapies to the vagina may lead to serious adverse events, including vaginal burns, scarring, pain during sexual intercourse, and recurring/chronic pain.[12]

And a 2019 literature review on the safety and efficacy of laser treatments for pussies concluded: "Based on the available scientific evidence and on the lack of long term follow-up, the use of LASER should, so far, not be recommended for the treatment of vaginal atrophy, vulvodynia, lichen sclerosus, stress urinary incontinence, vaginal prolapse, or vaginal laxity."[13] (Did you know *laser* was an acronym? Stands for "light amplification by stimulated emission of radiation.")

Pussy Prerogative and Pussy Prison

Some people say that everyone has the right to have plastic surgery if they want, and who is anybody to tell anybody else what to do with their body, because actually that's exactly what feminism is trying to stop, isn't it?!

Well . . . yes! And as Jia Tolentino wrote in a 2019 article about plastic surgery: "In a world where women are rewarded for youth and beauty in a way that they are rewarded for nothing else—and where a strain of mainstream feminism teaches women that self-objectification is progressive because it's profitable—cosmetic work might seem like one of the few guaranteed high-yield projects that a woman could undertake."[14]

After all, a few studies suggest that FGCS can indeed improve how people feel about their pussies and improve their sexual satisfaction (though other studies have found the opposite), so why shouldn't people do that?[15,16]

I've said many times in this very book that our bodies are ours, and we should do with them what we please. But I don't see resorting to FGCS to alleviate cruelly and intentionally, culturally imposed shame as "doing what we please." I see it as bribing a prison guard with your own flesh for an hour of yard time. And while I understand feeling like you'd do *anything* for some yard time, we shouldn't be in pussy prison in the first place.

Still, we should not judge or shame people who elect to have these surgeries. Nor should we assume that the bullshit is lost on them. As Lih-Mei Liao and Sarah M. Creighton wrote in the introduction to their 2019 book, *Female Genital Cosmetic Surgery: Solution to What Problem?*, some people with pussies "say explicitly that their desire to have the interventions is shaped by normative pressures. However, such awareness is not always enough to defend against the unrelenting feelings of being not good enough."[17]

Yes, we should all feel amazing about our bodies. And yes, that can be extremely hard to accomplish—harder than getting surgery. In a 2019 article about her labiaplasty, Allison Penner wrote:

> Even though I underwent the labiaplasty to address my physical pain, the insecurity I felt around my vulva's appearance has also disappeared, which I feel a lot of guilt about. I wish I could have been a better representative for the spectrum of vulva appearances and been as comfortable and confident with its former appearance as I am now.[18]

I feel that. I wish I loved my chubby belly. I definitely don't. That's OK, though, because I'm trying. The process is the point. Let's not turn escaping body standards into yet another standard that we can fail to meet. That's just another form of pussy prison. One FGCS-provider website listed, among the supposed benefits of these procedures, "a sense of freedom."[11]

If you're considering or have already gotten FGCS because, despite fully knowing the bullshit and the risks, you can't or couldn't live with your body as it is or was, I get it. I support you! I sincerely hope you get or got a reprieve from your suffering.

I just hope people don't confuse a "sense" of freedom for the real thing. Because if we lose sight of where we are and where we want to go, we're gonna be stuck here forever.

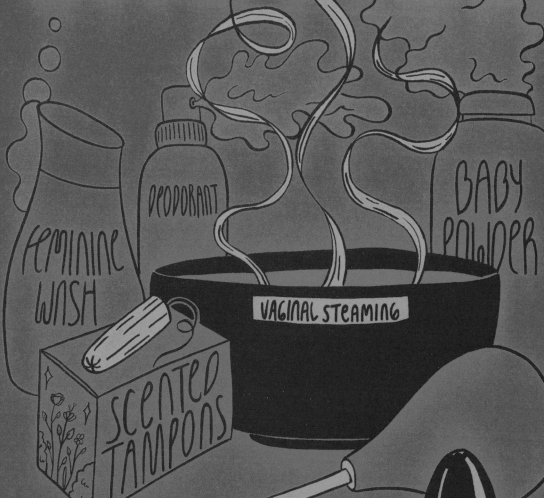
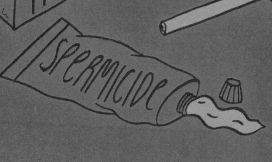
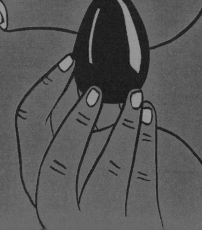

32
Shit You Should Never Use

HERE I HAVE COMPILED A LIST OF SOME THINGS THAT I WOULD ADVISE YOU NOT TO buy or use for/on/in/around your pussy. Of course, everyone should buy and use whatever they like and want to, as long as they're making informed decisions. Really, you do you. I'm trying to help you do that by giving you information, but I'm also going to give you my opinions because I have a lot of those!

Anything Scented

Anything scented or with fragrance/perfume is not a good idea. Fragrances are legally allowed to be trade secrets, so companies don't have to disclose what's in them to regulatory agencies like the FDA.[1] Products like scented toilet paper or scented "intimate wipes" often have ingredients that can irritate skin, that could mess up your hormones, and even that could cause cancer.[2] And since your vulva is extremely sensitive skin, it is prone to getting irritated and itchy from all those fun secret ingredients.[3,4] Also, your vagina is quick to absorb chemicals into your bloodstream, so if you put something like a scented tampon in there, whatever toxic stuff is in there will really get into your body.[3] Plus, have you ever smelled a bloody scented tampon? It's definitely fucking disgusting, which I would not say about a good old-fashioned bloody unscented tampon.

Douches

If your pussy smells bad all the sudden or just markedly different than usual, that's probably a sign of infection, which a douche will absolutely not heal and might actually make worse. Douches disrupt your microbiome's bacterial balance, which can lead to irritation, dryness, and infections like yeast and bacterial vaginosis (BV).[5] When your microbiome gets thrown off balance, your pH level gets less acidic, which makes it easier to get STIs.[6] As Hannah Silver wrote for our "Douches" article on Pussypedia.net, "Using a douche for a 'fresh and clean' vagina is a douchey thing to do to your vagina and your body." Selling douches is also a douchey thing to do. Let's not give our money to the people who try to convince us that our pussies are gross to sell us products that they know harm us.

Vaginal Steaming a.k.a. V-Steaming a.k.a. Yoni Steam a.k.a. Chai-Yok

There are no studies showing that this practice is harmful, but nor are there legitimate studies showing that it's safe. A few people have sent me a study called "Fourth Trimester Vaginal Steam Study." But if you go to the study's about section, the first person on their team is the self-professed owner of the largest distributor of vaginal-steam supplies in the United States. Their team is comprised of young people who are beautiful and diverse looking and have impressive educational backgrounds and amazing hair and outfits, and their team looks very trustworthy and feminist. I bet they are! But they have a vested interest in the success of the treatment they were studying, and therefore I don't trust that study. Also, their sample size was tiny. Poke around on the interwebs and you can find people sharing stories of trying to steam and getting burns on their vulvas. At least one burn incident has been documented in a medical journal.[7] Don't look it up; the picture is scary. Dr. Jen Gunter gives a hard no to steaming because "we don't know the effect of steam on the lower reproductive tract, but the lactobacilli strains that keep vaginas healthy are very finicky about their environment and raising the temperature with steam . . . is potentially harmful."[8] Same problem as douching. You don't want to mess up your microbiome . . . or spend money and time on something pointless.

Yoni Eggs

In 2018, Gwyneth Paltrow (who also made steaming a fad), through her company Goop, was promoting and selling "yoni eggs" made of jade and rose quartz, claiming that they were basically *ancient Chinese secrets*. No, literally, her language was "a strictly guarded secret of Chinese royalty in antiquity." The product descriptions claimed that these polished, egg-shaped rocks could "balance hormones, increase bladder control and regulate menstrual cycles." Surprise. There is absolutely no evidence that they can do any of those things. Also, jade is porous, and porous sex toys are literally considered impossible to disinfect, so I would think the same would apply (see Chapter 16 for more about disinfecting different materials). Anything unclean you're sticking in your vagina poses a risk of infection.

Just because something is ancient, alternative, or coming from another culture does not mean it is good or even OK for your pussy. There is definitely a colonialist global history of discarding a lot of valuable ancient knowledge. But that does not mean all ancient medicine is good. Or that modern (mostly white) depictions of ancient medicine are accurate. Look what Goop was doing—using *ancient* and *Chinese* as a way to capitalize on our collective (and kinda extractivist and orientalist) belief that ancient or Other = better. Eastern and Western, alternative and pharmaceutical health solutions merit equal skepticism.

Goop ultimately paid $145,000 in civil penalties for false claims in 2018.[9] And still! As of September 2020, they still sell them . . . for $66 . . . just now with fewer claims in the product descriptions about what the eggs do. One study by (again) Dr. Jen Gunter (who writes a lot about Goop's pseudo-medicinal mishegoss) shows that there is no evidence that jade eggs ever existed in ancient China.[10] All the sites I've found that tell this story do not cite their information and probably got it from Goop, whose team probably pulled it out of their asses as a marketing ploy. Goop can shove their yoni eggs up that same hole as far as I'm concerned.

"Feminine" Wash

Women's Voices for the Earth is a national nonprofit that, for almost three decades, has worked to raise awareness of and accountability for toxic chemicals, especially in products that go in and around pussies. They have a "Hall of Shame" of products, which includes the feminine washes by Summer's Eve, Equate, Vagisil, CVS, Intimore, and Lemisol. They say it's a no-go on these products because they contain potentially harmful things like fragrances, parabens, methylchloroisothiazolinone, methylisothiazolinone, DMDM hydantoin, D&C Red No. 33, Ext D&C Violet No. 2, and FD&C Yellow No. 5, which can mess with hormone levels and cause irritation, allergic reactions, and even asthma.[11] I say these products are a no-go because you don't need to waste your money on them! Your vagina cleans itself, and soaps can throw off the vagina's microbiome. And for your vulva, normal, fragrance-free soap will do.[12] Many sources, like Healthline and even Dr. Gunter, say you don't even need to use soap on your vulva.[13,14] I have a sweaty crotch, and that sounds entirely unrealistic to me, but, hey, try it for yourself!

Vaginal Deodorants

Vaginal deodorant as a concept makes me mad. PUSSIES HAVE A SMELL. Not only is this shit unnecessary, it's harmful. Vaginal deodorants often contain fragrance, parabens, and benzethonium chloride, which can (again!) cause irritation, messed-up hormones, harm to your reproductive abilities, and allergic reactions.[2] This has been known for quite some time. In a 1976 *New York Times* article about an FDA investigation into vaginal deodorants, Leonard H. Lavin, the president of a company that made them, argued that there was no reason to condemn products simply because they are not vital to human existence.[15]

Oh, but sometimes there is.

Even if vaginal deodorants weren't toxic chemically, the very existence of these products is toxic; it condemns the natural state of pussies and causes shame. It suggests that there is something wrong with what pussies smell like normally and that you should try to deodorize that natural smell. Advertisements for these products reiterate old, tired narratives that pussies are gross to make us ashamed, then capitalize on that shame by selling us products that are, at best, unnecessary and, at worst, really bad for us. Lavin also said that criticism against his products came from "negative-minded consumerist groups who would subject our entire economy to a Marxist purge of everything they object to." Lol. Boi, bye.

Baby Powder with Talc

Talc is a mineral and when it is mined it is sometimes mixed with asbestos, a known carcinogen—something that can cause cancer. Internal documents that came out in 2018 during a series of lawsuits show that Johnson & Johnson, a massive corporation that produces body products and pharmaceuticals, has known about this and even been worried about it for over 50 years.[16] But not worried enough to stop selling talc. After the World Health Organization started in 2006 to classify talc-based baby powder as a possible carcinogen when used on the genitals, Johnson & Johnson began an aggressive marketing campaign specifically aimed at selling the product to "curvy Southern women 18–49 skewing African American."[17] In March 2020, after at least 19,400 lawsuits related to talc body powders—many from people who developed ovarian cancer after heavy use of the product—Johnson & Johnson stopped selling talc-based baby powder . . . but only in the United States.[16] Evil fucks. Anyway, if you're determined to powder down there, reach for a non-talc-based powder.

Spermicide and Condoms with Spermicide

There is ample evidence that spermicide—specifically, an ingredient in it called *nonoxynol-9*, can mess up your microbiome and cause skin irritation, which can increase your chance of getting an STI.[18,19,20,21,22,23] There's also a wealth of studies that link spermicide to urinary tract infections.[24,25,26,27,28] There are just way better contraception options out there (see Chapter 20).

Learning to Fish . . . for Pussy Products

This is not an exhaustive list. There will be new fads, new Goops, new discoveries, and new useless and harmful products forever, or until capitalism and The Patriarchy collapse. So here are a few rules of thumb to help you decide what you might or might not want to buy and/or use in and around your pussy:

1. Be skeptical and critical. People tend to pick a side—alternative medicine or Western medicine—and trust one over the other. While both have a lot to offer, both also have a lot of bullshit. Picking a side does not make sense. Be skeptical of all marketing, of all people recommending anything, of all products. Think about who stands to gain from selling you

something. Is it the same person or organization giving you information about that something?

2. No matter who is providing the information, do your own research. Really, just google the product and look for things written about it and check that those things are not written by people who are selling the product. WomensVoices.org is a great resource for learning about different pussy-product chemicals. Go in neutral and let your research decide for you; it's easier to do better research if you don't have any hope or expectation beforehand of any product or practice turning out to be good or bad. Try to seek information both for and against what you're researching, without rooting for any particular outcome. Try to consider the whole landscape of information available when you make decisions.

3. Your pussy is probably fine. Vaginas have mechanisms to keep themselves clean. And again, it's normal for them to have a smell. It is not normal for that smell to be "tropical fresh"! If your pussy smells different from how it usually does, go to the doctor instead of reaching for a product. If you're just living your life and your pussy feels normal, leave it alone and let it do its gloriously perfect thing.

A Letter to Our Readers

Dear You,

We hope this book was helpful. We just want the best for you, no matter who you are. We wish you all the good things we have, the things that took us too long to get, the things we're still working on.

We hope you like yourself. And love and respect yourself. We hope you feel respected and loved and liked by others. And that you find the joy in loving, liking, and respecting others as well.

We hope you feel safe being exactly who you are. We hope you feel safe trying new things, even big things, and also feel safe making mistakes and failing.

We hope you are able to recognize your accomplishments, and to credit yourself for them. And we also hope that your love for yourself is not contingent on "accomplishments" and that your definition of success is broad and takes into consideration that just simply living is really fucking hard. We hope you feel proud of yourself.

We hope you have the kind of friends and lovers who feel proud of you too, who see you, who don't judge you, who help you see that the weirdest part of you is also the best part. The kinds of friends and lovers who you can laugh at all of the pain with and who you can dance with too. We hope you dance.

And we hope in the moments when you can't dance because of shame or fear or doubt that you can remember that those feelings are just the bullshit designed to keep you down, and that they are not really yours to bear. And we hope that you and your friends and lovers will find ways to beat back the bullshit with your love for yourselves and one another and your creativity and the fire in your hearts. We hope you feel, at least in moments, like your heart can move mountains.

We hope you feel peaceful and strong. We hope that your body brings you at least as much joy as consternation. We hope you feel entitled to the space your body takes up and more than that. We hope you feel entitled to take up lots of space, actually—all the space you need.

We hope you feel like you deserve it. Because you do.

We hope you have so much fun.

With love,
Zoe and María

Acknowledgments

Acknowledgments from Zoe

First and always, thank you to my partner in crime, María Conejo. We did it, you sexy bitch! I'm still the president of your fan club (and still not in a Selena kind of way). *Me inspiras, cabrona. Te admiro un chingo.*

Thank you to all of the friends and strangers who gave their time, money, labor, and expertise toward building Pussypedia.net and made all of this possible.

Thank you, Joseph Thomas, Michael Yap, and Dr. Jackie Jahn. You are each true masters of your crafts. Thank you for your friendship and for your work. Our collaboration has been one of the most meaningful experiences of my life.

Thank you, Lauren Marino, our brave editor, for believing in this book, for having a long view, for making it better. Thank you to the entire marketing and publicity team at Hachette.

Elianna Kan, our Russian agent, thank you for believing this book would work when I was too scared to hope and for not giving up even when I was mad at you for trying to convince me. Thank you for seeing my fear and the hope underneath it well enough to be able to pull me around so gently and delicately that I almost didn't notice it had happened. Thank you for being our champion, for your patience (×1000), for your diplomacy, for your dinners, for your unparalleled poetry selections, and most importantly for your friendship.

Melina Gaze and Tarah Knaresboro, I could so extremely literally not have done this without you two, your expertise, your generosity, and your support.

You saw my life very close up and decided that I deserved both your help and a few luxuries even when you both were busy AF, too. That was not lost on me. Thank you. Thank you for teaching me what you worked so hard to learn. Thank you for being SO THOROUGH and careful and detailed and thoughtful. Thank you for being people I could come to both with earnest existential crises and pure petulance and find warmth and encouragement. Your votes of confidence mean everything to me. You two made this book possible and beyond that, you made it fun.

Laura Lee Burks, thank you for knowing how to write good, where, commas, go, *which* versus *that*, and, what a real ellipsis is. Thank you for editing so carefully so quickly and with such a sharp eye for clarity and for remembering all the so many different tiny random stylistic things that need to stay consistent in a book that are wow, so, many. You really made this book so much better in so many ways.

Thank you, Charlie Blanc and Hannah Silver, for being so dang competent and capable and on it and organized, for helping me knock this fucker out and for the ongoing encouragement, which I really did need. You were dream research assistants. But you also are both, like, really good at *thinking*, and so I would also like to thank you for being amazing thinking assistants. I am so excited to watch you do Big Things. I can only hope to be able to help you as much as you helped me. Although you really won't need my help at all. I hope you know you are formidable.

Thank you, Meira Harris, Madeleine Wattenbarger, Lisa Giordono, Bryan Chanes, Oscar Mondragon, and Lauren Steury, for your thoughts, time, and precision. Thank you, Ellena Phillips, for the research and the spanking. And, Madeleine, also thank you for sitting next to me while I wrote this book in every way I could possibly mean that. And for the pickles.

Thank you to everyone who trusted me enough to talk to me about their post-birth pussies and pube-trimming strategies and period management in extreme detail.

Thank you, Debbie Millman, for encouraging and supporting this project every step of the way, for sharing your beautiful home with me.

Thank you, Amy Goldwasser, for opening every door you could for me and for always Getting It.

Thank you, Jessie Savin, for teaching me at a very young age that whoever gives the least fucks has the most power and for telling me hundreds of times to stop covering my belly. Rest in peace, sister.

Thank you, Elsa Mitsoglou, Esq., for alternately being my lawyerboo, boomom, teacherboo, and best friend. Thank you for never, ever letting me stop questioning everything, especially my beliefs about myself. Thank you for your companionship in joy and in heartbreak and in minor grievances. Thank you for always knowing when I actually did need you to TMWTD.

Thank you to my big, beautiful family for holding me always and reading this work all year and encouraging me. Thank you, Grandma Carol and Grampa Jimmy, for fostering my love of science. Thank you, Nana Barbara, for being a loving refuge for all of us. Thank you, Mama, for pushing me out of your pussy and for teaching me that playing hooky is healthy and that community takes work but that it's always worth it. Thank you, Marlee, for your lifelong insistence on utter emotional honesty from everyone. Nobody does that. *Gracias a Magda y Enrique por haberme acogido con tanto amor y a todas las Mujeres Rosas por haberle hecho entender a Dayron.*

Thank you, Dayron Lopez Rosas, for letting me put you so thoroughly on blast. Thank you for combing through every citation in this book to make sure they were in order. Thank you for listening. Thank you for teaching me that it is possible to have a relationship based in unflinching respect and kindness. Thank you for raising my standards for myself and others by being so goddamn fucking nice to everyone always. Thank you for making me laugh every single day even when you are sad. Thank you for taking such exquisite care of my body as my nurse, personal trainer, and sexual partner, and for loving it so unconditionally even when I can't. And thank you for saying I should never say thank you for that. You are an incomprehensible gift.

Lxs amo.

Acknowledgments from María

Thank you, Universe, for being aligned in such a way that Zoe and I got to know each other in this life. Thank you, Zoe, for believing in me, for making all your friends get to know and buy my art way before PP. You encouraged me to believe in myself as an artist and to be confident about my work. Thank you for coming with me further than I could ever imagined and for writing a book that already changed my life. I'm sure it will change many, many more.

Thank you, Mami Geli, for being my first home, for teaching me freedom as the most important thing above all things, for letting me always be myself. For being my teacher of perseverance, strength, resilience. For encouraging me since the first time you realized drawing was a thing for me, thank you for all the art and karate classes you signed me up to. Thank you for giving me the tools to fight back.

Thank you, Mamá María, for being the strongest and most loving human being this Earth has met. I'm very grateful I was lucky enough to get to listen to all the history of your life: the good, the bad, and the awful times. Thank you for being the bravest. Your bravery has motivated me my entire life to keep going and do whatever is, literally, in my hands to fight against the oppression of patriarchy and to encourage women to believe in themselves, to enjoy themselves. Thank you for showing up in my dreams wearing a Pussypedia T-shirt; I know you would be proud. I miss you every single day.

Thank you, Clau, for always being there, empowering me. I'm so grateful you are my sister. Thank you to all the women of my family for being brave and coming along in this journey with me. Thank you, Alex, for being my rock.

Thank you, friends, for being my compass, I love you all with all my heart.

Special thanks to my sexual partners for joining me in the pleasure quest and for helping me understand, love, and get to know my own body.

Thanks to all the amazing artists that helped us illustrate the platform and to all the female, nonbinary, intersex, trans artists out there creating art in the world.

You inspire me.

Thanks to all the people that supported this project.

Forever thankful to you, Elianna, for helping us make this book possible.

Thank you, Lauren and the Hachette team, for believing in us.

Thank you.

Thank you.

Thank you.

Notes

Introduction

1. Lorde, Audre. *Sister Outsider*. Berkeley: Crossing Press, 1984.

2. Wynn, Natalie. "Men." ContraPoints. August 23, 2019. Video, 30:34. https://www.you tube.com/watch?v=S1xxcKCGljY.

3. Crenshaw, Kimberlé. "Demarginalizing the Intersection of Race and Sex: A Black Feminist Critique of Antidiscrimination Doctrine, Feminist Theory and Antiracist Politics." *University of Chicago Legal Forum* 1989, no. 1 (1989): 8. https://chicagounbound.uchicago .edu/uclf/vol1989/iss1/8.

4. Irby, Samantha. "Body Negativity." In *Wow, No Thank You*. New York: Vintage Books, 2020.

5. Wallace, Sophia. "A Case for Cliteracy." Filmed October 2014 at TEDxSalford, Salford, England. Video, 23:17. https://www.ted.com/talks/sophia_wallace_a_case_for_cliteracy.

6. Jean Moore, Lisa, and Adele Clarke. "Clitoral Conventions and Transgressions: Graphic Representations in Anatomy Texts, 1900–1991." *Feminist Studies* 21, no. 2 (Summer 1995): 255–301. https://doi.org/10.2307/3178262.

7. Hoppe, A. Travis, Aviva Litovitz, Kristine A. Willis, et al. "Topic Choice Contributes to the Lower Rate of NIH Awards to African-American/Black Scientists." *Science Advances* 5, no. 10 (October 2019): eaaw7238. https://doi.org/10.1126/sciadv.aaw7238.

8. National Institutes of Health. "Estimates of Funding for Various Research, Condition, and Disease Categories (RCDC)." February 24, 2020. https://report.nih.gov/categorical _spending.aspx#legend11.

9. Parasar, Parveen, Pinar Ozcan, and Kathryn L. Terry. "Endometriosis: Epidemiology, Diagnosis and Clinical Management." *Current Obstetrics and Gynecology Reports* 6, no. 1. (January 2017): 34–41. https://doi.org/10.1007/s13669-017-0187-1.

10. Nutten, Sophie. "Atopic Dermatitis: Global Epidemiology and Risk Factors." *Annals of Nutrition and Metabolism* 66, suppl 1 (April 2015): 8–16. https://doi.org/10.1159 /000370220.

11. Washington, Harriet A. *Medical Apartheid: The Dark History of Medical Experimentation on Black Americans from Colonial Times to the Present*. New York: Anchor Books, 2008.

Pussy Parts

Chapter 1: Anus, Ass Crack, and Rectum

1. Feher, Joseph. *Quantitative Human Physiology: An Introduction*, 2nd ed. Cambridge: Elsevier, 2017.

2. National Cancer Institute. SEER Training Modules. "Anatomy of Colon and Rectum." Accessed November 2, 2020. https://training.seer.cancer.gov/colorectal/anatomy.

3. Ansari, Parswa. "Overview of the Anus and Rectum." *Merck Manual Consumer Version*. Last modified January 2020. https://www.merckmanuals.com/home/digestive-disorders /anal-and-rectal-disorders/overview-of-the-anus-and-rectum.

4. Cohen, Jeffrey, Camilo Fadul, Lawrence Jenkyn, et al. "Chapter 8—Reflex Evaluation." In *Disorders of the Nervous System*, edited by Alexander Reeves and Rand Swenson. Hanover: Dartmouth Medical School, 2008. https://www.dartmouth.edu/~dons/part_1 /chapter_8.html.

5. McBride, Kimberly R., and J. Dennis Fortenberry. "Heterosexual Anal Sexuality and Anal Sex Behaviors: A Review." *Journal of Sex Research* 47, no. 2–3 (March 2010): 123–36. https://doi.org/10.1080/00224490903402538.

6. Moali, Nazanin, and Tristan Taormino. "EP181—Your Ultimate Guide for Anal Pleasure with Tristan Taormino." *Sexology Podcast*. June 16, 2020. https://www.youtube.com /watch?v=fTkX94nEJF4.

7. Boston Women's Health Book Collective. *Our Bodies, Ourselves*. New York: Simon & Schuster, 2011.

8. Kaestle, Christine Elizabeth. "Sexual Insistence and Disliked Sexual Activities in Young Adulthood: Differences by Gender and Relationship Characteristics." *Perspectives on Sexual and Reproductive Health* 41, no. 1 (March 2009): 33–39. https://doi .org/10.1363/4103309.

9. Fahs, Breanne, Eric Swank, and Lindsay Clevenger. "Troubling Anal Sex: Gender, Power, and Sexual Compliance in Heterosexual Experiences of Anal Intercourse." *Gender Issues* 32, no. 1 (October 2014): 19–38. https://doi.org/10.1007/s12147-014-9129-7.

10. American College of Obstetricians and Gynecologists. "Problems of the Digestive System." FAQs. Last reviewed June 2020. https://www.acog.org/patient-resources/faqs /womens-health/problems-of-the-digestive-system.

11. Mayo Clinic Staff. "Anal Fissure." Mayo Clinic. Patient Care & Health Information. Diseases & Conditions. November 17, 2020. https://www.mayoclinic.org/diseases-conditions /anal-fissure/symptoms-causes/syc-20351424.

Chapter 2: The Clitoris

1. O'Connell, Helen E., Sanjeevan Kalavampara, et al. "Anatomy of the Clitoris." *Journal of Urology* 174, no. 4 (October 2005): 1189–95. https://doi.org/10.1097/01.ju.0000173639.38898 .cd.

2. O'Connell, Helen E., John M. Hutson, et al. "Anatomical Relationship Between Urethra and Clitoris." *Journal of Urology* 159, no. 6 (June 1998): 1892–97. https://doi.org/10.1016 /S0022-5347(01)63188-4.

3. Veale, David, Sarah Miles, et al. "Am I Normal? A Systematic Review and Construction of Nomograms for Flaccid and Erect Penis Length and Circumference in up to 15,521 Men." *BJU International* 115, no. 6 (June 2015): 978–86. https://doi.org/10.1111/bju.13010.

4. Chalker, Rebecca. *The Clitoral Truth: The Secret World at Your Fingertips*. New York: Seven Stories Press, 2002.

5. Boston University School of Sexual Medicine. "Female Genital Anatomy." For Health Care Professionals. Accessed December 4, 2020. https://www.bumc.bu.edu/sexualmedicine /physicianinformation/female-genital-anatomy/.

6. Gross, Rachel E., Jeffery DelViscio, and Dominic Smith. "The Clitoris: A Reveal Two Millennia in the Making." *Scientific American*. March 4, 2020. Video, 8:22. https://www .scientificamerican.com/video/the-clitoris-a-reveal-two-millennia-in-the-making/.

7. Deutsch, Maddie, and UCSF Transgender Care. "Information on Testosterone Hormone Therapy." July 2020. https://transcare.ucsf.edu/article/information-testosterone-hormone-therapy.

8. Sigurjónsson, Hannes, Caroline Möllerm, et al. "Long-Term Sensitivity and Patient-Reported Functionality of the Neoclitoris After Gender Reassignment Surgery." *Journal of Sexual Medicine* 14, no. 2 (February 2017): 269–73. https://doi.org/10.1016/j.jsxm.2016.12.003.

9. Laqueur, Thomas. *Making Sex: Body and Gender from the Greeks to Freud*. Cambridge: Harvard University Press, 1990.

10. Di Marino, Vincent, and Hubert Lepidi. *Anatomic Study of the Clitoris and the Bulbo-Clitoral Organ*. Boston: Springer, 2014. https://www.springer.com/gp/book/9783319048932.

11. Moore, Lisa J., and Adele E. Clarke. "Clitoral Conventions and Transgressions: Graphic Representations in Anatomy Texts, c1900–1991." *Feminist Studies* 21, no. 2 (Summer 1995): 255–301. https://doi.org/10.2307/3178262.

12. Sherfey, Mary Jane. "The Evolution and Nature of Female Sexuality in Relation to Psychoanalytic Theory." *Journal of the American Psychoanalytic Association* 14, no. 1 (January 1966): 28–128. https://doi.org/10.1177/000306516601400103.

13. "Women's Health Movement History." Women's Health in Women's Hands. Accessed December 4, 2020. http://womenshealthinwomenshands.com/about/our-history/.

14. Hite, Shere. *The Hite Report: A Nationwide Study of Female Sexuality*. New York: Seven Stories Press, 1976.

15. Seelye, Katharine Q. "Shere Hite, Who Challenged Myths of Female Sexuality, Dies at 77." *New York Times*, September 11, 2020. https://www.nytimes.com/2020/09/11/books/shere-hite-dead.html.

16. Fyfe, Melissa. "Get Cliterate: How a Melbourne Doctor Is Redefining Female Sexuality." *Sydney Morning Herald*, December 8, 2018. https://www.smh.com.au/lifestyle/health-and-wellness/get-cliterate-how-a-melbourne-doctor-is-redefining-female-sexuality-20181203-p50jvv.html.

17. Pin, Jessica. "The Senseless Omission of Clitoral Anatomy from Medical Textbooks." *Jessica Pin on Medium.com*, June 29, 2019. https://medium.com/@jessica86/the-needless-omission-of-clitoral-anatomy-from-medical-textbooks-87756656e8a6.

18. Puppo, Vincenzo, and Giulia Puppo. "Anatomy of Sex: Revision of the New Anatomical Terms Used for the Clitoris and the Female Orgasm by Sexologists." *Clinical Anatomy* 28, no. 3 (April 2015): 293–304. https://doi.org/10.1002/ca.22471.

19. "CLITERACY, 100 Natural Laws." Sophia Wallace—Art. Accessed December 4, 2020. https://www.sophiawallace.art/works#/cliteracy-100-natural-laws/.

Chapter 3: Liquids and Goops (Everything Except Pee and Blood)

1. Saltzman, William Mark, Michael L. Radomsky, et al. "Antibody Diffusion in Human Cervical Mucus." *Biophysical Journal* 66, no. 2 pt. 1 (February 1994): 508–15. https://doi.org/10.1016/s0006-3495(94)80802-1.

2. Brochmann, Nina, and Ellen Støkken Dahl. *The Wonder Down Under*. New York: Quercus, 2017.

3. World Health Organization. *WHO Laboratory Manual for the Examination and Processing of Human Semen*, 5th ed. Switzerland: WHO Press, 2010. https://www.who.int/publications/i/item/9789241547789.

4. Planned Parenthood. "Fertility Awareness." Learn. Birth Control. Accessed December 6, 2020. https://www.plannedparenthood.org/learn/birth-control/fertility-awareness.

5. Grande, G., D. Milardi, F. Vincenzoni, et al. "Proteomic Characterization of the Qualitative and Quantitative Differences in Cervical Mucus Composition During the Menstrual Cycle." *Molecular Omics* 11, no. 6 (June 2015): 1717–25. https://doi.org/10.1039/c5mb00071h.

6. Mayo Clinic Staff. "Masculinizing Hormone Therapy." Mayo Clinic. Patient Care & Health Information. Diseases & Conditions. Tests & Procedures. April 14, 2020. https://www.mayoclinic.org/tests-procedures/ftm-hormone-therapy/about/pac-2038509.

7. Rivera, Y., I. Yacobson, and D. Grimes. "The Mechanism of Action of Hormonal Contraceptives and Intrauterine Contraceptive Devices." *American Journal of Obstetrics and Gynecology* 181, no. 5 pt. 1 (November 1999): 1263–69. https://doi.org/10.1016/s0002-9378(99)70120-1.

8. Ferris, Daron, Paul Nyirjesy, Jack Sobles, et al. "Over-the-Counter Antifungal Drug Misuse Associated with Patient-Diagnosed Vulvovaginal Candidiasis." *Obstetrics & Gynecology* 99, no. 3 (August 2002): 419–25. https://www.sciencedirect.com/science/article/abs/pii/S0029784401017598.

9. Nagoski, Emily. *Come as You Are: The Surprising New Science That Will Transform Your Sex Life*. New York: Simon & Schuster, 2015.

10. Boston University School of Medicine. "Female Genital Anatomy." Sexual Medicine. For Health Care Professionals. Accessed December 6, 2020. https://www.bumc.bu.edu/sexualmedicine/physicianinformation/female-genital-anatomy/.

11. Pastor, Zlatko, and Roman Chmel. "Differential Diagnostics of Female 'Sexual' Fluids: A Narrative Review." *International Urogynecology Journal* 29 (November 2018): 621–29. https://doi.org/10.1007/s00192-017-3527-9.

12. Dwyer, Peter. "Skene's Gland Revisited: Function, Dysfunction and the G Spot." *International Urogynecology Journal* 23, no. 2 (September 2012): 135–37. https://doi.org/10.1007/s00192-011-1558-1.

13. Chalker, Rebecca. *The Clitoral Truth*. New York: Seven Stories Press, 2002.

14. Salama, Samuel, Florence Boitrelle, Amélie Gauquelin, et al. "Nature and Origin of 'Squirting' in Female Sexuality." *Journal of Sexual Medicine* 12, no. 3 (March 2015): 661–66. https://doi.org/10.1111/jsm.12799.

15. Schubach, Gary. "Urethral Expulsions During Sensual Arousal and Ladder Catheterization in Seven Human Females." *Electronic Journal of Human Sexuality* 4 (August 2001). http://www.ejhs.org/volume4/Schubach/abstract.html.

16. Rubio-Casillas, Alberto, and Emmanuele Jannini. "New Insights from Case of Female Ejaculation." *The Journal of Sexual Medicine* 8, no. 12 (December 2011): 3500–04. https://doi.org/10.1111/j.1743-6109.2011.02472.x.

17. Herbenick, Debra, Michael Reece, Devon Hensel, *et al.* "Association of Lubricant Use with Women's Sexual Pleasure, Sexual Satisfaction, and Genital Symptoms: A Prospective Daily Diary Study." *The Journal of Sexual Medicine* 8, no. 1 (January 2011): 202–212. https://doi.org/10.1111/j.1743-6109.2010.02067.x.

Chapter 4: The G-Spot

1. Jannini, Emmanuele, Odile Buisson, and Alberto Rubio-Casillas. "Beyond the G-Spot: Clitourethrovaginal Complex Anatomy in Female Orgasm." *Nature Reviews Urology* 11, no. 9 (Sep 2014): 531–38. https://doi.org/10.1038/nrurol.2014.193.

2. O'Connell, Helen, John M. Huston, Colin R. Anderson, et al. "Anatomical Relationship Between Urethra and Clitoris." *Journal of Urology* 159 (June 1998): 1892–97. https://doi.org/10.1016/S0022-5347(01)63188-4.

3. Kiefer, Elizabeth. "The G-Spot Doesn't Exist." *Cosmopolitan*, April 7, 2020. https://www.cosmopolitan.com/interactive/a32037401/g-spot-not-real.

4. Gosselin, Sophia. "Dr. Ernst Gräfenberg—Remembered by One of His Patients." Humboldt-Universität zu Berlin. December 23, 2006. Accessed via Internet Archive Wayback Machine. https://web.archive.org/web/20061223234326/http://www2.hu-berlin.de/sexology/BIB/grafen.htm.

5. Whipple, Beverly. "Ernst Gräfenberg: From Berlin to New York." *Scandinavian Journal of Sexology* 3, no. 2 (Aug 2000): 43–49. https://web.archive.org/web/20061216120809/http://www2.hu-berlin.de/sexology/GESUND/ARCHIV/GRAFENBERG.HTM.

6. Gräfenberg, Ernest. "The Role of Urethra in Female Orgasm." *International Journal of Sexology* 3, no. 3 (February 1950): 145–48. Accessed via Internet Archive Wayback Machine December 6, 2020. https://web.archive.org/web/20061205033615/http://doctorg.com/Grafenberg.htm.

7. Addiego, Frank, Edwin G. Belzer, Jill Comolli, et al. "Female Ejaculation: A Case Study." *The Journal of Sex Research* 17, no. 1 (Jan 1981): 13–21. https://doi.org/10.1080/00224498109551094.

8. Kahn Ladas, Alice, Beverly Whipple, and John D. Perry. *The G Spot and Other Recent Discoveries About Human Sexuality.* New York: Owl Books, 1982.

9. Nagoski, Emily. *Come as You Are: The Surprising New Science That Will Transform Your Sex Life.* New York: Simon & Schuster, 2015.

Chapter 5: The Urinary Tract and Peeing

1. National Institute of Diabetes and Digestive and Kidney Disease. "The Urinary Tract & How It Works." Health Information. Urologic Diseases. June 2020. https://www.niddk.nih.gov/health-information/urologic-diseases/urinary-tract-how-it-works.

2. Bergamin, Paul A., and Anthony J. Kiosoglous. "Non-Surgical Management of Recurrent Urinary Tract Infections in Women." *Translational Andrology and Urology* 6, no. 2 (July 2017): 142–52. https://doi.org/10.21037/tau.2017.06.09.

3. Foxman, Betsy. "Epidemiology of Urinary Tract Infections: Incidence, Morbidity, and Economic Costs." *American Journal of Medicine* 113, no. 1 (July 2002): 5–13. https://doi.org/10.1016/s0002-9343(02)01054-9.

4. Foxman, Betsy. "The Epidemiology of Urinary Tract Infection." *Nature Reviews Urology* 7, no. 12 (December 2010): 653–60. https://doi.org/10.1038/nrurol.2010.190.

5. Luber, Karl M. "The Definition, Prevalence, and Risk Factors for Stress Urinary Incontinence." *Reviews in Urology* 6, suppl. 3 (2004): S3–9. https://www.ncbi.nlm.nih.gov/pmc/articles/PMC1472862/#!po=76.6667.

6. Lasak, Anna Maria, Marjorie Jean-Michel, Phuong Uyen Le, et al. "The Role of Pelvic Floor Muscle Training in the Conservative and Surgical Management of Female Stress Urinary Incontinence: Does the Strength of the Pelvic Floor Muscles Matter?" *PM & R: The Journal of Injury, Function, and Rehabilitation* 10, no. 11 (May 2018): 1198–10. https://doi.org/10.1016/j.pmrj.2018.03.023.

7. Dallosso, Hellen M., Catherine McGrother, Ruth Matthews, et al. "The Association of Diet and Other Lifestyle Factors with Overactive Bladder and Stress Incontinence: A Longitudinal Study in Women." *British Journal of Urology International* 92, no. 1 (Jul 2003): 69–77. https://doi.org/10.1046/j.1464-410x.2003.04271.x.

8. de Oliveira, Maria Clara Eugênia, Larissa R. Varella, et al. "The Relationship Between the Presence of Lower Urinary Tract Symptoms and Waist Circumference." *Diabetes, Metabolic Syndrome and Obesity: Targets and Therapy* 9 (July 2016): 207–11. doi:10.2147/DMSO.S106221.

9. Højberg, Karen-Elise, Jannie Dalby Salvig, Nitnoi Albertsen Winsløw, et al. "Urinary Incontinence: Prevalence and Risk Factors at 16 Weeks of Gestation." *British Journal of*

Obstetrics and Gynaecology 106, no. 8 (August 1999): 842–50. https://doi.org/10.1111/j.1471
-0528.1999.tb08407.x.

10. Thom, David H., and Guri Rortveit. "Prevalence of Postpartum Urinary Incontinence:
A Systematic Review." *Acta Obstetricia et Gynecologica Scandinavica* 89, no. 12 (January
2010): 1511–22. https://doi.org/10.3109/00016349.2010.526188.

11. National Collaborating Centre for Women's and Children's Health (UK). "Urinary Incontinence in Women: The Management of Urinary Incontinence in Women." *NICE Clinical
Guidelines* 171, no. 123 (September 2013). Last modified April 2019. https://www.ncbi.nlm
.nih.gov/books/NBK328053/.

12. Eapen, Renu S., and Sidney B. Radomski. "Review of the Epidemiology of Overactive
Bladder." *Research and Reports in Urology* 8 (June 2016): 71–76. https://doi.org/10.2147/RRU
.S102441.

13. James, Sandy, Jody L. Herman, Susan Rankin, et al. *The Report of the 2015 U.S.
Transgender Survey.* US National Center for Transgender Equality. 2016. https://www.trans
equality.org/sites/default/files/docs/USTS-Full-Report-FINAL.PDF.

14. Bryce, Emma. "Why Do Some of Us Shiver When We Pee?" Live Science, July 28, 2018.
https://www.livescience.com/63197-why-pee-shivers.html.

15. Hilt, Evann E., Kathleen McKinley, Megan M. Pierce, et al. "Urine Is Not Sterile: Use of
Enhanced Urine Culture Techniques to Detect Resident Bacterial Flora in the Adult Female
Bladder." *Journal of Clinical Microbiology* 52, no. 3 (2014): 871–76. https://doi.org/10.1128
/JCM.02876-13.

Chapter 6: The Uterine Tubes and Ovaries

1. Boston Women's Health Book Collective. *Our Bodies, Ourselves.* New York: Simon &
Schuster, 2011.

2. Azziz, R. "Polycystic Ovary Syndrome." *Obstetrics & Gynecology* 132, no. 2 (2018):
321–36. https://doi.org/10.1097/aog.0000000000002698.

3. Baba, T., T. Endo, H. Honnma, Y. Kitajima, et al. "Association Between Polycystic
Ovary Syndrome and Female-to-Male Transsexuality." *Human Reproduction* 22, no. 4 (April
2007): 1011–16. https://doi.org/10.1093/humrep/del474.

4. Mueller, A., L. J. Gooren, S. Naton-Schötz, et al. "Prevalence of Polycystic Ovary Syndrome and Hyperandrogenemia in Female-to-Male Transsexuals." *Journal of Clinical Endocrinology & Metabolism* 93, no. 4 (April 2008): 1408–11. https://doi.org/10.1210/jc.2007
-2808.

5. Chan, K. J., J. J. Liang, J. D. Jolly, et al. "Exogenous Testosterone Does Not Induce or
Exacerbate the Metabolic Features Associated with PCOS Among Transgender Men." *Endocrinology Practice* 24, no. 6 (2018): 565–72. https://doi.org/10.4158/EP-2017-0247.

6. Knaresboro, Tarah. "Polycystic Ovary Syndrome." Pussypedia. Accessed January 30,
2021. https://www.pussypedia.net/articles/polycystic-ovary-syndrome-pcos.

7. Mayo Clinic Staff. "Ovarian Cysts." Mayo Clinic. Patient Care & Health Information.
Diseases & Conditions. August 26, 2020. https://www.mayoclinic.org/diseases-conditions
/ovarian-cysts/symptoms-causes/syc-20353405.

Chapter 7: The Uterus

1. Brochmann, Nina, and Ellen Støkken Dahl. *The Wonder Down Under.* New York: Quercus, 2017.

2. Bernstein, Matthew T., Lesley Graff, Lisa Avery, et al. "Gastrointestinal Symptoms Before and During Menses in Healthy Women." *BMC Women's Health* 14, no. 14 (January 2014).
https://doi.org/10.1186/1472-6874-14-14.

3. Tasca, Cecilia, Mariangela Rapetti, Mauro Giovanni Carta, et al. "Women and Hysteria in the History of Mental Health." *Clinical Practice & Epidemiology in Mental Health* 8, no. 1 (October 2012): 110–19. https://doi.org/10.2174/1745017901208010110.

4. Micale, Mark S. *Approaching Hysteria: Disease and Its Interpretations*. Princeton, NJ: Princeton University Press, 1995.

5. McVean, Ada. "The History of Hysteria." McGill University. Office for Science and Society. July 31, 2017. https://www.mcgill.ca/oss/article/history-quackery/history-hysteria.

6. Winstead, Barbara Ann. "Hysteria." In *Sex Roles and Psychopathology*, edited by Cathy Spatz Widom, 73–100. Boston: Springer, 1984. https://doi.org/10.1007/978-1-4684-4562 -6_4.

7. Johnson, Paula A., Lee Goldman, E. John Orav, et al. "Gender Differences in the Management of Acute Chest Pain." *Journal of General Internal Medicine* 11, no. 4 (April 1996): 209–17. https://doi.org/10.1007/BF02642477.

8. Kaul, Padma, Wei-Ching Chang, Cynthia M. Westerhout, et al. "Differences in Admission Rates and Outcomes Between Men and Women Presenting to Emergency Departments with Coronary Syndromes." *Canadian Medical Association Journal* 177, no. 10 (November 2007): 1193–99. https://doi.org/10.1503/cmaj.060711.

9. Sabin, Janice A. "How We Fail Black Patients in Pain." Association of American Medical Colleges. January 6, 2020. https://www.aamc.org/news-insights/how-we-fail -black-patients-pain.

10. Guidone, Heather C. "The Womb Wanders Not: Enhancing Endometriosis Education in a Culture of Menstrual Misinformation." In *The Palgrave Handbook of Critical Menstruation Studies*, edited by Chris Bobel, Inga T. Winkler, Breanne Fahs, et al. Singapore: Palgrave Macmillan, 2020. https://doi.org/10.1007/978-981-15-0614-7_22.

11. Parasar, Parveen, Pinar Ozcan, and Kathryn L. Terry. "Endometriosis: Epidemiology, Diagnosis and Clinical Management." *Current Obstetrics and Gynecology Reports* 6, no. 1 (March 2017): 34–41. https://doi.org/10.1007/s13669-017-0187-1.

12. Nnoaham, Kelechi E., Lone Hummelshoj, Premila Webster, et al. "Impact of Endometriosis on Quality of Life and Work Productivity: A Multicenter Study Across Ten Countries." *Fertility and Sterility* 96, no. 2 (August 2011): 366–73. https://doi.org/10.1016 /j.fertnstert.2011.05.090.

13. Clark, Michelle. "Experiences of Women with Endometriosis: An Interpretative Phenomenological Analysis" no. 114. Edinburgh, Queen Margaret University, Professional Doctorate Thesis, 2012. https://eresearch.qmu.ac.uk/handle/20.500.12289/7722.

14. Boston Women's Health Book Collective. *Our Bodies, Ourselves*. New York: Simon & Schuster, 2011.

15. American Association of Gynecologic Laparoscopists. "AAGL Practice Report: Practice Guidelines for the Diagnosis and Management of Endometrial Polyps." *Journal of Minimally Invasive Gynecology* 19, no. 1 (January–February 2012): 3–10. https://doi.org/10.1016 /j.jmig.2011.09.003.

16. Dreisler, Eva, Soren Stampe Sorensen, P. H. Ibsen, et al. "Prevalence of Endometrial Polyps and Abnormal Uterine Bleeding in a Danish Population Aged 20–74 years." *Ultrasound in Obstetrics and Gynecology: The Official Journal of the International Society of Ultrasound in Obstetrics and Gynecology* 33, no. 1 (December 2009): 102–08. https://doi .org/10.1002/uog.6259.

17. Anastasiadis, Paul, N. G. Koutlaki, G. C. Galazios, et al. "Endometrial Polyps: Prevalence, Detection, and Malignant Potential in Women with Abnormal Uterine Bleeding." *European Journal of Gynaecological Oncology* 21, no. 2 (1999): 180–83. https://pubmed.ncbi .nlm.nih.gov/10843481/.

18. Stewart, Elizabeth A., C. L. Cookson, Renate Schulze-Rath. "Epidemiology of Uterine Fibroids: A Systematic Review." *BJOG: An International Journal of Obstetrics and Gynaecology* 124, no. 10 (September 2017): 1501–12. https://doi.org/10.1111/1471-0528.14640.

19. Stewart, Elizabeth, Wanda Nicholson, Linda Bradley, et al. "The Burden of Uterine Fibroids for African-American Women: Results of a National Survey." *Journal of Women's Health* 22, no. 10 (October 2013): 807–16. https://www.ncbi.nlm.nih.gov/pmc/articles/PMC3787340/.

20. Mayo Clinic Staff. "Uterine Artery Embolization." Patient Care & Health Information. Tests & Procedures. June 08, 2019. https://www.mayoclinic.org/tests-procedures/uterine-artery-embolization/about/pac-20384713.

21. Hers Foundation. "HERS Historic Nationwide Protest." Accessed December 6, 2020. https://www.hersfoundation.org/protest/.

22. National Women's Health Network. "Hysterectomy." Last modified 2015. https://nwhn.org/hysterectomy/.

23. Obedin-Maliver, Juno. "Hysterectomy." University of California San Francisco Transgender Care. June 17, 2016. https://transcare.ucsf.edu/guidelines/hysterectomy.

24. National Center for Transgender Equality. "What Does Medicare Cover for Transgender People?" Accessed December 6, 2020. https://transequality.org/know-your-rights/medicare.

Chapter 8: The Vaginal Corona, Formerly Known as the Hymen (and the Virginity Myth)

1. Brochmann, Nina, and Ellen Støkken Dahl. *The Wonder Down Under*. New York: Quercus, 2017.

2. Nagoski, Emily. *Come as You Are: The Surprising New Science That Will Transform Your Sex Life*. New York: Simon & Schuster, 2015.

3. Ferrel Pokorny, Susan. "Configuration of the Prepubertal Hymen." *American Journal of Obstetrics and Gynecology* 157, no. 4 (October 1987): 950–56. https://doi.org/10.1016/s0002-9378(87)80094-7.

4. Mishori, Ranit, Hope Ferdowsian, Karen Naimer, et al. "The Little Tissue That Couldn't—Dispelling Myths About the Hymen's Role in Determining Sexual History and Assault." *Reproductive Health* 16, no. 74 (June 2019). https://doi.org/10.1186/s12978-019-0731-8.

5. Heger, Astrid H., Lynne Ticson, Lisa Guerra, et al. "Appearance of the Genitalia in Girls Selected for Nonabuse." *Journal of Pediatric and Adolescent Gynecology* 15, no. 1 (February 2002): 27–35. https://doi.org/10.1016/s1083-3188(01)00136-x.

6. Berenson, Abbey, Astrid Heger, and Sally Andrews. "Appearance of the Hymen in Newborns." *Official Journal of the American Academy of Pediatrics* 87, no. 4 (April 1991): 458–65. https://pediatrics.aappublications.org/content/87/4/458/tab-article-info.

7. Knöfel Magnusson, Anna. Swedish Association for Sexuality Education. *The Vaginal Corona*. Stockholm: Brommatryck & Brolins, 2009. https://www.rfsu.se/globalassets/pdf/vaginal-corona-english.pdf.

8. Swedish Association for Sexuality Education. "Vaginal Corona." Om RFSU. Om oss. In English. National Work. Sex and Relations. December 12, 2017. https://www.rfsu.se/om-rfsu/om-oss/in-english/national-work/sex-and-relations/the-vaginal-corona/.

9. Dølvik Brochmann, Nina, and Ellen Støkken Dahl. "The Virginity Fraud." May 18, 2017. TEDxOslo. Video, 12:18. https://www.youtube.com/watch?v=fBQnQTkhsq4.

Chapter 9: The Vulva and Vagina

1. Lyons, Jack, and Brian Catlin. "Etymology of Abdominal Visceral Terms." Dartmouth Medical School. Basic Human Anatomy. 2008. http://www.dartmouth.edu/~humananatomy/resources/etymology/Pelvis.htm#.

2. Chalker, Rebecca. *The Clitoral Truth*. New York: Seven Stories Press, 2002.

3. Nagoski, Emily. *Come as You Are: The Surprising New Science That Will Transform Your Sex Life*. New York: Simon & Schuster, 2015.

4. Gunter, Jen. *The Vagina Bible*. New York: Citadel Press, 2019.

5. Ramsey, Sara, Clare Sweeney, Michael Fraser, et al. "Pubic Hair and Sexuality: A Review." *Journal of Sexual Medicine* 6, no. 8 (August 2009): 2102–10. https://doi.org/10.1111/j.1743-6109.2009.01307.x.

6. Luster, Jamie, Abigail Norris Turner, John P. Henry Jr., et al. "Association Between Pubic Hair Grooming and Prevalent Sexually Transmitted Infection Among Female University Students." *PLOS ONE* 14, no. 9 (September 2019): e0221303. https://doi.org/10.1371/journal.pone.0221303.

7. Osterberg, E. Charles, Thomas W. Gaither, Mohannad A. Awad, et al. "Correlation Between Pubic Hair Grooming and STIs: Results from a Nationally Representative Probability Sample." *Sexually Transmitted Infections* 93, no. 3 (December 2016): 162–66. https://doi.org/10.1136/sextrans-2016-052687.

8. Gaither, Thomas W., Kirkpatrick Fergus, Siobhan Sutcliffe, et al. "Pubic Hair Grooming and Sexually Transmitted Infections: A Clinic-Based Cross-Sectional Survey." *Sexually Transmitted Diseases* 47, no. 6 (June 2020): 419–25. https://doi.org/10.1097/OLQ.0000000000001176.

9. Barnhart, Kurt E., Scott Pretorius, and Daniel Malamud. "Lesson Learned and Dispelled Myths: Three-Dimensional Imaging of the Human Vagina." *Fertility and Sterility* 81, no. 5 (May 2004): 1383–84. https://doi.org/10.1016/j.fertnstert.2004.01.016.

10. Boston University School of Medicine. "Female Genital Anatomy." Sexual Medicine. For Health Care Professionals. Accessed October 7, 2020. https://www.bumc.bu.edu/sexualmedicine/physicianinformation/female-genital-anatomy/.

11. Anderson, Deborah J., Jai Marathe, and Jeffrey Pudney. "The Structure of the Human Vaginal *Stratum Corneum* and Its Role in Immune Defense." *American Journal of Reproductive Immunology* 71, no. 6 (June 2014): 618–23. https://doi.org/10.1111/aji.12230.

12. Pastor, Zlatko, and Roman Chmel. "Differential Diagnostics of Female 'Sexual' Fluids: A Narrative Review." *International Urogynecology Journal* 29, no. 5 (December 2018): 621–29. https://doi.org/10.1007/s00192-017-3527-9.

13. Amabebe, Emmanuel, and Dilly O. C. Anumba. "The Vaginal Microenvironment: The Physiologic Role of *Lactobacilli*." *Frontiers in Medicine* 5 (June 2018): 181. https://doi.org/10.3389/fmed.2018.00181.

14. Alexander, Nancy, Edward Baker, Marc Kaptein, Ulrich Karck, Leslie Miller, et al. "Why Consider Vaginal Drug Administration?" *Fertility and Sterility* 82, no. 1 (July 2014): 1–12. https://doi.org/10.1016/j.fertnstert.2004.01.025.

15. Center for Transgender Health. "FAQ: Vaginoplasty." Johns Hopkins Medicine. Accessed October 7, 2020. https://www.hopkinsmedicine.org/center-transgender-health/services-appointments/faq/vaginoplasty.

16. Meltzer, Toby. "Vaginoplasty Procedures, Complications and Aftercare." University of California San Francisco Transgender Care. June 17, 2016. https://transcare.ucsf.edu/guidelines/vaginoplasty.

17. Alvisi, Stefania, Giulia Gava, Isabella Orsili, et al. "Vaginal Health in Menopausal Women." *Medicina* 55, no. 10 (September 2019): 615. https://doi.org/10.3390/medicina55100615.

18. Anderson, Deborah J., Jai Marathe, and Jeffrey Pudney. "The Structure of the Human Vaginal *Stratum Corneum* and Its Role in Immune Defense." *American Journal of Reproductive Immunology* 71, no. 6 (March 2014): 618–23. https://doi.org/10.1111/aji.12230.

19. Farage, Miranda, and Howard Maibach. "Lifetime Changes in the Vulva and Vagina." *Archives of Gynecology and Obstetrics* 273, no. 4 (January 2005): 195–202. https://doi.org/10.1007/s00404-005-0079-x.

20. Land, Emily. "Q&A: Gynecologic and Vaginal Care for Trans Men." San Francisco AIDS Foundation. July 23, 2019. https://www.sfaf.org/collections/beta/qa-gynecologic-and-vaginal-care-for-trans-men/.

21. National Health Service. "Vagina Changes After Childbirth." Live Well. Sexual Health. Last reviewed October 23, 2018. https://www.nhs.uk/live-well/sexual-health/vagina-changes-after-childbirth/.

22. O'Malley, Deirdre, Agnes Higgins, Cecily Begley, et al. "Prevalence of and Risk Factors Associated with Sexual Health Issues in Primiparous Women at 6 and 12 Months Postpartum; a Longitudinal Prospective Cohort Study (the MAMMI Study)." *BMC Pregnancy and Childbirth* 18, no. 196 (May 2018). https://doi.org/10.1186/s12884-018-1838-6.

23. Gleichert, James E. "Étienne Joseph Jacquemin, Discoverer of 'Chadwick's Sign.'" *Journal of the History of Medicine and Allied Sciences* 26, no. 1 (January 1971): 75–80. https://doi.org/10.1093/jhmas/XXVI.1.75.

24. Barad, David H. "Vaginal Discharge." MSD Manual Consumer Version. Last modified April 2020. https://www.msdmanuals.com/home/women-s-health-issues/symptoms-of-gynecologic-disorders/vaginal-discharge.

25. Gonçalves, Bruna, Carina Ferreira, Carlos Tiago Alves, Mariana Henriques, Joana Azeredo, et al. "Vulvovaginal Candidiasis: Epidemiology, Microbiology and Risk Factors." *Critical Reviews in Microbiology* 42, no. 6 (December 2016): 905–27. https://doi.org/10.3109/1040841x.2015.1091805.

26. *Diagnostic and Statistical Manual of Mental Disorders: DSM-5.* Arlington, VA: American Psychiatric Association, 2013.

27. Dias-Amaral, Ana, and Marques-Pinto, A. "Female Genito-Pelvic Pain/Penetration Disorder: Review of the Related Factors and Overall Approach." *Revista Brasileira de Ginecologia e Obstetrícia* 40, no. 12 (2018): 787–93. https://doi.org/10.1055/s-0038-1675805.

28. Bergeron, Sophie, Barbara D. Reed, Ursula Wesselmann, et al. "Vulvodynia." *Nature Reviews Disease Primers* 6, no. 36 (2020). https://doi.org/10.1038/s41572-020-0164-2.

29. Crowley, Tessa, David Goldmeier, and Janice Hiller. "Diagnosing and Managing Vaginismus." *BMJ* 338 (June 2009): b2284. https://doi.org/10.1002/ca.22495.

30. Özen, Beliz, Y. Ozay Özdemir, and E. Emrem Beştepe. "Childhood Trauma and Dissociation Among Women with Genito-Pelvic Pain/Penetration Disorder." *Neuropsychiatric Disease and Treatment* 23, no. 14 (February 2018): 641–46. https://doi.org/10.2147/NDT.S151920.

31. Meana, Marta, Evan Fertel, and Caroline Maykut. "Treating Genital Pain Associated with Sexual Intercourse." In *The Wiley Handbook of Sex Therapy*, edited by Zoë D. Peterson, 98–114. Chichester: Wiley Blackwell, 2017.

32. Brochmann, Nina, and Ellen Støkken Dahl. *The Wonder Down Under.* New York: Quercus, 2017.

33. Ghizzani, Anna, Stefano Luisi, Alessandra Cortocci, et al. "Genitopelvic Pain: Retrospective Evaluation of a Multimodal Treatment Efficacy." *Minerva Ginecologica* 72, no. 3 (June 2020): 123–31. https://doi.org/10.23736/S0026-4784.20.04555-4.

34. Haefner, Hope K., Michael E. Collins, Gordon D. Davis, et al. "The Vulvodynia Guideline." *Journal of Lower Genital Tract Disease* 9, no. 1 (January 2005): 40–51. https://doi.org/10.1097/00128360-200501000-00009.

35. Graziottin, Alessandra. "Dyspareunia and Vaginismus: Review of the Literature and Treatment." *Current Sexual Health Reports* 5, no. 1 (March 2008): 43–50. https://doi.org/10.1007/s11930-008-0008-7.

36. Murina, Fillipo, Roberto Bernorio, and Rosanna Palmiotto. "The Use of Amielle Vaginal Trainers as Adjuvant in the Treatment of Vestibulodynia: An Observational Multicentric Study." *Medscape Journal of Medicine* 10, no. 1 (January 2008): 23. https://pubmed.ncbi.nlm.nih.gov/18324333/.

37. Anderson, Alexandra B., Natalie O. Rosen, Lisa Price, et al. "Associations Between Penetration Cognitions, Genital Pain, and Sexual Well-Being in Women with Provoked Vestibulodynia." *Journal of Sexual Medicine* 13, no. 3 (2016): 444–52. https://doi.org/10.1016/j.jsxm.2015.12.024.

38. Bergeron, Sophie, Wendy M. Likes, and Marc Steben. "Psychosexual Aspects of Vulvovaginal Pain." *Best Practice & Research: Clinical Obstetrics & Gynaecology* 28, no. 7 (October 2014): 991–99. https://doi.org/10.1016/j.bpobgyn.2014.07.007.

39. Rosen, Natalie O., Sophie Bergeron, Gentiana Sadikaj, et al. "Impact of Male Partner Responses on Sexual Function in Women with Vulvodynia and Their Partners: A Dyadic Daily Experience Study." *Health Psychology* 33, no. 8 (August 2014): 823–31. https://doi.org/10.1037/a0034550.

40. Davis, Seth N., Sophie Bergeron, Gentiana Sadikaj, et al. "Partner Behavioral Responses to Pain Mediate the Relationship Between Partner Pain Cognitions and Pain Outcomes in Women with Provoked Vestibulodynia." *Journal of Pain* 16, no. 6 (June 2015): 549–57. https://doi.org/10.1016/j.jpain.2015.03.002.

41. Schimpf, Megan O., Heidi S. Harvie, Tola B. Omotosho, et al. "Does Vaginal Size Impact Sexual Activity and Function?" *International Urogynecology Journal* 21, no. 4 (December 2010): 447–52. htpps://doi.org/10.1007/s00192-009-1051-2.

42. Koedt, Anne. "Myth of the Vaginal Orgasm." Somerville, MA: New England Free Press, 1970. Accessed via CUNY Academic Commons. https://wgs10016.commons.gc.cuny.edu/the-myth-of-the-vaginal-orgasm-by-anne-koedt-1970/.

43. Levin, Roy J. "Recreation and Procreation: A Critical View of Sex in the Human Female." *Clinical Anatomy* 28, no. 3 (December 2014): 339–54. https://doi.org/10.1002/ca.22495.

44. Shafik, Ahmed, Olfat El Sibai, Ali A. Shafik, et al. "The Electrovaginogram: Study of the Vaginal Electric Activity and Its Role in the Sexual Act and Disorders." *Archives of Gynecology and Obstetrics* 169, no. 4 (May 2004): 282–86. htpps://doi.org/10.1007/s00404-003-0571-0.

Hormones and the Menstrual Cycle

Chapter 11: The Menstrual Cycle: Gender Narratives from Menarche to Menopause

1. Corinna, Heather. *What Fresh Hell Is This? Perimenopause, Menopause, Other Indignities, and You.* New York: Hachette, 2021.

2. Wharton, W., C. E. Gleason, S. R. Olson, et al. "Neurobiological Underpinnings of the Estrogen—Mood Relationship." *Current Psychiatry Reviews* (August 2012): 247–56. https://www.ncbi.nlm.nih.gov/pmc/articles/PMC3753111/.

3. Cappelletti, Maurand, and Kim Wallen. "Increasing Women's Sexual Desire: The Comparative Effectiveness of Estrogens and Androgens." *Hormones and Behavior* 78 (February 2016): 178–93. https://doi.org/10.1016/j.yhbeh.2015.11.003.

4. Albert, Kimberly, Jens Pruessner, and Paul Newhouse. "Estradiol Levels Modulate Brain Activity and Negative Responses to Psychosocial Stress Across the Menstrual Cycle." *Psychoneuroendocrinology* 59 (September 2015): 14–24. https://doi.org/10.1016/j.psyneuen.2015.04.022.

5. Jordan-Young, Rebecca, and Katrina Karkazis. *Testosterone: An Unauthorized Biography.* Boston: Harvard University Press, 2019.

6. Irwig, M. S., M. Fleseriu, J. Jonklaas, et al. "Off-Label Use and Misuse of Testosterone, Growth Hormones, Thyroid Hormone, and Adrenal Supplements: Risks and Costs of a Growing Problem." *Endocrine Practice* 26, no. 3 (March 2020): 340–53. https://doi.org/10.4158/PS-2019-0540.

7. Butler Tobah, Yvonne. "Testosterone Therapy in Women: Does It Boost Sex Drive?" Mayo Clinic. Patient Care & Health Information. Diseases & Conditions.. Menopause. Expert Answers. June 19, 2019. https://www.mayoclinic.org/diseases-conditions/menopause/expert-answers/testosterone-therapy/faq-20057935.

8. National Health Service. "Periods and Fertility in the Menstrual Cycle." Conditions. Periods. Last reviewed August 5, 2019. https://www.nhs.uk/conditions/periods/fertility-in-the-menstrual-cycle.

9. Brochmann, Nina, and Ellen Støkken Dahl. *The Wonder Down Under.* New York: Quercus, 2017.

10. Wood, Jill M. "(In)Visible Bleeding: The Menstrual Concealment Imperative." In *The Palgrave Handbook of Critical Menstruation Studies*, edited by Chris Bobel, Inga T. Winkler, Breanne Fahs, et al., 319–36. Singapore: Palgrave Macmillan, 2020. https://doi.org/10.1007/978-981-15-0614-7_25.

11. Punzi, Maria Carmen, and Mirjam Werner. "Challenging the Menstruation Taboo One Sale at a Time: The Role of Social Entrepreneurs in the Period Revolution." In *The Palgrave Handbook of Critical Menstruation Studies*, edited by Chris Bobel, Inga T. Winkler, Breanne Fahs, et al., 319–336. Singapore: Palgrave Macmillan, 2020. https://doi.org/10.1007/978-981-15-0614-7_60.

12. Frank, S. E., and Jac Dellaria. "Navigating the Binary: A Visual Narrative of Trans and Genderqueer Menstruation." In *The Palgrave Handbook of Critical Menstruation Studies*, edited by Chris Bobel, Inga T. Winkler, Breanne Fahs, et al., 319–36. Singapore: Palgrave Macmillan, 2020. https://doi.org/10.1007/978-981-15-0614-7_7.

13. Deutsch, Maddie. "Information on Testosterone Hormone Therapy." UCSF Transgender Care. For Patients. Hormone Therapy. July 2020. https://transcare.ucsf.edu/article/information-testosterone-hormone-therapy.

14. Ahmad, Shazia, and Matthew Leinung. "The Response of the Menstrual Cycle to Initiation of Hormonal Therapy in Transgender Men." *Transgender Health* 2, no. 1 (2017): 176–79. https://doi.org/10.1089/trgh.2017.0023.

15. Derntl, Brigit, Ramona L. Hack, Ilse Kyrspin-Exner, et al. "Association of Menstrual Cycle Phase with the Core Components of Empathy." *Current Psychiatry Review* 8, no. 3 (January 2012): 247–56. https://doi.org/10.1016/j.yhbeh.2012.10.009.

16. Alvergne, A., and V. Högqvist Tabor. "Is Female Health Cyclical? Evolutionary Perspectives on Menstruation." *Trends in Ecology & Evolution* 33, no. 6 (June 2018): 399–14. https://doi.org/10.1016/j.tree.2018.03.006.

17. OBOS Anatomy and Menstruation Contributors. "Internal Organs: Uterus, Fallopian Tubes, Ovaries," Our Bodies Ourselves, March 31, 2014. https://www.ourbodiesourselves.org/book-excerpts/health-article/internal-organs-uterus-fallopian-tubes-ovaries.

18. OBOS Anatomy and Menstruation Contributors. "Stages in the Menstrual Cycle." Our Bodies Ourselves, April 1, 2014. https://www.ourbodiesourselves.org/book-excerpts/health-article/stages-in-the-menstrual-cycle.

19. Mayo Clinic Staff. "Mittelschmerz." Patient Care & Health Information. Diseases & Conditions. September 25, 2020. https://www.mayoclinic.org/diseases-conditions/mittelschmerz/symptoms-causes/syc-20375122.

20. Case, Alison M., and Robert Reid. "Effects of the Menstrual Cycle on Medical Disorders." *Archives of Internal Medicine* 158, no. 3 (August 1998): 1405–12. https://doi.org/10.001/archinte.158.13.1405.

21. Spencer, S. J., C. M. Steele, and D. M. Quinn. "Stereotype Threat and Women's Math Performance." *Journal of Experimental Social Psychology* 35, no. 1 (January 1999): 4–28. https://doi.org/10.1006/jesp.1998.1373.

22. Spencer, S. J., C. Logel, and P. G. Davies. "Stereotype Threat." *Annual Review of Psychology* 67, no. 1 (January 2016): 415–37. https://doi.org/10.1146/annurev-psych-073115-103235.

23. Nguyen, H. H. D., and A. M. Ryan. "Does Stereotype Threat Affect Test Performance of Minorities and Women? A Meta-Analysis of Experimental Evidence." *Journal of Applied Psychology* 93, no. 6 (December 2008): 1314–34. https://doi.org/10.1037/a0012702.

24. Dalton, Katharina, and Raymond Greene. "The Premenstrual Syndrome." *British Medical Journal* 4818, no. 1 (May 1953): 1007–14. https://doi.org/10.1136/bmj.1.4818.1007.

25. Hawes, Ellen, and Tian P. S. Oei. "The Menstrual Distress Questionnaire: Are the Critics Right?" *Current Psychology* 11 (September 1992): 264–81. https://doi.org/10.1007/BF02686846.

26. McFarlane, J., C. L. Martin, and T. M. Williams. "Mood Fluctuations: Women Versus Men and Menstrual Versus Other Cycles." *Psychology of Women Quarterly* 12 (1998): 201–23.

27. McFarlane, J. M., and T. M. Williams. "Placing Premenstrual Syndrome in Perspective." *Psychology of Women Quarterly* 18, no. 3 (September 1994): 339–73. https://doi.org/10.1111/j.1471-6402.1994.tb00460.x.

28. Cosgrove, L., and B. Riddle. "Constructions of Femininity and Experiences of Menstrual Distress." *Women Health* 38, no. 3 (2003): 37–58. https://doi.org/10.1300/J013v38n03_04.

29. Romans, S., R. Clarkson, G. Einstein, M. Petrovic, and D. Stewart. "Mood and the Menstrual Cycle: A Review of Prospective Data Studies." *Gender Medicine* 9, no. 5 (October 2012): 361–84. https://doi.org/10.1016/j.genm.2012.07.003.

30. King, Sally. "Premenstrual Syndrome (PMS) and the Myth of the Irrational Female." In *The Palgrave Handbook of Critical Menstruation Studies*, edited by Chris Bobel, Inga T. Winkler, Breanne Fahs, et al., 287–302. Singapore: Palgrave Macmillan, 2020. https://doi.org/10.1007/978-981-15-0614-7_23.

31. Gottlieb, Alma. "Menstrual Taboos: Moving Beyond the Curse." In *The Palgrave Handbook of Critical Menstruation Studies*, edited by Chris Bobel, Inga T. Winkler, Breanne Fahs, et al., 143–62. Singapore: Palgrave Macmillan, 2020. https://doi.org/10.1007/978-981-15-0614-7_14.

32. Osório, Flávia L., Juliana M. de Paula Cassis, João P. Machado de Sousa, et al. "Sex Hormones and Processing of Facial Expressions of Emotion: A Systematic Literature Review." *Frontiers in Psychology* 9 (April 2018): 529. https://doi.org/10.3389/fpsyg.2018.00529.

33. Yonkers, Kimberly, and Robert F. Casper. "Epidemiology and Pathogenesis of Premenstrual Syndrome and Premenstrual Dysphoric Disorder." Up to Date. Last updated

October 22, 2019. https://www.uptodate.com/contents/epidemiology-and-pathogenesis-of
-premenstrual-syndrome-and-premenstrual-dysphoric-disorder.

34. Chisholm, Andrea. "Premenstrual Dysphoria Disorder: It's Biology, Not a Behavior Choice." *Harvard Health* (blog). Harvard Health Publishing. Harvard Medical School. May 30, 2017. https://www.health.harvard.edu/blog/premenstrual-dysphoria
-disorder-its-biology-not-a-behavior-choice-2017053011768.

35. Biggs, Ashley. "Premenstrual Dysphoric Disorder." Pussypedia. Accessed February 4, 2020. https://www.pussypedia.net/articles/premenstrual-dysphoric-disorder-pmdd.

36. Dubey, N., J. F. Hoffman, K. Schuebel, et al. "The ESC/E(Z) Complex, an Intrinsic Cellular Molecular Pathway Differentially Responsive to Ovarian Steroids in Premenstrual Dysphoric Disorder." *Molecular Psychiatry* 22 (January 2017): 1172–84. https://doi.org/10.1038/mp.2016.229.

37. Cassels, Alan, and Roy Moynihan. *Selling Sickness: How the World's Biggest Pharmaceutical Companies Are Turning Us All into Patients.* New York: Nation Books, 2005.

38. Vedantam, Shankar. "Renamed Prozac Fuels Women's Health Debate." *Washington Post*, April 29, 2001. https://www.washingtonpost.com/archive/politics/2001/04/29/renamed-prozac-fuels-womens-health-debate/b05311b4-514a-4e65-aaa5-434cb2934271.

39. Cosgrove, L., S. Krimsky, M. Vijayaraghavan, et al. "Financial Ties Between DSM-IV Panel Members and the Pharmaceutical Industry." *Psychotherapy and Psychosomatics* 75, no. 3 (April 2006): 154–60. https://doi.org/10.1159/000091772.

40. PLOS Medicine Editors. "Does Conflict of Interest Disclosure Worsen Bias?" *PLOS Medicine* 9, no. 4 (April 2012): e1001210. https://doi.org/10.1371/journal.pmed.1001210.

41. Yellowlees, Douglas. "Does Conflict of Interest Bias Psychiatric Research?" Psychiatry Advisor, March 27, 2020. https://www.psychiatryadvisor.com/home/topics/general-psychiatry/does-conflict-of-interest-bias-psychiatric-research.

42. Perlis, Roy H., and S. Clifford. "Industry Sponsorship and Financial Conflict of Interest in the Reporting of Clinical Trials in Psychiatry." *American Journal of Psychiatry* 162, no. 10 (October 2005): 1957–60. https://doi.org/10.1176/appi.ajp.162.10.1957.

43. Fiedman, L. S., and E. D. Richter. "Relationship Between Conflicts of Interest and Research Results." *Journal of General Internal Medicine* 19, no. 1 (January 2004): 51–56. https://doi.org/10.1111/j.1525-1497.2004.30617.x.

44. Choudhry, N. K. "Relationships Between Authors of Clinical Practice Guidelines and the Pharmaceutical Industry." *JAMA* 287, no. 5 (February 2002): 612. https://doi.org/10.1001/jama.287.5.612.

45. Fresques, Hannah. "Doctors Prescribe More of a Drug If They Receive Money from a Pharma Company Tied to It." ProPublica, December 20, 2019. https://www.propublica.org/article/doctors-prescribe-more-of-a-drug-if-they-receive-money-from-a-pharma-company
-tied-to-it.

46. Ornstein, Charles, Mike Tigas, and Ryann Grochowski Jones. "Now There's Proof: Docs Who Get Company Cash Tend to Prescribe More Brand-Name Meds." ProPublica, March 17, 2016. https://www.propublica.org/article/doctors-who-take-company
-cash-tend-to-prescribe-more-brand-name-drugs.

47. Hantsoo, Liisa, and C. Neill Epperson. "Premenstrual Dysphoric Disorder: Epidemiology and Treatment." *Women's Mental Health* 17, no. 11 (September 2015): 87. https://doi.org/10.1007%2Fs11920-015-0628-3.

48. Shanmugan S., W. Cao, T. D. Satterthwaite, et al. "Impact of Childhood Adversity on Network Reconfiguration Dynamics During Working Memory in Hypogonadal Women." *Psychoneuroendocrinology* 119 (September 2020): 104710. https://doi.org/10.1016/j.psyneuen.2020.104710.

Chapter 12: Period Products and the Earth

1. Munoz Boudet, Ana Maria, Paola Buitrago, Benedicte Leroy De La Briere, et al. "Gender Differences in Poverty and Household Composition Through the Life-Cycle: A Global Perspective." World Bank Policy Research Working Paper no. 8360 (March 2018). http://hdl .handle.net/10986/29426.

2. United Nations Climate Change. "Introduction to Gender and Climate Change." Topics. Accessed December 6, 2020. https://unfccc.int/gender.

3. International Union for Conservation of Nature. "Gender and Climate Change." Issues Brief. Accessed December 6, 2020. https://www.iucn.org/resources/issues-briefs /gender-and-climate-change.

4. Gammon, Crystal. "Pollution, Poverty and People of Color: Asthma and the Inner City." *Scientific American*, June 20, 2012. https://www.scientificamerican.com/article /pollution-poverty-people-color-asthma-inner-city/.

5. Alam, Mayesha, Rukmani Bhatia, and Briana Mawby. "Women and Climate Change—Impact and Agency in Human Rights, Security, and Economic Development." Georgetown Institute for Women, Peace, and Security. 2015. https://giwps.georgetown.edu/wp-content /uploads/2017/09/Women-and-Climate-Change.pdf.

6. Gelin, Martin. "The Misogyny of Climate Deniers." *New Republic*, August 28, 2019. https://newrepublic.com/article/154879/misogyny-climate-deniers.

7. Kim, Susan, and Elissa Stein. *Flow: The Cultural Story of Menstruation*. London: St. Martin's Griffin, 2009.

8. Borunda, Alejandra. "How Tampons and Pads Became so Unsustainable." *National Geographic*, September 6, 2019. https://www.nationalgeographic.com/environment/2019/09 /how-tampons-pads-became-unsustainable-story-of-plastic/.

9. Duffin, Erin. "Resident Population of the United States by Sex and Age as of July 1, 2019." Statista, November 5, 2020. https://www.statista.com/statistics/241488 /population-of-the-us-by-sex-and-age/.

10. Spinks, Rosie. "Why Do American Women Prefer Applicator Tampons, While the Rest of the World's Women Don't?" Quartz, March 8, 2018. https://qz.com/quartzy/1224531 /why-american-women-use-applicator-tampons-and-european-women-dont/.

11. Jennings-Edquist, Grace. "American Women Are Completely Freaked by Australian Tampons." MamaMia, November 6, 2020. https://www.mamamia.com.au /non-applicator-tampons/.

12. Butler, Kiera. "Stop Using Plastic Tampon Applicators!" *Mother Jones*, March–April 2016. https://www.motherjones.com/environment/2016/03/plastic-tampon -applicator-beach-pollution/.

13. Mazgaj, Marta, Katsiaryna Yaramenka, and Oleksandra Malovana. "Comparative Life Cycle Assessment of Sanitary Pads and Tampons." Life Cycle Assessment Course Paper, Royal Institute of Technology Stockholm, May 22, 2006. https://docplayer.net/39797321 -Comparative-life-cycle-assessment-of-sanitary-pads-and-tampons.html.

14. Davidson, Ana. "Narratives of Menstrual Product Consumption: Convenience, Culture, or Commoditization?" *Bulletin of Science Technology & Society* 32, no. 1 (June 2012): 56–70. http://dx.doi.org/10.1177/0270467612444579.

15. Women's Voices for the Earth. "New Tampon Testing Reveals Undisclosed Carcinogens and Reproductive Toxins." June 5, 2018. https://www.womensvoices.org/2018/06 /05/new-tampon-testing-reveals-undisclosed-carcinogens-and-reproductive-toxins/.

16. Women's Voices for the Earth. "Always Pads Testing Results." August 2014. https://www .womensvoices.org/menstrual-care-products/detox-the-box/always-pads-testing-results/.

17. DeVito, Michael J., and Arnold Schecter. "Exposure Assessment to Dioxins from the Use of Tampons and Diapers." *Environmental Health Perspectives* 110, no. 1 (February 2002): 23–28. https://doi.org/10.1289/ehp.0211023.

18. Abrams, Rachel. "Under Pressure, Feminine Product Makers Disclose Ingredients." *New York Times*, October 26, 2015. https://www.nytimes.com/2015/10/27/business/under-pressure-feminine-product-makers-disclose-ingredients.html.

19. Women's Voices for the Earth. "What's in Your Tampon?" 2018. https://www.womensvoices.org/menstrual-care-products/whats-in-your-tampon/.

20. Mayo Clinic Staff. "Toxic Shock Syndrome." Mayo Clinic. Patient Care & Health Information. Diseases & Conditions. March 18, 2020. https://www.mayoclinic.org/diseases-conditions/toxic-shock-syndrome/symptoms-causes/syc-20355384.

21. Choy, Jessian. "My Menstrual Underwear Has Toxic Chemicals in It." *Sierra*, January 7, 2020. https://www.sierraclub.org/sierra/ask-ms-green/my-menstrual-underwear-has-toxic-chemicals-it.

22. Carlsen Bach, Cathrine, Anne Vested, Kristian Tore Jørgensen, et al. "Perfluoroalkyl and Polyfluoroalkyl Substances and Measures of Human Fertility: A Systematic Review." *Critical Reviews in Toxicology* 46, no. 9 (October 2016): 735–55. https://doi.org/10.1080/10408444.2016.1182117.

23. Segran, Elizabeth. "Report: Thinx Menstrual Underwear Has Toxic Chemicals in the Crotch." Fast Company, January 13, 2020. https://www.fastcompany.com/90450618/report-thinx-menstrual-underwear-has-toxic-chemicals-in-the-crotch.

24. Thinx. "How We Ensure Thinx Are Body-Safe." January 14, 2020. https://www.shethinx.com/blogs/thinx-piece/how-we-ensure-thinx-are-body-safe.

25. Smith, Charles B., Vici Noble, Rhonda Bensch, et al. "Bacterial Flora of the Vagina During the Menstrual Cycle—Findings in Users of Tampons, Napkins, and Sea Sponges." *Annals of Internal Medicine* 96, no. 6 (June 1, 1982): 948–51. https://doi.org/10.7326/0003-4819-96-6-948.

26. Food and Drug Administration. "CPG Sec. 345.300 Menstrual Sponges." August 24, 2018. https://www.fda.gov/regulatory-information/search-fda-guidance-documents/cpg-sec-345300-menstrual-sponges.

27. Plumer, Bradford. "The Origins of Anti-Litter Campaigns." *Mother Jones*, May 22, 2006. https://www.motherjones.com/politics/2006/05/origins-anti-litter-campaigns/.

28. Griffin, Paul. "The Carbon Majors Database—CDP Carbon Majors Report 2017." CDP. July 2017. https://6fefcbb86e61af1b2fc4-c70d8ead6ced550b4d987d7c03fcdd1d.ssl.cf3.rackcdn.com/cms/reports/documents/000/002/327/original/Carbon-Majors-Report-2017.pdf?1501833772.

29. Whitney, A. K. "Is the 'Green' Menstrual Movement Ableist?" *Dame*, July 2, 2019. https://www.damemagazine.com/2019/07/02/is-the-green-menstrual-movement-ableist/.

Sex and Masturbation
Chapter 13: Consent

1. May, Emmeline, and Blue Seat Studios. "Tea Consent." May 12, 2017. Video, 2:51. https://www.youtube.com/watch?v=oQbei5JGiT8.

2. Friedman, Jaclyn. "Sex & Consent: It's Time to Go Beyond the Rules." Refinery29, September 6, 2018. https://www.refinery29.com/en-us/sex-consent-laws-yes-means-yes-Jaclyn-Friedman.

3. Williams, D. J., Jeremy Thomas, Emily Prior, et al. "From 'SSC' and 'RACK' to the '4Cs:' Introducing a New Framework for Negotiating BDSM Participation." *Electronic Journal of Human Sexuality* 17 (July 2014). http://www.ejhs.org/volume17/BDSM.html.

4. Switch, Gary. "Origin of RACK: RACK vs. SSC." Iron Gate. Accessed July 19, 2020. https://www.the-iron-gate.com/essays/138.

5. Fischel, Joseph. *Screw Consent: A Better Politics of Sexual Justice.* Oakland: University of California Press, 2019.

6. Lorde, Audre. "Uses of the Erotic: The Erotic as Power." *Sister Outsider.* New York: Crown Publishing Group, 1984. https://fredandfar.com/blogs/ff-blog/the-erotic-as-power-by-audre-lorde.

Chapter 14: Masturbation: Yes

1. Fahs, Breanne, and Elena Frank. "Notes from the Back Room: Gender, Power, and (In) Visibility in Women's Experiences of Masturbation." *Journal of Sex Research* 51, no. 3 (April 2013): 241–52. https://doi:10.1080/00224499.2012.745474.

2. Hogarth, Harriet, and Roger Ingham. "Masturbation Among Young Women and Associations with Sexual Health: An Exploratory Study." *Journal of Sex Research* 46, no. 6 (April 2009): 558–67. https://doi:10.1080/00224490902878993.

3. Carvalheira, Ana, and Isabel Leal. "Masturbation Among Women: Associated Factors and Sexual Response in a Portuguese Community Sample." *Journal of Sex & Marital Therapy* 39, no. 4 (February 2013): 347–67. https://doi.org/10.1080/0092623X.2011.628440.

4. Safron, Adam. "What Is Orgasm? A Model of Sexual Trance and Climax via Rhythmic Entrainment." *Socioaffective Neuroscience & Psychology* 6, no. 1 (October 2016). https://doi.org/10.3402/snp.v6.31763.

5. Planned Parenthood. "Masturbation. Is it Good for You?" Learn. For Teens. Sex. Masturbation. Accessed November 15, 2020. https://www.plannedparenthood.org/learn/teens/sex/masturbation/masturbation-good-you.

6. Komisaruk, Barry R., and Beverly Whipple. "The Suppression of Pain by Genital Stimulation in Females." *Annual Review of Sex Research* 6, no. 1 (1995): 151–86. https://doi.org/10.1080/10532528.1995.10559904.

7. Rowland, David, Krisztina Hevesi, Gabrielle R. Conway, et al. "Relationship Between Masturbation and Partnered Sex in Women: Does the Former Facilitate, Inhibit, or Not Affect the Latter?" *Journal of Sexual Medicine* 17, no. 1 (January 2019): 37–47. https://doi.org/10.1016/j.jsxm.2019.10.012.

8. Burri, Andrea V., Lynn M. Cherkas, and Tim D. Spector. "Emotional Intelligence and Its Association with Orgasmic Frequency in Women." *Journal of Sexual Medicine* 6, no. 7 (July 2009): 1930–37. https://doi.org/10.1111/j.1743-6109.2009.01297.x.

9. López, Canela. "Vibrators Should be Covered by Health Insurance, Says Former US Surgeon General Joycelyn Elders." Insider, May 6, 2020. https://www.insider.com/former-us-surgeon-general-vibrators-should-be-covered-by-insurance-2020-5.

10. "100 Women of the Year. 1994: Joyselyn Elders." *Time*, March 5, 2020. https://time.com/5793727/joycelyn-elders-100-women-of-the-year/.

11. Jehl, Douglas. "Surgeon General Forced to Resign by White House." *New York Times*, December 10, 1994. https://www.nytimes.com/1994/12/10/us/surgeon-general-forced-to-resign-by-white-house.html.

12. Ross, Sami. "Feel Yourself to Heal Yourself." Pussypedia. Accessed November 15, 2020. https://www.pussypedia.net/articles/masturbation-as-self-care.

13. Hodges, Frederick M. "History of Sexual Medicine: The Antimasturbation Crusade in Antebellum American Medicine." *Journal of Sexual Medicine* 2, no. 5 (September 2005): 722–31. https://doi.org/10.1111/j.1743-6109.2005.00133.x.

14. Salam, Maya. "Sex Sells, but When It Comes to Female Pleasure, the New York Subway Isn't So Sure." *New York Times*, June 25, 2019.

15. Davidson, J. Kenneth, and Nelwyn B. Moore. "Masturbation and Premarital Sexual Intercourse Among College Women: Making Choices for Sexual Fulfillment." *Journal of Sex & Marital Therapy* 20, no. 3 (1994): 178–99. https://doi.org/doi:10.1080/00926239408403429.

16. brown, adrienne maree. *Pleasure Activism*. Chico, CA: AK Press, 2020.

17. Michael, Reece, Debby Herbenick, J. Fortenberry, et al. "National Survey of Sexual Health and Behavior." Center for Sexual Health Promotion at the Indiana University School of Public Health. Accessed December 6, 2020. http://www.nationalsexstudy.indiana.edu/.

18. Nagoski, Emily. *Come as You Are: The Surprising New Science That Will Transform Your Sex Life*. New York: Simon & Schuster, 2015.

Chapter 16: Sex Toys

1. Grand View Research. "Sex Toys Market Size, Share & Trends Analysis Report by Type (Male, Female), by Distribution Channel (E-commerce, Specialty Stores, Mass Merchandizers), by Region (North America, Europe, APAC, LATAM, MEA), and Segment Forecasts, 2020–2027." Market Analysis Report. 2020. https://www.grandviewresearch.com/industry-analysis/sex-toys-market.

2. Statista. "How Often Do You Use Sex Toys?" 2020. https://www.statista.com/forecasts/744534/use-frequency-of-sex-toys-by-female-consumers-in-the-us.

3. Herbenick, Debra, Michael Reece, Stephanie Sanders, et al. "Prevalence and Characteristics of Vibrator Use by Women in the United States: Results from a Nationally Representative Study." *Journal of Sexual Medicine* 6, no. 7 (July 2009): 1857–66. https://doi.org/10.1111/j.1743-6109.2009.01318.x.

4. Marin, Vanessa. "Are Vibrators Addictive?" *Bustle*, May 12, 2014. https://www.bustle.com/articles/24049-are-vibrators-addictive-or-numbing-our-sex-therapist-has-your-answer.

5. Miller, Korin. "Can You Get Addicted to Your Vibrator?" *Glamour*, April 12, 2016. https://www.glamour.com/story/vibrator-addiction.

6. Barnes, Zahra. "Ob/Gyns Explain If You Can Actually Get 'Addicted' to Your Vibrator." *Self*, January 15, 2016. https://www.self.com/story/obgyns-explain-if-you-can-actually-get-addicted-to-your-vibrator.

7. Rubin, Elizabeth, Neha A. Deshpande, Peter J. Vasquez, et al. "A Clinical Reference Guide on Sexual Devices for Obstetrician-Gynecologists." *Obstetrics and Gynecologist* 133, no. 6 (June 2019): 1259–68. https://doi.org/10.1097/AOG.0000000000003262.

8. Cinar, H., M. Berkesoglu, M. Derebey, E. Karadeniz, C. Yildirim, et al. "Surgical Management of Anorectal Foreign Bodies." *Nigerian Journal of Clinical Practice* 2, no. 6 (June 2018): 721–25. httsp://doi.org/10.4103/njcp.njcp_172_17.

9. Pinto, Valdir Monteiro, Mariza Vono Tancredi, Antonio Tancredi Neto, et al. "Sexually Transmitted Disease / HIV Risk Behaviour Among Women Who Have Sex with Women." *AIDS* 4 (October 2005): 64–69. https://doi.org/10.1097/01.aids.0000191493.43865.2a.

10. Kwakwa, Helena A., and M. W. Ghobrial. "Female-to-Female Transmission of Human Immunodeficiency Virus." *Clinical Infectious Diseases* 36, no. 3 (February 2003): 40–41. https://doi.org/10.1086/345462.

11. Marrazzo, Jeanne M., Laura A. Koutsky, David A. Eschenbach, et al. "Characterization of Vaginal Flora and Bacterial Vaginosis in Women Who Have Sex with Women." *Journal of Infectious Diseases* 185, no. 9 (May 2002): 1307–13. https://doi.org/10.1086/339884.

12. Sloat, Sarah. "America Has an Extremely Disturbing Sex Toy Problem." *Inverse*, September 14, 2017. https://www.inverse.com/article/30641-sex-toys-testing-regulations.

13. Dangerous Lilly. "Sex Toy Cleaning & Material Information Guide." Accessed December 6, 2020. http://dangerouslilly.com/sex-toy-reviews/sex-toy-care-and-maintenance/.

14. Agency for Toxic Substances and Disease Registry. "Toxicological Profile for Vinyl Chloride." US Department of Health and Human Services, Public Health Service. Toxic Substances Portal—Vinyl Chloride. July 2006. https://www.atsdr.cdc.gov/phs/phs .asp?id=280&tid=51.

15. Danish Environmental Protection Agency. "Survey and Health Assessment of Chemicals Substances in Sex Toys." *Survey of Chemical Substances in Consumer Products* no. 77 (2006). https://www2.mst.dk/udgiv/publications/2006/87-7052-227-8/html/helepubl _eng.htm.

16. Solovey, Matthew. "Popular Disinfectants Do Not Kill HPV." *Penn State News*, February 12, 2014. https://news.psu.edu/story/303743/2014/02/12/research /popular-disinfectants-do-not-kill-hpv.

Chapter 18: Types of Orgasms

1. Nagoski, Emily. *Come as You Are: The Surprising New Science That Will Transform Your Sex Life.* New York: Simon & Schuster, 2015.

2. Gunter, Jen. *The Vagina Bible.* New York: Citadel Press, 2019.

3. Komisaruk, Barry, and Beverly Whipple. "Non-Genital Orgasms." *Sexual and Relationship Therapy* 26, no. 4 (Dec 2012): 356–72. https://doi.org/10.1080/14681994.2011 .649252.

4. Tepper, Mitchell. *Living Your Life: Sexuality Following Spinal Cord Injury.* New York: United Spinal Association, 2018. https://www.unitedspinal.org/pdf/SexualityFollowing SCIBooklet.pdf.

5. Brochmann, Nina, and Ellen Støkken Dahl. *The Wonder Down Under.* New York: Quercus, 2017.

6. Deutsch, Maddie. "Information on Testosterone Hormone Therapy." 2020. University of California San Francisco Transgender Care. https://transcare.ucsf.edu/article /information-testosterone-hormone-therapy.

Abortion and Contraception
Chapter 19: Abortion

1. Jones, Rachel, and Jenna Jerman. "Population Group Abortion Rates and Lifetime Incidence of Abortion: United States, 2008–2014." *American Journal of Public Health* 107, no. 12 (November 2017): 1904–09. https://doi.org/10.2105/AJPH.2017.304042.

2. Corinna, Heather. "All About Abortion." Scarleteen. Last updated January 10, 2020. Excerpted from *S.E.X.: The All-You-Need-To-Know Sexuality Guide to Get You Through Your Teens and Twenties*, 2nd ed. Boston: Da Capo Lifelong Books, 2016. https://www.scarleteen .com/article/bodies/all_about_abortion.

3. New York Times Editorial Board. "A Woman's Rights: Part 4. Slandering the Unborn." *New York Times*, December 28, 2018. https://www.nytimes.com/interactive/2018/12/28 /opinion/crack-babies-racism.html.

4. Bartz, Deborah, and Paul D. Blumenthal. "First-Trimester Pregnancy Termination: Medication Abortion." *UpToDate.* Last reviewed November 2020. https://www.uptodate.com /contents/first-trimester-pregnancy-termination-medication-abortion.

5. Raymond, Elizabeth, Margo Harrison, and Mark Weaver. "Efficacy of Misoprostol Alone for First-Trimester Medical Abortion: A Systematic Review." *Obstetrics and Gynecology* 137, no. 1 (January 2019): 137–47. https://doi.org/10.1097/AOG.0000000000 003017.

6. von Hertzen, Helena, Gilda Piaggio, Nguyen Thi My Huong, Karine Arustamyan, Evelio Cabezas, et al. "Efficacy of Two Routes of Administration of Misoprostol for Termination

of Early Pregnancy: A Randomised Controlled Equivalence Trial." *Lancet* 369 (June 2007): 1938–46. https://doi.org/10.1016/S0140-6736(07)60914-3.

7. Chen, Melissa, and Mitchell Creinin. "Mifepristone with Buccal Misoprostol for Medical Abortion: A Systematic Review." *Obstetrics & Gynecology* 126, no. 1 (July 2015): 12–21. https://uttmacher.org/uc/item/0v4749ss.

8. National Academies of Sciences Engineering Medicine. *The Safety and Quality of Abortion Care in the United States*. Washington: National Academies Press US, 2018. https://www.nap.edu/read/24950/chapter/4#54.

9. Aiken, Abigail, Irena Digol, James Trussell, and Rebecca Gomperts. "Self Reported Outcomes and Adverse Events After Medical Abortion Through Online Telemedicine: Population Based Study in the Republic of Ireland and Northern Ireland." *BMJ* 357 (May 2017). https://doi.org/10.1136/bmj.j2011.

10. World Health Organization. *Clinical Practice Handbook for Safe Abortion*. WHO Library Cataloguing-in-Publication Data, 2014. https://apps.who.int/iris/bitstream/handle/10665/97415/9789241548717_eng.pdf;jsessionid=FAFDB89E9069D66C495181A842B82D0E?sequence=1.

11. OBOS Abortion Contributors. "Aspiration Abortion." Our Bodies Ourselves, 2014. https://www.ourbodiesourselves.org/book-excerpts/health-article/vacuum-aspiration-abortion/.

12. OBOS Abortion Contributors. "Dilation and Evacuation Abortion." Our Bodies Ourselves, April 2, 2014. https://www.ourbodiesourselves.org/book-excerpts/health-article/dilation-and-evacuation-abortion/.

13. OBOS Abortion Contributors. "Induction Abortion." Our Bodies Ourselves, April 2, 2014. https://www.ourbodiesourselves.org/book-excerpts/health-article/induction-abortion/.

14. The SIA Legal Team. "Decriminalizing Self-Managed and Supported Non-Clinical Abortion." If/When/How, 2018. https://www.ifwhenhow.org/resources/roes-unfinished-promise/.

15. ReproAction. "Understanding and Advocating for Self-Managed Abortion." Accessed December 7, 2020. https://reproaction.org/campaign/self-managed-abortion/.

16. Herold, Steph. "Need an Abortion? There's an App for That." Bitchmedia, January 22, 2020. https://www.bitchmedia.org/article/abortion-apps-spreading-misinformation.

Chapter 20: Contraception: Options and Phantom Side Effects

1. Corinna, Heather. "Birth Control Bingo." Scarleteen. Last updated August 28, 2019. https://www.scarleteen.com/article/sexual_health/birth_control_bingo.

2. Faculty of Sexual and Reproductive Healthcare. "FSRH CEU Statement: Contraceptive Choices and Sexual Health for Transgender and Non-binary People." October 16, 2017. https://www.fsrh.org/documents/fsrh-ceu-statement-contraceptive-choices-and-sexual-health-for/.

3. Corinna, Heather. "Birth Control Bingo: Condoms." Scarleteen. Last updated October 8, 2018. https://www.scarleteen.com/birth_control_bingo_condoms.

4. Sanders, Stephanie A., William L. Yarber, Erin L. Kaufman, et al. "Condom Use Errors and Problems: A Global View." *Sexual Health* 9, no. 1 (February 2012): 81–95. https://doi.org/10.1071/SH11095.

5. Corinna, Heather. "Birth Control Bingo: The Contraceptive Patch." Scarleteen. Last updated November 20, 2020. https://www.scarleteen.com/birth_control_bingo_the_contraceptive_patch.

6. Institute for Quality and Efficiency in Health Care. "Contraception: Hormonal Contraceptives." InformedHealth.org. Cologne: Institute for Quality and Efficiency in Health Care. Last updated June 29, 2017. https://www.ncbi.nlm.nih.gov/books/NBK441576/.

7. Washington, Harriet. *Medical Apartheid*. New York: Anchor Books, 2006.

8. Bedsider. "The Pill." Birth Control Methods. Last modified November 2020. https://www.bedsider.org/methods/the_pill.

9. Corinna, Heather. "Birth Control Bingo: The Combination Pill." Scarleteen. Last updated June 13, 2016. https://www.scarleteen.com/birth_control_bingo_the_combination_pill.

10. Bedsider. "The Ring." Birth Control Methods. Last modified January 7, 2021. https://www.bedsider.org/methods/the_ring.

11. Bedsider. "The Shot." Birth Control Methods. Last modified November 2020. https://www.bedsider.org/methods/the_shot.

12. Corinna, Heather. "Birth Control Bingo: Depo-Provera." Scarleteen. Last updated June 13, 2016. https://www.scarleteen.com/birth_control_bingo_depo_provera.

13. Bedsider. "Implant." Birth Control Methods. Last modified November 2020. https://www.bedsider.org/methods/implant.

14. Corinna, Heather. "Birth Control Bingo: The Contraceptive Implant." Scarleteen. Last updated November 19, 2020. https://www.scarleteen.com/birth_control_bingo_the_contraceptive_implant.

15. Bedsider. "The Patch." Birth Control Methods. Last modified November 2020. https://www.bedsider.org/methods/the_patch.

16. Bedsider. "IUD." Birth Control Methods. Last modified November 2020. https://www.bedsider.org/methods/iud.

17. Corinna, Heather. "Birth Control Bingo: Intrauterine Devices (IUD)." Scarleteen. Last updated November 19, 2020. https://www.scarleteen.com/birth_control_bingo_intrauterine_devices_iud.

18. Corbett, Megan. "A History: The IUD." Reproductive Health Access Project. January 17, 2013. https://www.reproductiveaccess.org/2013/01/a-history-the-iud/.

19. Lotfy Fayed, Hala, Hatem H. Eleishi, Heba A. Kamal, et al. "Rheumatoid Arthritis Activity and Severity in Relation to Commonly Used Contraceptive Methods in a Cohort of Egyptian Female Patients." *International Journal of Clinical Rheumatology* 12, no. 6 (January 2017): 168–82. https://doi.org/10.4172/1758-4272.1000153.

20. Bedsider. "Emergency Contraception." Birth Control Methods. Last modified September 2020. https://www.bedsider.org/methods/emergency_contraception.

21. Corinna, Heather. "Birth Control Bingo: Emergency Contraception." Scarleteen. Last updated November 20, 2020. https://www.scarleteen.com/birth_control_bingo_emergency_contraception.

22. Van Damme, L., V. Chandeying, G. Ramjee, et al. "Safety of Multiple Daily Applications of COL-1492, a Nonoxynol-9 Vaginal Gel, Among Female Sex Workers. COL-1492 Phase II Study Group." *AIDS* 14, no. 1 (January 2000): 85–88. https://doi.org/10.1097/00002030-200001070-00010.

23. Kreiss J., E. Ngugi, K. Holmes, et al. "Efficacy of Nonoxynol 9 Contraceptive Sponge Use in Preventing Heterosexual Acquisition of HIV in Nairobi Prostitutes." *JAMA* 268, no. 4 (July 1992): 477–82. https://doi.org/10.1001/jama.1992.03490040053025.

24. Roddy R. E., L. Zekeng, K. A. Ryan, et al. "A Controlled Trial of Nonoxynol 9 Film to Reduce Male-to-Female Transmission of Sexually Transmitted Diseases." *New England Journal of Medicine* 339, no. 8 (August 1998): 504–10. https://doi.org/10.1056/NEJM199808203390803.

25. Cone, R. A., T. Hoen, X. Wong, et al. "Vaginal Microbicides: Detecting Toxicities in Vivo That Paradoxically Increase Pathogen Transmission." *BMC Infectious Diseases* 1, no. 6 (June 2006): 90. https://doi.org/10.1186/1471-2334-6-90.

26. Fields, Scott, Benben Song, Bareza Rasoul, et al. "New Candidate Biomarkers in the Female Genital Tract to Evaluate Microbicide Toxicity." *PLOS ONE* 9, no. 10 (October 2014): e110980. https://doi.org/10.1371/journal.pone.0110980.

27. Fihn, Stephan D., Edward J. Boyko, Chi-Ling Chen, et al. "Use of Spermicide-Coated Condoms and Other Risk Factors for Urinary Tract Infection Caused by Staphylococcus saprophyticus." *JAMA Internal Medicine* 158, no. 3 (February 1998): 281–87. https://doi.org/10.1001/archinte.158.3.281.

28. Fihn, Stephan, Edward J. Boyko, Chi-Ling Chen, et al. "Association Between Use of Spermicide-Coated Condoms and Escherichia Coli Urinary Tract Infection in Young Women." *American Journal of Epidemiology* 144, no. 5 (September 1996): 512–20. https://doi.org/10.1093/oxfordjournals.aje.a008958.

29. Dienye, Paul O., and Precious K. Gbeneol. "Contraception as a Risk Factor for Urinary Tract Infection in Port Harcourt, Nigeria: A Case Control Study." *African Journal of Primary Health Care & Family Medicine* 3, no. 1 (June 2011): 207. https://doi.org/10.4102/phcfm.v3i1.207.

30. Handley, Margaret Ann, Arthur L. Reingold, Stephen Shiboski, et al. "Incidence of Acute Urinary Tract Infection in Young Women and Use of Male Condoms with and Without Nonoxynol-9 Spermicides." *Epidemiology* 13, no. 4 (July 2002): 432–36. https://doi.org/0.1097/00001648-200207000-00011.

31. Foxman, Betsy, and J. W. Chi. "Health Behavior and Urinary Tract Infection in College-Aged Women." *Journal of Clinical Epidemiology* 43, no. 4 (January 1990): 329–37. https://doi.org/10.1016/0895-4356(90)90119-a.

32. Bedsider. "Diaphragm." Birth Control Methods. Last modified November 2020. https://www.bedsider.org/methods/diaphragm.

33. Corinna, Heather. "Birth Control Bingo: Cervical Barriers." Scarleteen. Last updated November 19, 2020. https://www.scarleteen.com/birth_control_bingo_cervical_barriers.

34. Bedsider. "Cervical Cap." Birth Control Methods. Last modified November 2020. https://www.bedsider.org/methods/cervical_cap.

35. Planned Parenthood. "How Do I Use a Diaphragm?" Learn. Birth Control. Accessed January 17, 2020. https://www.plannedparenthood.org/learn/birth-control/diaphragm/how-do-i-use-a-diaphragm.

36. Planned Parenthood. "Birth Control." Learn. Birth Control. Accessed January 17, 2020. https://www.plannedparenthood.org/learn/birth-control.

37. Caya. "Use of Lubricants Based on Silicone Oil." Press Releases. Accessed January 17, 2020. https://www.caya.eu/footer/press-releases/use-of-lubricants-based-on-silicone-oil.

38. Fihn, Stephan D., Robert H. Latham, Pacita Roberts, et al. "Association Between Diaphragm Use and Urinary Tract Infection." *Journal of the American Medical Association* 254, no. 2 (July 1985): 240–45. https://doi.org/10.1001/jama.1985.03360020072027.

39. Foxman, Betsy, and Ralph R. Frerichs. "Epidemiology of Urinary Tract Infection: I. Diaphragm Use and Sexual Intercourse." *American Journal of Public Health* 75, no. 11 (November 1985): 1308–13. https://doi.org/0.2105/ajph.75.11.1308.

40. Peddie, Barbara A., Vicki A. Bishop, Elspeth E. Blake, et al. "Association Between Diaphragm Use and Asymptomatic Bacteriuria." *Australian and New Zealand Journal of Obstetrics and Gynaecology* 26, no. 3 (August 1986): 225–27. https://doi.org/10.1111/j.1479-828x.1986.tb01572.x.

41. Vessey, M. P., M. A. Metcalfe, K. McPherson, et al. "Urinary Tract Infection in Relation to Diaphragm Use and Obesity." *International Journal of Epidemiology* 16, no. 3 (September 1987): 441–44. https://doi.org/10.1093/ije/16.3.441.

42. Corinna, Heather. "Birth Control Bingo: Contraceptive Sponge." Scarleteen. Last updated November 19, 2020. https://www.scarleteen.com/birth_control_bingo_contraceptive_sponge.

43. Bedsider. "Fertility Awareness." Birth Control Methods. Last modified November 2020. https://www.bedsider.org/methods/fertility_awareness.

44. Corinna, Heather. "Birth Control Bingo: Fertility Awareness." Scarleteen. Last updated November 19, 2020. https://www.scarleteen.com/birth_control_bingo_fertility_awareness.

45. Bedsider. "Withdrawal." Birth Control Methods. Last modified November 2020. https://www.bedsider.org/methods/withdrawal.

46. Casey, Frances E. "Permanent Contraception." *Merck Manual Consumer Version.* Last updated May 2020. https://www.merckmanuals.com/home/women-s-health-issues /family-planning/permanent-contraception.

47. Kaiser, R., M. Kusche, and H. Würz. "Hormone Levels in Women After Hysterectomy." *Archives of Gynecology and Obstetrics* 244, no. 3 (September 1989): 169–73. https://doi .org/10.1007/BF00931295.

48. Castelo-Branco, C., M. J. Martínez de Osaba, J. A. Vanrezc, et al. "Effects of Oophorectomy and Hormone Replacement Therapy on Pituitary-Gonadal Function." *Maturitas* 17, no. 2 (September 1993): 101–11. https://doi.org/10.1016/0378-5122(93)90005-3.

49. National Health Service. "Female Sterilisation." Conditions. Contraception. Last modified February 22, 2018. https://www.nhs.uk/conditions/contraception/female -sterilisation/.

50. Schaffir, Johnathan, Brett L. Worly, and Tamar L. Gur. "Combined Hormonal Contraception and Its Effects on Mood: A Critical Review." *European Journal of Contraception & Reproductive Health Care* 21, no. 5 (August 2016): 347–55. https://doi.org/10.1080/13625187 .2016.1217327.

51. Fruzzetti, Franca, and Tiziana Fidecicchi. "Hormonal Contraception and Depression: Updated Evidence and Implications in Clinical Practice." *Clinical Drug Investigation* 40 (September 2020): 1097–106. https://doi.org/10.1007/s40261-020-00966-8.

52. Skovlund, Wessel Charlotte, Lina Steinrud Mørch, Lars Vedel Kessing, et al. "Association of Hormonal Contraception with Depression." *JAMA Psychiatry* 73, no. 11 (November 2016): 1154–62. https://doi.org/10.1001/jamapsychiatry.2016.2387.

53. Larsson, Gerd, Febe Blohm, Gunilla Sundell, et al. "A Longitudinal Study of Birth Control and Pregnancy Outcome Among Women in a Swedish Population." *Contraception* 56, no. 1 (July 1997): 9–16. https://doi.org/10.1016/S0010-7824(97)00068-1.

54. Rosenberg, Michael J., and Michael S. Waugh. "Oral Contraceptive Discontinuation: A Prospective Evaluation of Frequency and Reasons." *American Journal of Obstetrics and Gynecology* 179, no. 3 (September 1998): 577–82. https://doi.org/10.1016/S0002-9378(98) 70047-X.

55. Sanders, Stephanie A., Cynthia A. Graham, Jennifer L. Bass, et al. "A Prospective Study of the Effects of Oral Contraceptives on Sexuality and Well-Being and Their Relationship to Discontinuation." *Contraception* 64, no. 1 (July 2001): 51–58. https://doi.org/10.1016 /S0010-7824(01)00218-9.

56. Poromaa, Inger Sundström, and Birgitta Segebladh. "Adverse Mood Symptoms with Oral Contraceptives." *Acta Obstetricia et Gynecologica Scandinavica* 91, no. 4 (December 2011): 420–27. https://doi.org/10.1111/j.1600-0412.2011.01333.x.

57. Rapkin, Andrea J., Giovanni Biggio, and Alessandra Concas. "Oral Contraceptives and Neuroactive Steroids." *Pharmacology Biochemistry and Behavior* 84, no. 4 (August 2006): 628–34. https://doi.org/10.1016/j.pbb.2006.06.008.

58. O'Connell, Katharine, Anne R. Davis, and Jennifer Kerns. "Oral Contraceptives: Side Effects and Depression in Adolescent Girls." *Contraception* 75, no. 4 (April 2007): 299–304. https://doi.org/10.1016/j.contraception.2006.09.008.

59. Redmond, Geoffrey, Amy J. Godwin, William Olson, et al. "Use of Placebo Controls in an Oral Contraceptive Trial: Methodological Issues and Adverse Event and Incidence."

Contraception 60, no. 2 (August 1999): 81–85. https://doi.org/10.1016/S0010-7824(99)00069-4.

60. Graham, Cynthia A., and Barbara B. Sherwin. "The Relationship Between Mood and Sexuality in Women Using an Oral Contraceptive as Treatment for Premenstrual Symptoms." *Psychoneuroendocrinology* 18, no. 4 (January 1993): 273–81. https://doi.org/10.1016/0306-4530(93)90024-F.

61. Graham, Cynthia, Rebecca Ramos, John Bancroft, et al. "The Effects of Steroid Contraceptives on the Well-Being and Sexuality of Women: A Double Blind, Placebo-Controlled, Two-Centre Study of Combined and Progestogen-Only Methods." *Contraception* 52, no. 6 (December 1995): 363–69. https://doi.org/10.1016/0010-7824(95)00226-X.

62. Duke, Janine, David W. Sibbritt, and Anne F. Young. "Is There an Association Between the Use of Oral Contraception and Depressive Symptoms in Young Australian Women?" *Contraception* 75, no. 1 (January 2007): 27–31. https://doi.org/10.1016/j.contraception.2006.08.002.

63. Keyes, Katherine M., Keely Cheslack-Postava, Carolyn Westhoff, et al. "Association of Hormonal Contraceptive Use with Reduced Levels of Depression Symptoms: National Study of Sexually Active Women in the United States." *American Journal of Epidemiology* 178, no. 9 (November 2013): 1378–88. https://doi.org/10.1093/aje/kwt188.

64. Lewis, Carolin, Ann-Christin S. Kimmig, Rachel G. Zsido, et al. "Effects of Hormonal Contraceptives on Mood: A Focus on Emotion Recognition and Reactivity, Reward Processing, and Stress Response." *Current Psychiatry Reports* 21, no. 115 (November 2019): P27–31. https://doi.org/10.1007/s11920-019-1095-z.

65. Wimberly, Yolanda H., Sian Cotton, Abbey M. Wanchick, et al. "Attitudes and Experiences with Levonorgestrel 100 µg/ethinyl estradiol 20 µg Among Women During a 3-Month Trial." *Contraception* 65, no. 6 (July 2002): 403–6. https://doi.org/10.1016/S0010-7824(02)00314-1.

66. Brochmann, Nina, and Ellen Støkken Dahl. *The Wonder Down Under.* New York: Quercus, 2017.

Chapter 21: The Other Kind of Birth Control

1. Davis, Angela. *Women, Race, & Class.* New York: Random House, 1983.

2. Washington, Harriet A. *Medical Apartheid: The Dark History of Medical Experimentation on Black Americans from Colonial Times to the Present.* New York: Harlem Moon, 2006.

3. Sanger, Margaret. "The Eugenic Value of Birth Control Propaganda (1921)." Public Writings and Speeches of Margaret Sanger. New York University. Accessed December 4, 2020. https://www.nyu.edu/projects/sanger/webedition/app/documents/show.php?sangerDoc=238946.xml.

4. Gross, Terry. "The Supreme Court Ruling That Led to 70,000 Forced Sterilizations." *Fresh Air.* National Public Radio. March 7, 2016. https://www.npr.org/sections/health-shots/2016/03/07/469478098/the-supreme-court-ruling-that-led-to-70-000-forced-sterilizations.

5. Ordover, Nancy. *American Eugenics, Race, Queer Anatomy, and the Science of Nationalism.* Minneapolis: University of Minnesota Press, 2003.

6. Pendergrass, Drew C., and Michelle Y. Raji. "The Bitter Pill: Harvard and the Dark History of Birth Control." *Harvard Crimson*, September 28, 2017. https://www.thecrimson.com/article/2017/9/28/the-bitter-pill/.

7. Lopez, Iris. *Matters of Choice: Puerto Rican Women's Struggle for Reproductive Freedom.* New Brunswick, NJ: Rutgers University Press, 2008.

8. Marks, Lara. "Human Guinea Pigs? The History of the Early Oral Contraceptive Clinical Trials." *History and Technology* 15, no. 4 (1999): 263–88. https://doi.org/10.1080/07341519908581949.

9. Southern Poverty Law Center. "Landmark Case: Relf v. Weinberger. Sterilization Abuse." Seeking Justice. Case Docket. Accessed December 4, 2020, https://www.splcenter.org/seeking-justice/case-docket/relf-v-weinberger.

10. Roberts, Dorothy. "Forum: Black Women and the Pill." *Perspectives on Sexual and Reproductive Health* 32, no. 2 (2000). https://doi.org/10.1363/3209200.

11. Torpy, Sally. "Native American Women and Coerced Sterilization: On the Trail of Tears in the 1970s." *American Indian Culture and Research Journal* 24, no. 2 (2000): 1–22. https://doi.org/10.17953/aicr.24.2.7646013460646042.

12. Minna, Alessandra. "STERILIZED in the Name of Public Health Race, Immigration, and Reproductive Control in Modern California." *American Public Health Association* 95, no. 7 (October 2004): 1128–38. https://doi.org/10.2105/AJPH.2004.041608.

13. Borrero, Sonia, Nikki Zite, Joseph E. Potter, et al. "Medicaid Policy on Sterilization—Anachronistic or Still Relevant?" *New England Journal of Medicine* 370, no. 2 (January 2014): 102–04. https://doi.org/10.1056/NEJMp1313325.

14. Benson, Rachel. "Guarding Against Coercion While Ensuring Access: A Delicate Balance." *Guttmacher Policy Review* 17, no. 3 (April 2017). https://doi.org/10.1080/23293691.2018.1556424.

15. Downing, Roberta A., Thomas A. La Veist, and Heather E. Bullock. "Intersections of Ethnicity and Social Class in Provider Advice Regarding Reproductive Health." *National Library of Medicine. National Center for Biotechnology Information* 97, no. 10 (October 2007): 1903–07. https://doi.org/10.2105/AJPH.2006.092585.

16. Christopherson, Sarah. "NWHN-SisterSong Joint Statement of Principles on LARCs." National Women's Health Network. February 8, 2017. https://www.nwhn.org/wp-content/uploads/2017/02/LARCStatementofPrinciples.pdf.

17. Johnson, Corey G. "Female Inmates Sterilized in California Prisons Without Approval." *Reveal News*, July 7, 2013. https://revealnews.org/article/female-inmates-sterilized-in-california-prisons-without-approval/.

18. Manian, Maya. "Immigration Detention and Coerced Sterilization: History Tragically Repeats Itself." News-American Civil Liberties Union. September 29, 2020. https://www.aclu.org/news/immigrants-rights/immigration-detention-and-coerced-sterilization-history-tragically-repeats-itself/.

19. SisterSong Women of Color Reproductive Justice Collective. "Web Home." Accessed August 7, 2020. https://www.sistersong.net/.

20. Ross, Loretta J. "CLPP Conference 2014." Civil Liberties and Public Policy. Video, 10:24. December 21, 2014. https://www.youtube.com/watch?v=mPhI45jIsYU.

Infections

Chapter 22: Safer/Funner Sex

1. Sanchez, T. Diana, Jennifer Cocker, and Karlee R. Boike. "Doing Gender in the Bedroom: Investing in Gender Norms and the Sexual Experience." *Personality and Social Psychology Bulletin* 31, no. 10 (October 2005): 1445–55. https://doi.org/10.1177/0146167205277333.

2. Curtin, Nicola L., Monique Ward, Ann Merriweather, et al. "Femininity Ideology and Sexual Health in Young Women: A Focus on Sexual Knowledge, Embodiment, and Agency." *International Journal of Sexual Health* 23, no. 1 (March 2011): 48–62. https://doi.org/10.1080/19317611.2010.524694.

3. Sanchez, Diana T., and Amy K. Kiefer. "Body Concerns In and Out of the Bedroom: Implications for Sexual Pleasure and Problems." *Archives of Sexual Behavior* 36, no. 6 (December 2007): 808–20. https://doi.org/10.1007/s10508-007-9205-0.

4. Shearer, Cindy L., Shelley J. Hosterman, Mariama Gillen, et al. "Are Traditional Gender Role Attitudes Associated with Risky Sexual Behavior and Condom-Related Beliefs?" *Sex Roles* 52, no. 5 (March 2005): 311–24. https://doi.org/10.1007/s11199-005-2675-4.

5. Grose, Rose Grace, Shelly Grabe, and Danielle Kohfeldt. "Sexual Education, Gender Ideology, and Youth Sexual Empowerment." *Journal of Sex Research* 51, no. 7 (September 2013): 742–53. https://doi.org/10.1080/00224499.2013.809511.

6. Schick, Vannessa, Alyssa N. Zucker, and Laina Bay-Cheng. "Safer, Better Sex Through Feminism: The Role of Feminist Ideology in Women's Sexual Well-Being." *Psychology of Women Quarterly* 32, no. 3 (September 2008): 225–32. https://doi.org/10.1111/j.1471-6402.2008.00431.x.

7. Rowen, Tami S., Benjamin N. Breyer, Tzu-Chin Lin, et al. "Use of Barrier Protection for Sexual Activity Among Women Who Have Sex with Women." *International Journal of Gynecology & Obstetrics* 120, no. 1 (January 2013): 42–45. https://doi.org/10.1016/j.ijgo.2012.08.011.

8. Valle, Giuseppina Holway, and Stephanie M. Hernandez. "Oral Sex and Condom Use in a U.S. National Sample of Adolescents and Young Adults." *Journal of Adolescent Health* 62, no. 4 (April 2018): P402–10. https://doi.org/10.1016/j.jadohealth.2017.08.022.

9. Copen, Casey E. "Condom Use During Sexual Intercourse Among Women and Men Aged 15–44 in the United States: 2011–2015 National Survey of Family Growth." *National Health Statistics Reports* no. 105. Centers for Disease Control and Prevention. August 10, 2017. https://www.cdc.gov/nchs/data/nhsr/nhsr105.pdf.

10. Hess, Amanda. "Bill Gates Wants to Build a Condom That Feels Good. That's Not 'Pervy.'" *Slate*, March 25, 2013. https://slate.com/human-interest/2013/03/bill-gates-funds-condoms-gates-pledges-100000-for-a-more-pleasurable-condom.html.

11. Global Advisory Board for Sexual Health and Wellbeing. "SEXUAL PLEASURE: The Forgotten Link in Sexual and Reproductive Health and Rights." 2018. https://www.gab-shw.org/resources/training-toolkit/.

12. Pleasure Project. https://thepleasureproject.org/.

13. The Participants of the 24th World Congress of the World Association for Sexual Health. "Mexico City World Congress of Sexual Health Declaration on Sexual Pleasure." October 15, 2019. https://worldsexualhealth.net/declaration-on-sexual-pleasure/.

14. Cornwall, Andrea. *The Power of Pleasure*. London: Zeb Books, 2013.

15. Holland, J., C. Ramazonoglu, S. Scott, et al. "Risk, Power and the Possibility of Pleasure: Young Women and Safer Sex." *AIDS Care* 4, no. 3 (1992): 273–83. httsp://doi.org/10.1080/09540129208253099.

16. National Institutes of Health. National Institute of Allergy and Infectious Disease. "HIV Undetectable=Untransmittable (U=U), or Treatment as Prevention." Diseases & Conditions. HIV/AIDS. Prevention. Last reviewed May 21, 2019. https://www.niaid.nih.gov/diseases-conditions/treatment-prevention.

17. San Francisco AIDS Foundation. "Living Positively: Your Roadmap to Living with HIV." January 2019. https://www.sfaf.org/wp-content/uploads/2019/04/Living-Positively-Print-version.pdf.

18. American Sexual Health Association. "Your Safer Sex Toolbox." Accessed January 20, 2019. https://www.ashasexualhealth.org/safer-sex-toolbox.

19. Warner, Lee, Markus Steiner, and Katherine Stone. "Male Condoms." *UpToDate*. Last updated April 7, 2020. https://www.uptodate.com/contents/male-condoms.

Chapter 23: STI Stigma and Shame

1. Cuatrecasas, Pedro. "Drug Discovery in Jeopardy." *Journal of Clinical Investigation* 116, no. 11 (November 2006): 2837–42. https://doi.org/10.1172/JCI29999.

2. Hubbard Burns, Diane. "Herpes Incidence Still on Increase." *South Florida Sun Sentinel*, July 20, 1986. https://www.sun-sentinel.com/news/fl-xpm-1986-07-20-8602120634-story.html.

3. Gruber, Franjo, Jasna Lipozencic, and Tatjana Kehler. "History of Venereal Diseases from Antiquity to the Renaissance." *Acta Dermatovenerologica Croatica* 23, no. 1 (December 2015): 1–11. https://pubmed.ncbi.nlm.nih.gov/25969906/.

4. Carney, Orla, Emma Ross, Chris Bunker, et al. (1994). "A Prospective Study of the Psychological Impact on Patients of a First Episode of Genital Herpes." *BMJ* 70, no. 1 (October 2002): 40–45. https://doi.org/10.1136/sti.70.1.40.

5. Cunningham, Scott, Jeanne M. Tschann, J. Gurvey, et al. "Adolescent Sexual Health. Attitudes About Sexual Disclosure and Perceptions of Stigma and Shame." *Sexually Transmitted Infections* 78, no. 5 (2002): 334–38. https://doi.org/10.1136/sti.78.5.334.

6. Fortenberry, J. Dennis. "Health Care Seeking Behaviors Related to Sexually Transmitted Diseases Among Adolescents." *American Journal of Public Health* 87, no. 3 (March 1997): 417–20. https://doi.org/10.2105/ajph.87.3.417.

7. Morris, Jessica, Sheri A. Lippman, Susan Philip, et al. "Sexually Transmitted Infection Related Stigma and Shame Among African American Male Youth: Implications for Testing Practices, Partner Notification, and Treatment." *AIDS Patient Care and STDs* 28, no. 9 (September 2014): 499–506. https://doi.org/10.1089/apc.2013.0316.

8. Denison, Hayley J., Collette Bromhead, Rebecca Grainger, et al. "Barriers to Sexually Transmitted Infection Testing in New Zealand: A Qualitative Study." *Australian and New Zealand Journal of Public Health* 41, no. 4 (August 2017): 327–28. https://doi.org/10.1111/1753-6405.12680.

9. Theunissen, Kevin, Arjan E. R. Boss, Christian J. P. A. Hoebe, et al. "Chlamydia Trachomatis Testing Among Young People: What Is the Role of Stigma?" *BMC Public Health* 15, no. 651 (July 2015). https://doi.org/10.1186/s12889-015-2020-y.

10. Malta, Monica, Francisco I. Bastos, Steffanie A Strathdee, et al. "Knowledge, Perceived Stigma, and Care-Seeking Experiences for Sexually Transmitted Infections: A Qualitative Study from the Perspective of Public Clinic Attendees in Rio de Janeiro, Brazil." *BMC Public Health* 7, no. 18 (February 2007). https://doi.org/10.1186/1471-2458-7-18.

11. Lieber, Eli, Li Zunyou Wu, et al. "HIV/STD Stigmatization Fears as Health Seeking Barriers in China." *AIDS and Behavior* 10 (December 2006): 463–71. https://doi.org/10.1007/s10461-005-9047-5.

12. Donohue, Caitlin. "Club Herpes. Would You Believe Me If I Said I'm Sometimes Happy I Have an STI?" *Rookie*, October 28, 2014. https://www.rookiemag.com/2014/10/the-sti-society/.

Chapter 24: The Usual Suspects

1. Gorgos, Linda M., and Jeanne M. Marrazzo. "Sexually Transmitted Infections Among Women Who Have Sex with Women." *Clinical Infectious Diseases* 53, no. 3 (December 2011): 84–91. https://doi.org/10.1093/cid/cir697.

2. Singh-Kurtz, Sangeeta, and Dan Kopf. "The Rise in Americans Saying they Are Bisexual Is Driven by Women." *Quartz*, April 23, 2019. https://qz.com/1601527/the-rise-of-bisexuals-in-america-is-driven-by-women/.

3. Centers for Disease Control and Prevention. "Chlamydia." Sexually Transmitted Disease Surveillance 2017. 2017. https://www.cdc.gov/std/stats17/chlamydia.htm.

4. Brochmann, Nina, and Ellen Støkken Dahl. 2019. *The Wonder Down Under*. New York: Quercus, 2017.

5. Centers for Disease Control and Prevention. "Table 10. Chlamydia—Reported Cases and Rates of Reported Cases by Age Group and Sex, United States, 2014–2018." Sexually Transmitted Disease Surveillance 2018. 2018. https://www.cdc.gov/std/stats18/tables/10.htm.

6. Chelimo, Carol, Trecia A. Wouldes, Linda D. Cameron, et al. "Risk Factors for and Prevention of Human Papillomaviruses (HPV), Genital Warts and Cervical Cancer." *Journal of Infection* 66, no. 3 (March 2013): 207–17. https://doi.org/10.1016/j.jinf.2012.10.024.

7. Planned Parenthood. "HPV Myths Versus Facts." Accessed December 6, 2020. https://www.plannedparenthood.org/files/3413/9611/7996/HPV_Myths_v_Facts.pdf.

8. Centers for Disease Control and Prevention. "Other STDs." Sexually Transmitted Disease Surveillance 2018. 2018. https://www.cdc.gov/std/stats18/other.htm#hpv.

9. American Cancer Society Medical and Editorial Content Team. 2020. "HPV and HPV Testing." HPV (HUMAN PAPILLOMAVIRUS). Last modified July 30, 2020. https://www.cancer.org/cancer/cancer-causes/infectious-agents/hpv/hpv-and-hpv-testing.html.

10. Centers for Disease Control and Prevention. "Questions and Answers on HPV." Human Papillomavirus (HPV). Last reviewed: May 24, 2019. https://www.cdc.gov/hpv/parents/questions-answers.html.

11. Patel, Harshila, Monika Wagner, Puneet Singhal, et al. "Systematic Review of the Incidence and Prevalence of Genital Warts." *BMC Infectious Diseases* 13, no. 39 (January 2013). https://10.1186/1471-2334-13-39.

12. Withers, Rachel. "People Ages 27 to 45 Can Now Get the HPV Vaccine. But Will It Be Covered by Insurance?" *Slate*, October 9, 2018. https://slate.com/technology/2018/10/hpv-vaccine-insurance-coverage-age-27-45.html.

13. Mayo Clinic Staff. "Colposcopy." Mayo Clinic. Patient Care & Health Information. Tests & Procedures. Accessed December 6, 2020. https://www.mayoclinic.org/tests-procedures/colposcopy/about/pac-20385036.

14. Planned Parenthood. "What Is Cryotherapy?" Learn. Cancer. Cervical Cancer. Accessed December 6, 2020. https://www.plannedparenthood.org/learn/cancer/cervical-cancer/what-cryotherapy.

15. Planned Parenthood. "What's LEEP?" Learn. Cancer. Cervical Cancer. Accessed December 6, 2020. https://www.plannedparenthood.org/learn/cancer/cervical-cancer/whats-leep.

16. Cendejas, Blanca R., Karen K. Smith-McCune, and Michelle J. Khan. "Does Treatment for Cervical and Vulvar Dysplasia Impact Women's Sexual Health?" *American Journal of Obstetrics and Gynecology* 212, no. 3 (March 2015): 291–297. http://doi.org/10.1016/j.ajog.2014.05.039.

17. Planned Parenthood. "What Are the Symptoms of Herpes?" Learn. Sexually Transmitted Infections (STDs). Oral & Genital Herpes. Accessed December 6, 2020. https://www.plannedparenthood.org/learn/stds-hiv-safer-sex/herpes/what-are-the-symptoms-of-herpes.

18. Xu, Fujie, Maya R. Sternberg, Benny J Kottiri, et al. "Trends in Herpes Simplex Virus Type 1 and Type 2 Seroprevalence in the United States." *JAMA* 296, no. 8 (August 2006): 964–73. https://doi.org/10.1001/jama.296.8.964.

19. Black, Finn. "The STI Files: Herpes." Scarleteen, November 10, 2020. https://www.scarleteen.com/article/sexual_health/the_sti_files_herpes.

20. McQuillan, Geraldine, Deanna Kruszon-Moran, Elaine W. Flagg, et al. "Prevalence of Herpes Simplex Virus Type 1 and Type 2 in Persons Aged 14–49: United States, 2015–2016." *NCHS Data Brief* 304 (February 2018). National Center for Health Statistics. Centers for Disease Control and Prevention. https://www.cdc.gov/nchs/data/databriefs/db304.pdf.

21. Kissinger, Patricia. "Epidemiology and Treatment of Trichomoniasis." *Current Infectious Disease Reports* 31, no. 17 (June 2015). https://doi.org/10.1007/s11908-015-0484-7.

22. Kissinger, Patricia, and Alys Adamski. "Trichomoniasis and HIV Interactions: A Review." *Sexually Transmitted Infections* 89, no. 6 (September 2013): 426–33. https://doi.org/10.1136/sextrans-2012-051005.

23. Centers for Disease Control and Prevention. "Trichomoniasis Treatment and Care." Trichomoniasis. Last reviewed January 4, 2017. https://www.cdc.gov/std/trichomonas/treatment.htm.

24. Centers for Disease Control and Prevention. "Gonorrhea." Sexually Transmitted Disease Surveillance 2018. Last reviewed July 30, 2019. https://www.cdc.gov/std/stats18/gonorrhea.htm.

25. HIV.gov. "U.S. Statistics." HIV Basics. Data & Trends. U.S. Statistics. Last updated June 30, 2020. https://www.hiv.gov/hiv-basics/overview/data-and-trends/statistics.

26. Centers for Disease Control and Prevention. "Syphilis." Sexually Transmitted Disease Surveillance 2017. Last reviewed July 24, 2018. https://www.cdc.gov/std/stats17/syphilis.htm.

27. Kruszon-Moran, Deanna, Ryne Paulose-Ram, Crescent B. Martin, et al. "Prevalence and Trends in Hepatitis B Virus Infection in the United States, 2015–2018." *NCHS Data Brief 361* (March 2020). National Center for Health Statistics. Centers for Disease Control and Prevention. https://www.cdc.gov/nchs/products/databriefs/db361.htm.

28. Centers for Disease Control and Prevention. "Surveillance for Viral Hepatitis—United States, 2017." Viral Hepatitis. Last reviewed November 14, 2019. https://www.cdc.gov/hepatitis/statistics/2017surveillance/index.htm.

Chapter 25: What to Get Tested For and When

1. Boston Women's Health Book Collective. *Our Bodies, Ourselves*. New York: Simon & Schuster, 2011.

2. Moon, Allison. *Girl Sex 101*. n.p.: Lunatick Ink, 2015.

3. Centers for Disease Control and Prevention. "Genital Herpes Screening FAQ." Sexually Transmitted Diseases (STDs) > Herpes. Last reviewed: February 9, 2017. https://www.cdc.gov/std/herpes/screening.htm.

4. Mayo Clinic Staff. "STD Testing: What's Right for You?" Mayo Clinic. Patient Care & Health Information. Diseases & Conditions. Sexually Transmitted Diseases. September 16, 2020. https://www.mayoclinic.org/diseases-conditions/sexually-transmitted-diseases-stds/in-depth/std-testing/ART-20046019?p=1.

5. Centers for Disease Control and Prevention. "Screening Recommendations and Considerations Referenced in Treatment Guidelines and Original Sources." 2015 Sexually Transmitted Diseases Treatment Guidelines. Last reviewed June 4, 2015. https://www.cdc.gov/std/tg2015/screening-recommendations.htm.

6. Planned Parenthood. "HPV Myths Versus Facts." Accessed December 6, 2020. https://www.plannedparenthood.org/files/3413/9611/7996/HPV_Myths_v_Facts.pdf.

7. Centers for Disease Control and Prevention. "About HPV." HPV Home. Last reviewed October 29, 2020. https://www.cdc.gov/hpv/parents/questions-answers.html.

8. American Cancer Society. "HPV and HPV Testing." HPV (HUMAN PAPILLOMAVIRUS). Last modified July 30, 2020. https://www.cancer.org/cancer/cancer-causes/infectious-agents/hpv/hpv-and-hpv-testing.html.

9. Curry, Susan, Alex H. Krist, Douglas K. Owens, et al. "Screening for Cervical Cancer: US Preventive Services Task Force Recommendation Statement." *JAMA* 320, no. 7 (August 2018): 674–86. https://doi.org/10.1001/jama.2018.10897.

10. American College of Obstetricians and Gynecologists. "Cervical Cancer Screening (Update)." Practice Advisory. Last affirmed June 2020. https://www.acog.org/clinical/clinical-guidance/practice-advisory/articles/2018/08/cervical-cancer-screening-update.

11. California STD/HIV Prevention Training Center and California Department of Public Health-STD Control Branch. "California STD Screening Recommendations." November 18, 2015. https://www.cdph.ca.gov/Programs/CID/DCDC/CDPH%20Document%20Library/CA_STD-Screening-Recs.pdf.

12. Corinna, Heather. *S.E.X.: The All-You-Need-To-Know Sexuality Guide to Get You Through Your Teens and Twenties*, 2nd ed. Boston: Da Capo Lifelong Books, 2016.

13. North Dakota Department of Health. "Time Periods of Interest. VIH, STDs Viral Hepatitis." Last modified July 2018. http://www.ndhealth.gov/hiv/Docs/CTR/TimePeriods Reference_HIVSTDsHep.pdf.

14. Centers for Disease Control and Prevention. "HIV Testing." HIV. HIV Public Health Partners. Last reviewed June 9, 2020. https://www.cdc.gov/hiv/testing/index.html.

Chapter 26: Your Vagina Party: The Microbiome, BV, and Yeast

1. Amabebe, Emmanuel, and Dilly O. C. Anumba. "The Vaginal Microenvironment: The Physiologic Role of *Lactobacilli*." *Frontiers in Medicine* 5, no. 181 (June 2018). https://doi.org/10.3389/fmed.2018.00181.

2. Mendling, Werner. "Guideline: Vulvovaginal Candidosis (AWMF 015/072), S2k (Excluding Chronic Mucocutaneous Candidosis)." *Mycoses* 58, no. S1 (March 2015): 1–15. https://doi.org/10.1111/myc.12292.

3. Mirmonsef, Paria, Anna L. Hotton, Douglas Gilbert, et al. "Free Glycogen in Vaginal Fluids Is Associated with Lactobacillus Colonization and Low Vaginal pH." *PLOS ONE* 9, no. 7 (July 2014). https://doi.org/10.1371/journal.pone.0102467.

4. Dasari, Subramanyam, Raju Naidu Devanaboyaina Shouri, Rajendra Wudayagiri, et al. "Antimicrobial Activity of Lactobacillus Against Microbial Flora of Cervicovaginal Infections." *Asian Pacific Journal of Tropical Disease* 4, no. 1 (February 2014): 18–24. https://doi.org/10.1016/S2222-1808(14)60307-8.

5. Planned Parenthood. "What Is Bacterial Vaginosis?" Learn. Health and Wellness. Accessed December 6, 2020. https://www.plannedparenthood.org/learn/health-and-wellness/vaginitis/what-bacterial-vaginosis.

6. Centers for Disease Control and Prevention. "Vaginal Candidiasis." Fungal Diseases. Last reviewed November 10, 2020. https://www.cdc.gov/fungal/diseases/candidiasis/genital/index.html.

7. Mayo Clinic Staff. "Vaginitis." Mayo Clinic. Patient Care & Health Information. Diseases & Conditions. November 13, 2019. https://www.mayoclinic.org/diseases-conditions/vaginitis/symptoms-causes/syc-20354707.

8. Planned Parenthood. "What Is a Yeast Infection?" Learn. Health and Wellness. Vaginitis. Accessed December 10, 2020. https://www.plannedparenthood.org/learn/health-and-wellness/vaginitis/what-yeast-infection.

9. Mayo Clinic Staff. "Bacterial Vaginosis." Mayo Clinic. Patient Care & Health Information. Diseases & Conditions. November 13, 2019. https://www.mayoclinic.org/diseases-conditions/bacterial-vaginosis/symptoms-causes/syc-20352279.

10. Sobel, Jack D. "Vulvovaginal Candidosis." *Lancet* 369, no. 9577 (June 2007): 1961–71. https://doi.org/10.1016/S0140-6736(07)60917-9.

11. Healthwise Staff. "Vaginal Yeast Infection: Should I Treat It Myself?" Michigan Medicine. November 7, 2019. https://www.uofmhealth.org/health-library/tn9593.

12. Healthwise Staff. "Bacterial Vaginosis." Michigan Medicine. November 7, 2019. https://www.uofmhealth.org/health-library/hw53097.

13. Centers for Disease Control and Prevention. "Bacterial Vaginosis." Sexually Transmitted Diseases. Last Reviewed February 10, 2020. https://www.cdc.gov/std/bv/stats.htm.

14. Sobel, Jack D. "Recurrent Vulvovaginal Candidiasis." *American Journal of Obstetrics and Gynecology* 214, no. 1 (July 8, 2015): 15–21. https://doi.org/10.1016/j.ajog.2015.06.067.

15. Gonçalves, Bruna, Carina Ferreira, Carlos Tiago Alves, et al. "Vulvovaginal Candidiasis: Epidemiology, Microbiology and Risk Factors." *Critical Reviews in Microbiology* 42, no. 6 (April 2016): 905–27. https://doi.org/10.3109/1040841X.2015.1091805.

16. Winston McPherson, Gabrielle, Thomas Long, Stephen J. Salipante, et al. "The Vaginal Microbiome of Transgender Men." *Clinical Chemistry* 65, no. 1 (January 2019): 199–207. https://doi.org/10.1373/clinchem.2018.293654.

17. Land, Emily. "Q&A: Gynecologic and Vaginal Care for Trans Men." San Francisco AIDS Foundation. Sexual Health. July 23, 2019. https://www.sfaf.org/collections/beta/qa-gynecologic-and-vaginal-care-for-trans-men/.

18. Calhoun Rice, Sandy. "Postmenopausal Atrophic Vaginitis." Healthline. March 7, 2019. https://www.healthline.com/health/atrophic-vaginitis#complications.

19. A.D.A.M. Editorial Team. "Aging Changes in the Female Reproductive System." MedlinePlus. U.S. National Library of Medicine. Medical Encyclopedia. Last updated December 22, 2020. https://medlineplus.gov/ency/article/004016.htm.

20. Alvisi, Stefania, Giulia Gava, Isabella Orsili, et al. "Vaginal Health in Menopausal Women." *Medicina (Kaunas)* 55, no. 10 (October 2019): 615. https://doi.org/10.3390/medicina55100615.

21. Harvard Women's Health Watch. "Ask the Doctor: Can I Get a Yeast Infection After Menopause?" Harvard Health Publishing. Harvard Medical School. July 2012. https://www.health.harvard.edu/womens-health/can-i-get-a-yeast-infection-after-menopause.

22. Cauci, Sabina, Silvia Driussi, Davide De Santo, et al. "Prevalence of Bacterial Vaginosis and Vaginal Flora Changes in Peri- and Postmenopausal Women." *Journal of Clinical Microbiology* 40, no. 6 (June 2002): 2147–52. https://doi.org/10.1128/JCM.40.6.2147-2152.2002.

23. Fischer, Gayle, and Jennifer Bradford. "Vulvovaginal Candidiasis in Postmenopausal Women: The Role of Hormone Replacement Therapy." *Journal of Lower Genital Tract Disease* 15, no. 4 (October 2011): 263–67. https://doi.org/10.1097/lgt.0b013e3182241f1a.

24. Dennerstein, Graeme J., and David H. Ellis. "Oestrogen, Glycogen, and Vaginal Candidiasis." *Australian and New Zealand Journal of Obstetrics and Gynaecology* 41, no. 3 (February 13, 2018): 326–28. https://doi.org/10.1111/j.1479-828X.2001.tb01238.x.

25. Vodstrcil, Lenka A., Sandra M. Walker, Jane S. Hocking, et al. "Incident Bacterial Vaginosis (BV) in Women Who Have Sex with Women Is Associated with Behaviors That Suggest Sexual Transmission of BV." *Clinical Infectious Diseases* 60, no. 7 (April 1, 2015): 1042–53. https://doi.org/10.1093/cid/ciu1130.

26. Barbone, Fabio, Harland Austin, William C. Louv, et al. "A Follow-Up Study of Methods of Contraception, Sexual Activity, and Rates of Trichomoniasis, Candidiasis, and Bacterial Vaginosis." *American Journal of Obstetrics and Gynecology* 163, no. 2 (August 1990): 510–14. https://doi.org/10.1016/0002-9378(90)91186-G.

27. Bradshaw, Catriona Susan, Anna N. Morton, Suzanne M. Garland, et al. "Higher-Risk Behavioral Practices Associated with Bacterial Vaginosis Compared with Vaginal Candidiasis." *Obstetrics & Gynecology* 106, no. 1 (July 2005): 105–14. https://doi.org/10.1097/01.AOG.0000163247.78533.7b.

28. Foxman, Betsy. "The Epidemiology of Vulvovaginal Candidiasis: Risk Factors." *American Journal of Public Health* 80, no. 3 (March 1, 1990): 329–31. https://doi.org/10.2105/AJPH.80.3.329.

29. Hooton, Thomas M., Pacita L. Roberts, and Walter E. Stamm. "Effects of Recent Sexual Activity and Use of a Diaphragm on the Vaginal Microflora." *Clinical Infectious Diseases* 19, no. 2 (August 1994): 274–78. https://doi.org/10.1093/clinids/19.2.274.

30. Reed, Barbara D., Philip Zazove, Carl L. Pierson, Daniel W. Gorenflo, and Julie Horrocks. "Candida Transmission and Sexual Behaviors as Risks for a Repeat Episode of Candida Vulvovaginitis." *Journal of Women's Health* 12, no. 10 (December 2003): 979–89. https://doi.org/10.1089/154099903322643901.

31. Ravel, Jacques, Pawel Gajer, Zaid Abdo, et al. "Vaginal Microbiome of Reproductive-Age Women." *Proceedings of the National Academy of Sciences* 108, suppl. 1 (March 11, 2015): 4680–87. https://doi.org/10.1073/pnas.1002611107.

32. Zhou, Xia, Celeste J. Brown, Zaid Abdo, et al. "Differences in the Composition of Vaginal Microbial Communities Found in Healthy Caucasian and Black Women." *International Society for Microbial Ecology* 1, no. 2 (June 2007): 121–33. https://doi.org/10.1038/ismej.2007.12.

33. M. Fettweis, Jennifer, J. Paul Brooks, Myrna G. Serrano, et al. "Differences in Vaginal Microbiome in African American Women Versus Women of European Ancestry." *Microbiology* 160, pt. 10 (October 2014): 2272–82. https://doi.org/10.1099/mic.0.081034-0.

34. MacIntyre, David A., Manju Chandiramani, Yun S. Lee, et al. "The Vaginal Microbiome During Pregnancy and the Postpartum Period in a European Population." *Scientific Reports* 5, no. 8988 (March 2015). https://doi.org/10.1038/srep08988.

35. Jahn, Jaquelyn L., Jarvis T. Chen, Madina Agénor, et al. "County-Level Jail Incarceration and Preterm Birth Among Non-Hispanic Black and White US Women, 1999–2015." *Social Science & Medicine* 250, no. 112856 (February 2020). https://doi.org/10.1016/j.socscimed.2020.112856.

36. Bailey, Zinzi D., Nancy Krieger, Madina Agénor, et al. "Structural Racism and Health Inequities in the USA: Evidence and Interventions." *Lancet* 389, no. 10077 (April 8, 2017): 1453–63. https://doi.org/10.1016/S0140-6736(17)30569-X.

37. Washington, Harriet A. *Medical Apartheid: The Dark History of Medical Experimentation on Black Americans from Colonial Times to the Present.* New York: Anchor Books, 2008.

38. National Health Service. "Keeping Your Vagina Clean and Healthy." Live Well. Sexual Health. Last reviewed October 18, 2020. https://www.nhs.uk/live-well/sexual-health/keeping-your-vagina-clean-and-healthy.

39. Khalesi, Saman, Nick Bellissimo, Corneel Vandelanotte, et al. "A Review of Probiotic Supplementation in Healthy Adults: Helpful or Hype?" *European Journal of Clinical Nutrition* 73, no. 1 (January 2019): 24–37. https://doi.org/10.1038/s41430-018-0135-9.

40. Bilodeau, Kelly. "Should You Use Probiotics for Your Vagina?" *Harvard Health* (blog), December 27, 2019. https://www.health.harvard.edu/blog/should-you-use-probiotics-for-your-vagina-2019122718592.

41. Mastromarino, Paola, Beatrice Vitali, and Luciana Mosca. "Bacterial Vaginosis: A Review on Clinical Trials with Probiotics." *New Microbiologica* 36, no. 3 (July 2013): 229–38. http://www.newmicrobiologica.org/PUB/allegati_pdf/2013/3/229.pdf.

42. Cohen, Pieter A. "Probiotic Safety—No Guarantees." *JAMA International Medicine* 178, no. 12 (December 2018): 1577–78. https://doi.org/10.1001/jamainternmed.2018.5403.

43. Green, David H., Phil R. Wakeley, Anthony Page, et al. "Characterization of Two Bacillus Probiotics." *Applied and Environmental Microbiology* 65, no. 9 (September 2019): 4288–91. https://doi.org/10.1128/AEM.65.9.4288-4291.1999.

44. Hoa, Ngo Thi, Loredana Baccigalupi, Ashley Huxham, et al. "Characterization of Bacillus Species Used for Oral Bacteriotherapy and Bacterioprophylaxis of Gastrointestinal Disorders." *Applied and Environmental Microbiology* 66, no. 12 (December 2000): 5241–47. https://doi.org/10.1128/AEM.66.12.5241-5247.2000.

45. Davis, Allison P. "Woman Made Possibly Delicious Yogurt from Her Vagina." *The Cut,* February 10, 2015. https://www.thecut.com/2015/02/vagina-yogurt-a-way-to-fight-the-patriarchy.html.

46. Djohan, Vincent, Kpongbo Etienne Angora, Henriette Bosson-Vanga, et al. "Recurrent Vulvo-Vaginal Candidiasis in Abidjan (Côte d'Ivoire): Aetiology and Associated Factors." *Journal de Mycologie Médicale* 29, no. 2 (June 2019): 127–31. https://doi.org/10.1016/j.mycmed.2019.04.002.

47. Brouillette, Monique. "Decoding the Vaginal Microbiome." *Scientific American*, February 28, 2020. https://www.scientificamerican.com/article/decoding-the-vaginal-microbiome.

Reproduction
Chapter 27: Birth

1. Yang, Y. Tony, Michelle M. Mello, S. V. Subramanian, et al. "Relationship Between Malpractice Litigation Pressure and Rates of Cesarean Section and Vaginal Birth After Cesarean Section." *Medical Care* 47, no. 2 (February 2009): 234–42. https://doi.org/10.1097/MLR.0b013e31818475de.

2. Johnson, Nathanael. "For-Profit Hospitals Performing More C-Sections." Kaiser Health News. September 13, 2010. https://khn.org/news/californiawatch-profit-hospitals-performing-more-c-sections.

3. Centers for Disease Control and Prevention. "Racial and Ethnic Disparities Continue in Pregnancy-Related Deaths." CDC Newsroom. September 5, 2019. https://www.cdc.gov/media/releases/2019/p0905-racial-ethnic-disparities-pregnancy-deaths.html.

4. United Health Foundation. "America's Health Rankings 2018 Annual Report." Accessed December 6, 2020. https://www.americashealthrankings.org/learn/reports/2018-annual-report/findings-international-comparison.

5. MacDorman, Marian, and Eugene Declercq. "Trends and State Variations in Out-of-Hospital Births in the United States, 2004–2017." *Birth* 42, no. 6 (2019): 279–88. https://doi.org/10.1111/birt.12411.

Chapter 28: How Babies Are Really Made: Reproduction Inc.

1. Martin, Robert D. "The Macho Sperm Myth." Aeon. August 23, 2018. https://aeon.co/essays/the-idea-that-sperm-race-to-the-egg-is-just-another-macho-myth.

2. Ellington, E. J., D. P. Evenson, and R. W. Wright Jr. "Higher-Quality Human Sperm in a Sample Selectively Attach to Oviduct (Fallopian Tube) Epithelial Cells in Vitro." *Fertility and Sterility* 71, no. 5 (May 1999): 924–29. https://doi.org/10.1016/s0015-0282(99)00095-3.

3. Boston Women's Health Book Collective. *Our Bodies, Ourselves.* New York: Simon & Schuster, 2011.

4. Barron, Mary Lee. "The Fertility Window." *American Journal of Nursing* 106, no. 5 (May 2006): 15. https://doi.org/10.1097/00000446-200605000-00003.

5. Zinaman, Michael, Sarah Johnson, Jayne Ellis, et al. "Accuracy of Perception of Ovulation Day in Women Trying to Conceive." *Current Medical Research and Opinion* 28, no. 5 (April 2012): 749–54. https://doi.org/10.1185/03007995.2012.681638.

6. Faust, Bradley. "Findings from a Mobile Application–Based Cohort Are Consistent with Established Knowledge of the Menstrual Cycle, Fertile Window, and Conception."

Fertility and Sterility 112, no. 3 (September 2019): 450–57.e3 https://doi.org/10.1016/j
.fertnstert.2019.05.008.

7. Reports and Data. "Assisted Reproductive Technology (ART) Market by Procedure (Fresh Donor), by Technology (In-Vitro Fertilization (IVF), Frozen Embryo Replacement (FER), by Type (Artificial Insemination, Surrogacy), and by End Use (Fertility Clinics) Forecasts to 2027." Diagnostics. Assisted Reproductive Technology Art Market. June 2020. https://www.reportsanddata.com/report-detail/assisted-reproductive-technology-art-market.

8. Centers for Disease Control and Prevention. "ART Success Rates." Assisted Reproductive Technology (ART). Last reviewed December 31, 2020. https://www.cdc.gov/art/artdata/index.html.

9. Grant, Rebecca. "How Egg Freezing Got Rebranded as the Ultimate Act of Self-Care." *Guardian*, September 30, 2020. https://www.theguardian.com/us-news/2020/sep/30/egg-freezing-self-care-pregnancy-fertility.

10. Belluck, Pam. "What Fertility Patients Should Know About Egg Freezing." *New York Times*, March 13, 2018. https://www.nytimes.com/2018/03/13/health/eggs-freezing-storage-safety.html.

11. National Health Service. "Overview IVF." Conditions. Last reviewed June 11, 2018. https://www.nhs.uk/conditions/ivf/.

12. Surrogacy360. "Key Questions." Considering Surrogacy. Accessed January 20, 2021. https://surrogacy360.org/considering-surrogacy/key-questions/.

13. Eunice Kennedy Shriver National Institute of Child Health and Human Development. National Institute of Health. "Assisted Reproductive Technology (ART)." Health. Infertility. Treatments. Last reviewed January 31, 2017. https://www.nichd.nih.gov/health/topics/infertility/conditioninfo/treatments/art.

14. Gurevich, Rachel. "How Much Does IVF Really Cost?" VeryWell Family. March 5, 2020. https://www.verywellfamily.com/how-much-does-ivf-cost-1960212.

15. MacMillan, Carrie. "Is Egg Freezing Right for You?" Yale Medicine. May 29, 2019. https://www.yalemedicine.org/news/egg-freezing-fertility.

16. Surrogate.com. "How Much Does Surrogacy Cost?" Intended Parents. Accessed January 20, 2021. https://surrogate.com/intended-parents/the-surrogacy-process/how-much-does-surrogacy-cost.

17. National Conference of State Legislatures. "State Laws Related to Insurance Coverage for Infertility Treatment." June 12, 2019. https://www.ncsl.org/research/health/insurance-coverage-for-infertility-laws.aspx.

18. Cobo, Ana, Juan A. Garcia-Velasco, Aila Coello, et al. "Oocyte Vitrification as an Efficient Option for Elective Fertility Preservation." *Fertility and Sterility* 105, no. 3 (March 2016): P755–64.E8. https://doi.org/10.1016/j.fertnstert.2015.11.027.

19. Doyle, Joseph O., Kevin S. Richter, Joshua Lim, et al. "Successful Elective and Medically Indicated Oocyte Vitrification and Warming for Autologous in Vitro Fertilization, with Predicted Birth Probabilities for Fertility Preservation According to Number of Cryopreserved Oocytes and Age at Retrieval." *Fertility and Sterility* 105, no. 2 (February 2016): P459–66.E2. https://doi.org/10.1016/j.fertnstert.2015.10.026.

20. Gupta, Jyotsna Agnihotri. "Towards Transnational Feminisms: Some Reflections and Concerns in Relation to the Globalization of Reproductive Technologies." *European Journal of Women's Studies* 13, no. 1 (February 2006): 23–38. https://doi.org/10.1177/1350506806060004.

21. Lewin, Tamar. "Egg Donors Challenge Pay Rates, Saying They Shortchange Women." *New York Times*, October 16, 2015. https://www.nytimes.com/2015/10/17/us/egg-donors-challenge-pay-rates-saying-they-shortchange-women.html.

22. *Lindsay Kamakahi v. American Society for Reproductive Medicine*. United States District Court. Northern District of California. 3:11-cv-01781-JCS. 2011. https://s3.amazonaws.com/pacer-documents/27/239565/03517948509.pdf.

23. Poirier, Marianne, and Carla Lam. "New Reproductive Technologies and Disembodiment: Feminist and Material Resolutions." *International Feminist Journal of Politics* 17, no. 4 (October 2015): 682–84. https://doi.org/10.1080/14616742.2015.1082861.

24. Throsby, Karen. *When IVF Fails: Feminism, Infertility and the Negotiation of Normality*. Basingstoke, UK: Palgrave Macmillan, 2004.

25. Storrow, Richard F. "Quests for Conception: Fertility Tourists, Globalization and Feminist Legal Theory." *Hastings Law Journal* 57 (2005): 295. https://repository.uchastings.edu/hastings_law_journal/vol57/iss2/2/.

26. Ryan, Maura A. "The Introduction of Assisted Reproductive Technologies in the 'Developing World': A Test Case for Evolving Methodologies in Feminist Bioethics." *Signs* 34, no. 4 (Summer 2009): 805–25. https://doi.org/10.1086/597133.

27. Franklin, Sarah B. *Biological Relatives: IVF, Stem Cells, and the Future of Kinship*. Durham, NC: Duke University Press, 2013.

28. Noyes, Nicole, E. Porcu, and A. Borini. "Over 900 Oocyte Cryopreservation Babies Born with No Apparent Increase in Congenital Anomalies." *Reproductive Biomedicine Online* 18, no. 6 (April 2009): 769–76. https://doi.org/10.1016/S1472-6483(10)60025-9.

29. Norsigian, Judy, and Timothy R. B. Johnson. "A Call for Protecting the Health of Women Who Donate Their Eggs." *Our Bodies, Our Blog*. Our Bodies, Ourselves. March 29, 2016. https://www.ourbodiesourselves.org/2016/03/a-call-for-protecting-the-health-of-women-who-donate-their-eggs.

30. Myers, Evan R. "Outcomes of Donor Oocyte Cycles in Assisted Reproduction." *JAMA* 310, no. 22 (December 2013): 2403–04. https://doi.org/10.1001/jama.2013.280925.

31. Brody, Jane E. "Do Egg Donors Face Long-Term Risks?" *New York Times*, July 10, 2017. https://www.nytimes.com/2017/07/10/well/live/are-there-long-term-risks-to-egg-donors.html.

32. Zuckerbrod, Samara. "Egg Donation." Pussypedia. Accessed January 20, 2021. https://www.pussypedia.net/articles/egg-donation.

Chapter 29: Miscarriage

1. American College of Nurse Midwives. "Share with Women: Miscarriage." *Journal of Midwifery and Women's Health* 58, no. 4 (August 2013): 479–80. https://doi.org/10.1111/jmwh.12084.

2. Mayo Clinic. "Miscarriage." Patient Care & Health Information. Diseases & Conditions. July 16, 2019. https://www.mayoclinic.org/diseases-conditions/pregnancy-loss-miscarriage/symptoms-causes/syc-20354298.

3. American College of Obstetricians and Gynecologists. "Frequently Asked Questions: Pregnancy: Early Pregnancy Loss." Last reviewed February 2020. https://www.acog.org/Patients/FAQs/Early-Pregnancy-Loss.

4. Boston Women's Health Book Collective. *Our Bodies, Ourselves*. New York: Simon & Schuster, 2011.

5. Brochmann, Nina, and Ellen Støkken Dahl. *The Wonder Down Under*. New York: Quercus, 2017.

6. Bardos, Jonah, Daniel Hercz, Jenna Friedenthal, et al. "A National Survey on Public Perceptions of Miscarriage." *Obstetrics & Gynecology* 125, no. 6 (June 2015): 1313–20. https://doi.org/10.1097/AOG.0000000000000859.

7. Harlan, Ash. "Miscarriage." Pussypedia. Accessed December 4, 2020. https://www.pussypedia.net/articles/miscarriage.

8. New York Times Editorial Board. "Slandering the Unborn. A Woman's Rights Prt. 4." *New York Times*, December 28, 2018. https://www.nytimes.com/interactive/2018/12/28/opinion/crack-babies-racism.html.

9. Haubursin, Christophe. "An Indiana Woman Is Facing 20 Years in Prison for 'Feticide.'" Vox. April 3, 2015. https://www.vox.com/2015/4/3/8336863/an-indiana-woman-is-facing-20-years-in-prison-for-feticide.

10. North, Anna. "She Had a Stillborn Baby. Now She's Being Charged with Murder." Vox. November 8, 2019. https://www.vox.com/identities/2019/11/8/20954980/stillbirth-miscarriage-murder-abortion-chelsea-becker-news.

11. "Woman Charged with Baby's Death After Police Say She Admitted to Drug Use During Pregnancy." WRTV Indianapolis. February 15, 2018. https://www.wrtv.com/news/local-news/madison-county/woman-charged-with-babys-death-after-police-say-she-admitted-to-drug-use-during-pregnancy.

12. *Help Christine Taylor* (blog). http://helpchristinetaylor.blogspot.com/.

13. Washington, Harriet A. *Medical Apartheid: The Dark History of Medical Experimentation on Black Americans from Colonial Times to the Present*. New York: Harlem Moon, 2006.

14. National Advocates for Pregnant Women. "About Us." Accessed Dec 4, 2020. https://www.nationaladvocatesforpregnantwomen.org/about-us/.

Shit The Patriarchy Tries to Sell You
Chapter 30: Intersex Surgery and the International Movement Against It

1. Human Rights Watch, InterACT. "'I Want to Be Like Nature Made Me' Medically Unnecessary Surgeries on Intersex Children in the US." Human Rights Watch. July 25, 2017. https://www.hrw.org/report/2017/07/25/i-want-be-nature-made-me/medically-unnecessary-surgeries-intersex-children-us#.

2. Office of the United Nations High Commissioner for Human Rights, UN Women, Joint United Nations Programme on HIV/AIDS, et al. "Eliminating Forced, Coercive and Otherwise Involuntary Sterilization. An Interagency Statement." World Health Organization. May 2014. https://www.who.int/reproductivehealth/publications/gender_rights/eliminating-forced-sterilization/en.

3. Elders, M. Joycelyn, David Satcher, and Richard Carmona. "Re-Thinking Genital Surgeries on Intersex Infants." Palm Center. June 20, 2017. https://www.palmcenter.org/publication/re-thinking-genital-surgeries-intersex-infants.

4. Office of the United Nations High Commissioner for Human Rights. "Intersex Awareness Day." OHCHR. October 24, 2016. https://www.ohchr.org/EN/NewsEvents/Pages/DisplayNews.aspx?NewsID=20739&LangID=E.

Chapter 31: Pussy Plastic Surgery

1. American College of Obstetricians and Gynecologists. "Elective Female Genital Cosmetic Surgery." *Obstetrics & Gynecology* 135, no. 1 (January 2020): e36–42. https://www.acog.org/clinical/clinical-guidance/committee-opinion/articles/2020/01/elective-female-genital-cosmetic-surgery.

2. Pariser, Joseph J., and Nicholas Kim. "Transgender Vaginoplasty: Techniques and Outcomes." *Translational Andrology and Urology* 8, no. 3 (June 2019): 241–47. https://doi.org/10.21037/tau.2019.06.03.

3. American Society for Aesthetic Plastic Surgery. "Cosmetic (Aesthetic) Surgery National Data Bank Statistics." Aesthetic Society. March 28, 2018. https://www.surgery.org/sites/default/files/ASAPS-Stats2018_0.pdf.

4. MBS Item Statistics Reports (Items 35533 and 35569 [from January 2000 to December 2011]). Medicare Australia. Accessed December 6, 2020. https://www.medicareaustralia.gov.au/statistics/mbs_item.shtml.

5. Liao, Lih Mei, and Sarah M. Creighton. "Requests for Cosmetic Genitoplasty: How Should Healthcare Providers Respond?" *BMJ* 334, no. 26 (May 2007): 1090–92. https://doi.org/10.1136/bmj.39206.422269.BE.

6. International Society of Aesthetic Plastic Surgery. "Plastic Surgeries Trends on the Rise." August 5, 2017. https://www.isaps.org/blog/plastic-surgeries-trends-rise/.

7. Zwier, Sandra. "'What Motivates Her': Motivations for Considering Labial Reduction Surgery as Recounted on Women's Online Communities and Surgeons' Websites." *Sexual Medicine* 2, no. 1 (April 1, 2014): 16–23. https://doi.org/10.1002/sm2.20.

8. Royal Australian College of General Practitioners. "Female Genital Cosmetic Surgery—a Resource for General Practitioners and Other Health Professionals." July 2015. https://www.racgp.org.au/download/Documents/Guidelines/Female-genital-cosmetic-surgery-toolkit.pdf.

9. Bramwell, R., C. Morland, and A. Garden. "Expectations and Experience of Labial Reduction: A Qualitative Study." *BJOG: An International Journal of Obstetrics & Gynaecology* 114, no. 12 (September 2007): 1493–99. https://doi.org/10.1111/j.1471-0528.2007.01509.x.

10. Crouch, N. S., R. Deana, L. Michala, L.-M. Liao, et al. "Clinical Characteristics of Women and Girls Seeking Labia Reduction Surgery." *BJOG: An International Journal of Obstetrics & Gynaecology* 118, no. 12 (August 2011): 1507–10. https://doi.org/10.1111/j.1471-0528.2011.03088.x.

11. Mowat, Hayley, Karalyn McDonald, Amy Shields Dobson, et al. "The Contribution of Online Content to the Promotion and Normalisation of Female Genital Cosmetic Surgery: A Systematic Review of the Literature." *BMC Women's Health* 15, no. 1 (November 25, 2015). https://doi.org/10.1186/s12905-015-0271-5.

12. Food and Drug Administration. "FDA Warns Against Use of Energy-Based Devices to Perform Vaginal 'Rejuvenation' or Vaginal Cosmetic Procedures: FDA Safety Communication." July 30, 2018. https://www.fda.gov/medical-devices/safety-communications/fda-warns-against-use-energy-based-devices-perform-vaginal-rejuvenation-or-vaginal-cosmetic.

13. Preti, Mario, Pedro Vieira-Baptista, Giuseppe Alessandro Digesu, et al. "The Clinical Role of LASER for Vulvar and Vaginal Treatments in Gynaecology and Female Urology: A Best Practice Document." *Journal of Lower Genital Tract Disease* 22, no. 3 (April 2019): 151–60. https://doi.org/10.1097/LGT.0000000000000462.

14. Tolentino, Jia. "The Age of Instagram Face." *New Yorker*, December 12, 2019. https://www.newyorker.com/culture/decade-in-review/the-age-of-instagram-face.

15. Goodman, Michael P., Otto J. Placik, David L. Matlock, et al. "Evaluation of Body Image and Sexual Satisfaction in Women Undergoing Female Genital Plastic/Cosmetic Surgery." *Aesthetic Surgery Journal* 36, no. 9 (April 15, 2016): 1048–57. https://doi.org/10.1093/asj/sjw061.

16. Sharp, Gemma, Julie Mattiske, and Kirsten I. Vale. "Motivations, Expectations, and Experiences of Labiaplasty: A Qualitative Study." *Aesthetic Surgery Journal* 36, no. 8 (February 23, 2016): 920–28. https://doi.org/10.1093/asj/sjw014.

17. Creighton, Sarah M., and Lih-Mei Liao. *Female Genital Cosmetic Surgery—Solution to What Problem?* London: Cambridge University Press, 2019. https://doi.org/10.1017/9781108394673.001.

18. Penner, Allison. "I Had Plastic Surgery on My Labia. Here's Why I Did It and What Happened After." *HuffPost,* May 7, 2019. www.huffpost.com/entry/labiaplasty-labia-surgery_n_5d1b824fe4b082e55370add2.

Chapter 32: Shit You Should Never Use

1. US Food & Drug Administration. "Fragrances in Cosmetics." FDA, August 24, 2020. https://www.fda.gov/cosmetics/cosmetic-ingredients/fragrances-cosmetics#labeling.

2. Women's Voices for the Earth. "Chemicals of Concern in Period Care Products." Accessed December 6, 2020. https://www.womensvoices.org/menstrual-care-products/chemicals-of-concern-in-feminine-care-products/.

3. Farage, Miranda. "Sensitive Skin in the Genital Area." *Frontiers in Medicine* 6, no. 96 (May 15, 2019). https://doi.org/10.3389/fmed.2019.00096.

4. American College of Obstetricians and Gynecologists. "Disorders of the Vulva: Common Causes of Vulvar Pain, Burning, and Itching." American College of Obstetricians and Gynecologists. February 2019. https://www.acog.org/patient-resources/faqs/gynecologic-problems/disorders-of-the-vulva-common-causes-of-vulvar-pain-burning-and-itching.

5. Centers for Disease Control and Prevention. "Douching." Office on Women's Health. January 19, 2015. https://www.womenshealth.gov/files/documents/fact-sheet-douching.pdf.

6. Cone, Richard. "Vaginal Microbiota and Sexually Transmitted Infections That May Influence Transmission of Cell-Associated HIV." *Journal of Infectious Diseases* 210, no. 3 (December 2014): 616–21. https://doi.org/10.1093/infdis/jiu459.

7. Robert, Magali. "Second-Degree Burn Sustained After Vaginal Steaming." *Journal of Obstetrics and Gynaecology Canada* 41, no. 6 (June 2019): 838–39. https://doi.org/10.1016/j.jogc.2018.07.013.

8. Gunter, Jen. "Gwyneth Paltrow Says Steam Your Vagina, an OB/GYN Says Don't." Dr. Jen Gunter. January 27, 2015. https://drjengunter.com/2015/01/27/gwyneth-paltrow-says-steam-your-vagina-an-obgyn-says-dont/.

9. Garcia, Sandra. "Goop Agrees to Pay $145,000 for 'Unsubstantiated' Claims About Vaginal Eggs." *New York Times*, September 5, 2018. https://www.nytimes.com/2018/09/05/business/goop-vaginal-egg-settlement.html.

10. Gunter, Jen, and Sarah Parcak. "Vaginal Jade Eggs: Ancient Chinese Practice or Modern Marketing Myth?" *Female Pelvic Medicine & Reconstructive Surgery* 25, no. 1 (February 2018): 1–2. https://doi.org/10.1097/spv.0000000000000643.

11. Women's Voices for the Earth. "Chem Fatale Report: Potential Health Effects of Toxic Chemicals in Feminine Care Products." Accessed December 6, 2020. https://www.womensvoices.org/menstrual-care-products/chem-fatale-report/.

12. National Health Service. "Keeping Your Vagina Clean and Healthy." Live Well. Sexual Health. Last modified October 18, 2018. https://www.nhs.uk/live-well/sexual-health/keeping-your-vagina-clean-and-healthy/.

13. Ferguson, Sian. "How to Clean Your Vagina and Vulva." Healthline. February 5, 2019. https://www.healthline.com/health/how-to-clean-your-vagina#how-to-wash.

14. Gunter, Jen. "How Should I Be Washing My Vulva on a Day-to-Day Basis?" *New York Times*, accessed Oct 25, 2020. https://www.nytimes.com/ask/answers/how-should-i-be-washing-my-vulva-day-to-day.

15. Lichtenstein, Grace. "U.S. Studies Feminine Sprays' Safety." *New York Times*, December 12, 1971. https://www.nytimes.com/1971/12/05/archives/us-studies-feminine-sprays-safety.html.

16. Hsu, Tiffany, and Roni Caryn Rabin. "Johnson & Johnson to End Talc-Based Baby Powder Sales in North America." *New York Times*, May 19, 2020. https://www.nytimes.com/2020/05/19/business/johnson-baby-powder-sales-stopped.html.

17. Kirkham, Chris, and Lisa Girion. "Special Report: As Baby Powder Concerns Mounted, J&J Focused Marketing on Minority, Overweight Women." Reuters. April 9, 2020. https://reut.rs/2In34UG.

18. Planned Parenthood. "What Are the Disadvantages of Using Spermicide?" Learn. Birth Control. Accessed Oct 25, 2020. https://www.plannedparenthood.org/learn/birth-control/spermicide/what-are-disadvantages-using-spermicide.

19. Van Damme, L., V. Chandeying, G. Ramjee, et al. "Safety of Multiple Daily Applications of COL-1492, a Nonoxynol-9 Vaginal Gel, Among Female Sex Workers. COL-1492 Phase II Study Group." *AIDS* 14, no. 1. (January 2000): 85–88. https://doi.org/10.1097/00002030-200001070-00010.

20. Kreiss J., E. Ngugi, K. Holmes, et al. "Efficacy of Nonoxynol 9 Contraceptive Sponge Use in Preventing Heterosexual Acquisition of HIV in Nairobi Prostitutes." *JAMA* 268, no. 4 (July 1992): 477–82. https://doi.org/10.1001/jama.1992.03490040053025.

21. Roddy R. E., L. Zekeng, K. A. Ryan, et al. "A Controlled Trial of Nonoxynol 9 Film to Reduce Male-to-Female Transmission of Sexually Transmitted Diseases." *New England Journal of Medicine* 339, no. 8 (August 1998): 504–10. https://doi.org/10.1056/NEJM199808203390803.

22. Cone, R. A., T. Hoen, X. Wong, et al. "Vaginal Microbicides: Detecting Toxicities in Vivo That Paradoxically Increase Pathogen Transmission." *BMC Infectious Diseases* 1, no. 6 (June 2006): 90. https://doi.org/10.1186/1471-2334-6-90.

23. Fields, Scott, Benben Song, Bareza Rasoul, et al. "New Candidate Biomarkers in the Female Genital Tract to Evaluate Microbicide Toxicity." *PLOS ONE* 9, no. 10 (October 2014): e110980. https://doi.org/10.1371/journal.pone.0110980.

24. Fihn, Stephan D., Edward J. Boyko, Chi-Ling Chen, et al. "Use of Spermicide-Coated Condoms and Other Risk Factors for Urinary Tract Infection Caused by Staphylococcus saprophyticus." *JAMA Internal Medicine* 158, no. 3 (February 1998): 281–87. https://doi.org/10.1001/archinte.158.3.281.

25. Fihn, Stephan, Edward J. Boyko, Chi-Ling Chen, et al. "Association Between Use of Spermicide-Coated Condoms and Escherichia Coli Urinary Tract Infection in Young Women." *American Journal of Epidemiology* 144, no. 5 (September 1996): 512–20. https://doi.org/10.1093/oxfordjournals.aje.a008958.

26. Dienye, Paul O., and Precious K. Gbeneol. "Contraception as a Risk Factor for Urinary Tract Infection in Port Harcourt, Nigeria: A Case Control Study." *African Journal of Primary Health Care & Family Medicine* 3, no. 1 (2011): 207. https://doi.org/10.4102/phcfm.v3i1.207.

27. Handley, Margaret Ann, Arthur L. Reingold, Stephen Shiboski, et al. "Incidence of Acute Urinary Tract Infection in Young Women and Use of Male Condoms with and Without Nonoxynol-9 Spermicides." *Epidemiology* 13, no. 4 (July 2002): 432–36. https://doi.org/0.1097/00001648-200207000-00011.

28. Foxman, Betsy, and J. W. Chi. "Health Behavior and Urinary Tract Infection in College-Aged Women." *Journal of Clinical Epidemiology* 43, no. 4 (1990): 329–37. https://doi.org/10.1016/0895-4356(90)90119-a.

Index

ejaculation, female, 15–16, 30–33, 42–44

ejaculation, male, 30–32, 203

Elders, Joycelyn, 144

Eli Lilly, 114

endometrial polyps, 66

endometriosis, 64–66, 71, 199

endometrium, 61–66, 105, 107

environmentalism, 119–128, 146, 220, 289, 302

episiotomy, 83, 273, 276–280

Epperson, Cynthia Neill, 116

Equal Pay Act, 211

erectile tissue, 11–13, 37–44, 81

erotic, 16, 32, 140, 146–148

erotic zones, 41–42, 146–148

estrogen
  birth control and, 194–199
  changes in, 82–83, 263–264
  gender-affirming therapy, 92–93
  levels of, 82–83, 263–264
  menstrual cycle and, 104–107, 112–114
  ovaries and, 55

"Eugenic Value of Birth Control Propaganda," 213

Everett, Annemarie, 49

Evolution and Nature of Female Sexuality in Relation to Psychoanalytic Theory (book), 18

experiments, 110, 214–215, 218

Facebook, 66

fallopian tubes, 14, 55–58, 286

Fallopius, Gabriel, 14–15, 58

Federation of Feminist Women's Health Centers (FFWHC), 20–21, 43, 78

"Female Ejaculation: A Case Study," 42

female genital cosmetic surgery (FGCS), 309–314

Female Genital Cosmetic Surgery: Solution to What Problem? (book), 313

"female prostate," 4–5, 30, 37, 43–45

"feminine" washes, 319–320

feminism, 119–128, 211–212, 226, 313

fertility awareness, 27, 203

Fertility Clinic Success Rates Report (2017), 287

fertilization
  assisted reproductive technology, 286–290
  conception and, 87, 107, 285–290
  of egg, 285–290
  reproduction and, 56, 107, 197, 285–286
  sperm and, 56, 87, 107–108, 285–287
  in vitro fertilization, 287–290

fetal development, 13, 17, 19, 295

fetal personhood, 295–296

Fiallo, Rafaella, 158

fibroids, 67–68, 216

Fischel, Joseph, 139

fissures, 8

fluids, types of, 15–16, 27–34, 47–52, 80

Food and Drug Administration (FDA), 105, 114, 123, 127, 188–189, 217, 268, 312, 317, 320

Forest Laboratories, 116

"Fourth Trimester Vaginal Steam Study," 318

Freud, Sigmund, 15, 18–19, 63, 182

Friedman, Jaclyn, 137

fungus, 83, 166, 261–264

G-spot
  anatomy of, 37–44
  clitoris and, 5, 30, 37–45
  erectile tissue, 37–44
  explanation of, 37–40

G Spot and Other Recent Discoveries About Human Sexuality (book), 42, 44

Galen, 14, 63

Gamble, Clarence, 213–214

Gardnerella, 261

Garnier, Pierre, 18

Gates, Bill, 227

Gates, Melinda, 227

sex toys (*continued*)
  lubricants for, 6, 164–166, 202
  masturbation and, 161–162, 176–178
  types of, 161–166
sexism, 93, 96, 99, 120, 221
Sexology (podcast), 5
sexting, 234–235
sexual assault, 134–136, 140, 153–155,
    171, 226, 235, 257
sexual harassment, 153
sexual identity, 91–100, 153–157, 174,
    303
sexual liberation, 215
"sexual revolution," 21
sexuality education, 75, 151–158, 169
sexually transmitted infections
    (STIs)
  barrier methods for, 225–235
  condoms, 225–232, 245, 256
  costs, 252, 257–258
  dormant periods, 257
  health insurance, 257–258
  lubricants and, 232–233
  masturbation and, 233–234
  preventing, 153–154, 164–165, 195,
    225–235, 245, 256
  resources on, 234–235, 258
  risk of, 6, 164–165, 225–235,
    237–240, 243–248, 251–265
  safer sex and, 138, 154, 164–165,
    225–235, 243–248
  spreading, 6, 164–165, 225–235,
    243–248, 251–256, 263–265
  stigma of, 228–232, 237–240, 246,
    253
  testing for, 228–231, 239–240,
    243–244, 247–248, 251–258
  treating, 228, 231, 238–240,
    244–247, 255–257
  types of, 225–235, 243–248, 252
  usual suspects, 243–248
  window period for, 257
She Represents: 44 Women Who Are
    Changing Politics and the World
    (book), 240

Sherfey, Mary Jane, 18–21
Shire Pharmaceuticals, 116
Sierra Club, 126
Silver, Hannah, 318
SisterSong, 218, 220–221
Skene's glands, 30
social justice, 151, 154, 157, 164, 216
social media
  anonymity and, 302–303
  Facebook, 66
  Instagram, 78
  Reddit, 70
  sex positivity and, 155
  Twitter, 22
  YouTube, 136, 196
Society for Assisted Reproductive
    Technology (SART), 289
Southern Poverty Law Center, 215
sperm
  birth control and, 29, 195–197,
    201–203, 321
  fertile periods, 27
  fertilization and, 56, 87, 107–108,
    285–287
  production of, 194
  reproduction and, 87, 285–287
spermicide, 195, 201–203, 321
sphincter, 5
sterilization laws, 213
sterilizations, 203–204, 211–221
stillbirth, 293. *See also* miscarriage
stratum corneum, 80
Streptococcus, 261
stress urinary incontinence (SUI),
    49–50, 312–313
Sun Sentinel (newspaper), 238
Supreme Court, 188, 213, 295–296
surgery
  clitoroplasty, 304
  female genital cosmetic surgery,
    309–314
  genital surgeries, 303–305
  hysterectomy, 62–63, 68–71, 104
  intersex surgery, 301–307
  labiaplasty, 309–311, 314

vaccines, 95–96, 245
vagina
    anatomy of, 77–87
    bacteria and, 29, 48–49, 80–83,
        261–269, 318
    bacterial vaginosis, 29, 261–269,
        318
    caring for, 267–269
    changes in, 82–83
    hymen, 73–75
    microbiome of, 82, 104, 201, 261–
        269, 318–321
    pain in, 84–86
    post-baby, 82–84
    pregnancy and, 82–84
    probiotics for, 267–269
    rejuvenation, 312
    sexually transmitted infections,
        225–235, 237–240, 243–248,
        252
    steaming, 267, 318–319
    stratum corneum, 80
    tenting, 87
    vaginal atrophy, 313
    vaginal ballooning, 87
    vaginal corona, 73–75
    vaginal discharge, 27–34, 80–83,
        107–108, 197–198, 203, 244, 247,
        256, 262–263
    vaginal laxity, 313
    vaginal mucosa, 80
    vaginal prolapse, 309, 313
    vaginoplasty, 29, 81–82, 304
    yeast infections, 83, 261–269, 318
vaginal atrophy, 313
vaginal ballooning, 87
vaginal corona, 73–75
vaginal deodorants, 267, 320
vaginal laxity, 313
vaginal microbiome, 82, 104, 201,
    261–269, 318–321
vaginal mucosa, 80
vaginal orgasms, 18–21, 37–39, 44,
    86–87, 181–182. See also
    orgasms

vaginal pacemaker, 87
vaginal prolapse, 309, 313
vaginal rejuvenation, 312
vaginal steaming, 267, 318–319
vaginal tenting, 87
vaginismus, 84–85
vaginitis, 262, 264
vaginoplasty, 29, 81–82, 304
Valenti, Jessica, 137
Vesalius, Andreas, 14
vestibular glands, 14–15, 22, 30
vestibulodynia, 84
"Virginity Fraud, The," 74
virginity myth, 73–75
VIRGO, 269
Vogue (magazine), 96
von Willebrand disease, 67
"Vos Sabés," 273
Vulgar.mx, 151, 157
vulva, 3, 11, 47, 50, 77–87, 124, 267,
    310–320
vulvar dysplasia, 245
vulvodynia, 84, 147, 312–313

Wallace, Sophia, 12, 23–24
warts, 244–245, 253
Washington, Harriet, 197, 212, 216,
    218, 266, 296
Westbrook, Cecilia, 268
What Fresh Hell Is This?:
    Perimenopause, Menopause, Other
    Indignities, and You (book), 104
Whipple, Beverly, 15, 39–42, 44
Whitman-Walker Health, 234
Whitney, A. K., 128
Williams, Tannis MacBeth, 110–111
Winship, Blanton, 214
Women of African Descent for
    Reproductive Justice, 220
Women of Color Sexual Health
    Network, 169
women's rights, 217–220, 295–296
"Women's Rights," 295
Women's Voices for the Earth,
    123–124

About the Author and Illustrator

MARÍA CONEJO
(1988, Morelos, México)
Lives and works in Mexico City

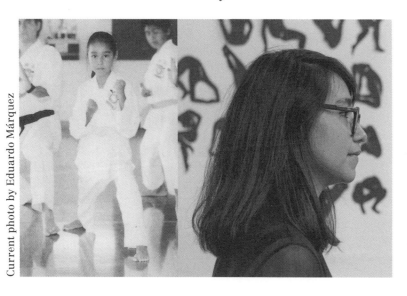

Current photo by Eduardo Márquez

A visual artist from Instituto Nacional de Bellas Artes' School of Design in Mexico, María's main media is drawing. Her work revolves around the body and its representation as a sign that communicates her existential concerns. María has been twice awarded the National Secretary of Culture's FONCA grant for young creators in 2014 and 2016. She was a finalist in the First Biennial of Illustration in Mexico, organized by Pictoline and the *New York Times* in 2018. Her work has been exhibited at SWAB Art Fair in Barcelona, De Kooning Studio in New York City in 2019, and in the Juxtapoz Clubhouse at Art Basel Miami in 2018 among many contemporary art fairs and illustrations shows in Mexico. Her work has been featured in such publications as the *Washington Post*, *Vice*, *Vogue*, and *Glamour LatAm*, *Revista de la Universidad*, *Revista Tierra Adentro*, *Revista Casa del Tiempo*, and *P Magazine* (NY), among others. She has collaborated with many feminist and human rights organizations to end gender violence.

@maria_conejo

http://mariaconejo.com/

ZOE MENDELSON

(1990, Chicago)

Lives and works in Mexico City

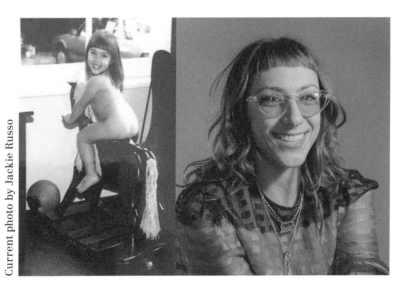

Current photo by Jackie Russo

Zoe is a writer, researcher, and content strategist. She tries to help people understand and care about important things. Past projects include a data narrative about drones, a civic engagement platform for millennials, and an official emoji pack for Mexico City. Current projects include a martial arts curriculum for dogs. Her writing has appeared in the *Washington Post*, *Los Angeles*

Times, *WIRED*, *Slate*, *Next City*, and elsewhere. Her projects have been covered by publications like the *New York Times en Español*, *Fast Company*, *BuzzFeed*, and *Vice i-D*. She has a BA from Barnard College of Columbia University in New York City.

@youngzokeziah

www.youngzo.com